Desmoid Tumors

Charisse Litchman
Editor

Desmoid Tumors

Springer

Editor
Dr. Charisse Litchman

Department of Neurology, The Stamford Hospital, Stamford, CT 06904

Assistant Clinical Professor, Department of Neurology, Columbia University

Co-Founder and Former Chair of the Scientific Advisory Board, The Desmoid Tumor Research Foundation

USA

cdlitchman@gmail.com

Office Address: 1290 Summer Street, Stamford, CT 06905

ISBN 978-94-007-1684-1 e-ISBN 978-94-007-1685-8
DOI 10.1007/978-94-007-1685-8
Springer Dordrecht Heidelberg London New York

Library of Congress Control Number: 2011933915

Printed on acid-free paper

Springer is part of Springer Science+Business Media (www.springer.com)

Preface

Desmoid tumors are currently amongst the rarest of rare tumors that afflict patients. The incidence of these tumors is not as low as is currently believed, however. Misdiagnosed by treating physicians and oncologists alike, especially in cases which remain stable or even regress over time, they may be labeled inaccurately or overlooked entirely. Indeed there are several different pathologic terms for desmoid tumors which confuse the diagnosis. Despite progress in molecular genetic profiling that would aid in precise identification, once designated as benign further efforts at identification are often abandoned.

Over the past decade, at major sarcoma centers, at high esteemed research institutions and at professional meetings such as the prestigious annual CTOS (Connective Tissue Oncology Society) meeting, the importance of understanding desmoid tumors has become increasingly more evident. More research projects were performed and publications submitted in the last 5 years than in the preceding 20 years. Much of this increasing awareness can be credited to the advent of vocal grass-root advocacy groups. Patient education has been heightened through contacts made on-line and powerful alliances forged between researchers, resulting in shared resources and improved outcomes. However, the majority of patients do not receive their care at dedicated sarcoma centers and many oncologists remain unfamiliar with the identification of and currently recommended treatments for desmoid tumors. This book will serve as the first comprehensive publication on the desmoid tumor. Although it may not answer all the questions, as most of these answers have not yet been found, it will introduce the reader, be he a scientist, physician or patient, to what a desmoid is and to the current important players who are leading the guest to find a cure.

Chapter 1 summarizes the increased recognition of the need to identify and treat desmoid tumors; Chap. 2 describes the clinical presentation and epidemiology of desmoid tumors; Chap. 3 discusses the pathology of desmoids; Chap. 4 describes the role of the APC gene and β-catenin in the genesis of desmoid tumors; Chap. 5 reviews the preferred imaging techniques to diagnose and monitor the disease; Chap. 6 outlines the surgical options; Chap. 7 describes current systemic therapy; Chap. 8 and 9 discuss the roles of traditional and interventional radiotherapy in the treatment of desmoid tumors; Chap. 10 describes desmoid tumors in the context of

Familial Adenomatous Polyposis; Chap. 11 addresses the unique features and challenges in treating children and adolescents with desmoid tumor; Chap. 12 details the role of microarrays in studying and distinguishing between desmoids and scar tissue and offers a glimpse into the new techniques of high-throughput sequencing; Chap. 13 outlines the difficulty in categorizing desmoids as benign or malignant and the implications of assigning either label; Chap. 14 examines the role of advocacy groups in promoting better recognition, patient-physician liaisons, researcher interest, desperately needed research funding and emerging patient support systems. Each of these chapters is followed by an extensive list of key references.

I would like to thank all the distinguished authors who enthusiastically agreed to contribute to this book and who without exception are working collaboratively to elucidate the etiology of and advance the search for a cure for this debilitating disorder.

Spring 2011 Charisse D. Litchman, MD

Contents

Contributors

Hani O. Al-Halabi Department of Radiation Oncology, McGill University, Montreal, Canada
e-mail: hani.elhalabi@mail.mcgill.ca

Benjamin Alman Department of Surgery, Division of Orthopedics, The Hospital for Sick Children, University of Toronto, Toronto ON, M5G 1L7. Toronto, Canada
e-mail: benjamin.alman@sickkids.ca

Yen-Lin Chen Department of Radiation Oncology, Massachusetts General Hospital, Boston, MA, USA

James Church Department of Colorectal Surgery, Cleveland Clinic Foundation, Cleveland, Ohio 44143, USA
e-mail: church@ccf.org

Chiara Colombo Department of Surgical Oncology and the Sarcoma Research Center, The University of Texas, MD Anderson Cancer Center, Houston, Texas 77030, USA
e-mail: ccolombo@mdanderson.org

Anastasia Constantinidou Sarcoma Unit, The Royal Marsden Hospital, London SW3 6JJ, UK
e-mail: anastasia.constantinidou@icr.ac.uk

Thomas F. DeLaney Department of Radiation Oncology, Massachusetts General Hospital, Boston, MA, USA
e-mail: tdelaney@partners.org

Paxton V. Dickson Department of Surgical Oncology, The University of Texas, MD Anderson Cancer Center, Houston, Texas 77030, USA
e-mail: PVDickson@mdanderson.org

Joseph P. Erinjeri Department of Interventional Radiology, NYU School of Medicine, New York, NY, USA
e-mail: erinjerj@mskcc.org

Wai Chin Foo Department of Pathology, The University of Texas, MD Anderson Cancer Center, Houston, Texas 77030, USA
e-mail: wfoo@mdanderson.org

Suzanne George Department of Medical Oncology, Center for Sarcoma and Bone Oncology, Dana-Farber Cancer Institute, Boston, MA, USA
e-mail: suzanne_george@dfci.harvard.edu

Francis J. Hornicek Department of Orthopaedic Oncology, Massachusetts General Hospital, Boston, MA, USA
e-mail: fhornicek@partners.org

Sinchun Hwang Department of Radiology, Memorial Sloan Kettering Cancer Center, New York, NY, USA
e-mail: hwangs@mskcc.org

Ian Judson Sarcoma Unit, The Royal Marsden Hospital, London SW3 6JJ, UK
e-mail: ian.judson@icr.ac.uk

Jonathan Landa Department of Radiology, Memorial Sloan Kettering Cancer Center, New York, NY, USA
e-mail: landaj@mskcc.org

Alexander J. Lazar Departments of Pathology and the Sarcoma Research Center, The University of Texas, MD Anderson Cancer Center, Houston, Texas 77030, USA
e-mail: alazar@mdanderson.org

Robert A. Lefkowitz Department of Radiology, Memorial Sloan Kettering Cancer Center, 1275 York Avenue, New York, NY 10065, USA
e-mail: lefkowir@mskcc.org

Dina Lev Department of Cancer Biology and the Sarcoma Research Center, The University of Texas, MD Anderson Cancer Center, Houston, Texas 77030, USA
e-mail: dlev@mdanderson.org

Charisse Litchman Department of Neurology, The Stamford Hospital, Stamford, CT 06904, USA
e-mail: cdlitchman@gmail.com

Andrea Marrari Department of Medical Oncology, Center for Sarcoma and Bone Oncology, Dana-Farber Cancer Institute, Boston, MA, USA
e-mail: andrea_marrari@dfci.harvard.edu

Anthony Montag Departments of Pathology and Surgery, The University of Chicago, Chicago, IL 06037, USA
e-mail: amontag@bsd.uchicago.edu

John T. Mullen Department of Surgical Oncology, Massachusetts General Hospital, Boston, MA, USA

Raphael Pollock Department of Surgical Oncology, The University of Texas, MD Anderson Cancer Center, Houston, Texas 77030, USA
e-mail: rpollock@mdanderson.org

David S. Pryluck Department of Interventional Radiology, Hospital of the University of Pennsylvania, Philadelphia, PA, USA
e-mail: david.pryluck@uphs.upenn.edu

Matt van de Rijn Department of Pathology, Stanford University Hospital and Clinics, Stanford, CA 94305, USA
e-mail: mrijn@stanford.edu

Oakleigh Ryan Whiton House, Janesville, WI 53545, USA
e-mail: Oakleigh@whitonhouse.com

Michelle Scurr Sarcoma Unit, The Royal Marsden Hospital, London SW3 6JJ, UK
e-mail: michellescurr@hotmail.com

Stephen X. Skapek Department of Pediatrics, Section of Hematology/Oncology and Stem Cell Transplantation, The University of Chicago, Chicago, 60637 IL, USA
e-mail: sskapek@peds.bsd.uchicago.edu

Robert T. Sweeney Department of Pathology, Stanford University Hospital and Clinics, Stanford, CA 94305, USA
e-mail: sskapek@peds.bsd.uchicago.edu

Aaron R. Weiss Department of Pediatrics, Division of Pediatric Hematology/ Oncology, The Cancer Institute of New Jersey, New Brunswick, NJ 08903, USA
e-mail: weissar@umdnj.edu

Sam S. Yoon Department of Surgical Oncology, Massachusetts General Hospital, Boston, MA, USA

Chapter 1
Introduction

Charisse Litchman

The desmoid tumor (DT) is a rare tumor that arises from connective tissues. The incidence of newly diagnosed tumors is only two to four per one million people per year. The clinical presentation varies depending on its anatomic location and the ensuing devastation can result in limb amputation, bowel obstruction, and even death. The clinical behavior can be just as variable, from locally aggressive with catastrophic potential to stable or even spontaneously regressive disease. The similarity in these nonuniform tumors is their origin in aberrations in the APC/β-catenin pathway, the difficulty in diagnosis, and the lack of well-established protocols for their treatment.

One question that would be appropriately posed is why dedicate an entire book to such a rare tumor, and, for that matter, why expend so much effort and so many research dollars. The obvious first answer is the simple one: because people are suffering and they need our help. The more impressive argument is that the advances made in understanding this benign but debilitating disorder can be extrapolated to more common malignant tumors as well as to the common scar. The fact that desmoid tumors arise as a result of only a few mutations, as compared to the many different mutations identified in breast and colon cancers, simply makes the scientific exploration more straightforward. Further, the pathway implicated in the genesis of DT, the APC/β-catenin pathway, is thought to play a role in many solid tumors. Similarly, highlighting both the similarities and differences between desmoid tumors and scar tissue may one day result in treatments that improve healing.

There are many obstacles to overcome in trying to effect a change that will translate into more successful treatment of such a rare disorder. The first, of course, is recognition of the disorder, both for the individual patient and as an entity worth diagnosing and treating. The overwhelming consensus is that all desmoid tumor patients should be seen at a dedicated sarcoma center. However, there is often much confusion about the diagnosis and without a diagnosis such a referral will not be made. The different pathologic designations assigned to it, such as aggressive fibro-

C. Litchman (✉)
Department of Neurology, The Stamford Hospital, Stamford, CT 06904, USA
e-mail: cdlitchman@gmail.com

1290 Summer Street, Stamford, CT 06905, USA

C. Litchman (ed.), *Desmoid Tumors*,
DOI 10.1007/978-94-007-1685-8_1, © Springer Science+Business Media B.V. 2012

matosis, deep fibromatosis, nonmetastasizing fibrosarcoma, Grade I fibrosarcoma, and musculoaponeurotic fibromatosis, add to the uncertainty. A very common story is that the patient is greeted in the recovery room by a smiling, confident surgeon who reassures the patient that there is no need for concern as it is just scar tissue or just some benign process.

After receiving such good news, many patients will not seek further medical followup until they become symptomatic. But even more horrifying than this benevolent neglect is the well-intentioned maiming of patients by surgeons who perform repeated resections in the hope of a cure. Repeated surgical trauma may make DT more aggressive and the pursuit of negative margins not justified in the face of great morbidity.

The disease entity as a whole suffers from the same lack of notoriety. Desmoid tumors are truly an orphan disease; even experts who dedicate their lives to combatting it cannot agree on whether it falls into the category of a sarcoma. Labeling it as benign or malignant creates false assumptions about its genesis and the natural course of this disease. One exciting development has been the acceptance of desmoid tumors into NORD, the National Organization of Rare Disorders. This organization is dedicated to advancing the cause of rare orphan diseases through education, lobbying of politicians, and promoting research. The quest for a cure has been further advanced by advocacy groups such as the Desmoid Tumor Research Foundation and SARC (Sarcoma Alliance for Research through Collaboration) in the US and Association S.O.S. Desmoide in Europe. Each year dozens of sarcoma advocacy groups exchange ideas and forge partnerships of collaboration at the CTOS (Connective Tissue Oncology Society) meeting.

The efforts expended in bringing together dedicated professionals and laypersons have translated into highly sophisticated and collaborative research in institutions across the world. The identification of Tumor Initiating Cells, or stem cells, in desmoid tumors may provide a therapeutic target. The elucidation of molecular pathways has already started to provide markers which will one day dictate the appropriate therapy individualized for each patient. Labs are sharing precious tissue samples and devising new techniques for amplification. Through the study of desmoid tumors, new forms of RNA have been identified that will have resounding ramifications throughout the research community.

Just as the number of desmoid patients is small, so is the community of professionals dedicated to finding a cure. Many of those brilliant clinicians and researchers contributed to this book. I would again like to thank each one of these contributors, all of whom did not hesitate to sign on, and challenge them to make the data presented in this first edition obsolete in the near future.

Part I
The Identification and Treatment of Desmoid Tumors

Chapter 2
Clinical Presentation of Desmoid Tumors

Anastasia Constantinidou, Michelle Scurr, Ian Judson and Charisse Litchman

Contents

Abstract Desmoid tumors (DT) constitute a rare fibroblastic proliferative disease. They present sporadically or as a manifestation of a hereditary syndrome such as Familial Adenomatous Polyposis (FAP). Despite the absence of metastatic potential, DT may cause debilitating symptoms and in some cases life-threatening organ damage because of their locally invasive nature. DT may range from small slow-growing masses to rapidly enlarging aggressive tumors. The clinical course of the disease is unpredictable but available data suggest an initial phase of growth may be followed by a long period of growth arrest with tumor stabilization or even regression. FAP-related DT are preferentially located in the abdomen whereas sporadic DT tend to involve mostly the extremities, although the abdomen and the thorax may also be affected. Antecedent trauma, pregnancy and estrogens play a role in the genesis of some desmoid tumors. Surgery is the favored current approach in the treatment of most desmoid tumors. Definitive protocols are not available as

C. Litchman (✉)
Department of Neurology, The Stamford Hospital, Stamford, CT 06904, USA
e-mail: cdlitchman@gmail.com

C. Litchman (ed.), *Desmoid Tumors*,
DOI 10.1007/978-94-007-1685-8_2,

most studies have been retrospective, small and comprised of mixed populations of FAP and non-FAP as well as of mixed populations of extra-abdominal and intra-abdominal patients.

Keywords FAP • Musculoaponeurotic • Sporadic • Primary tumor • β-catenin • Abdominal • Extra-abdominal • Intra-abdominal • Pregnancy • Head and neck • Trauma

2.1 Introduction

Desmoid tumors (DT) also known as aggressive fibromatosis (AF) constitute a rare fibroblastic proliferative disease. As suggested by their name (desmoid from the Greek word "*δεσμος*" meaning *band-like*) DT may occur in any musculoaponeurotic or fascial tissue [1]. Usually the masses are firm and fixed to surrounding tissue. It is uncommon to note lymphadenopathy, overlying skin changes, erythema, or dilated veins.

Desmoid tumors can occur anywhere in the body and are generally divided by anatomic designation as extra-abdominal, abdominal, or intra-abdominal (see Fig. 2.1). The behaviors of the tumors, including growth rates, age predilection and recurrence rates often vary with the location of the tumor [2, 3]. The most common locations are the extremities (around the limb girdles or the proximal extremities), the abdominal wall (most commonly in women during or after pregnancy), and intra-abdominal or mesenteric. Depending on their location, they tend to infiltrate adjacent organs, extend along fascial planes, compress blood vessels and nerves, erode bones or obstruct organs such as the bowel.

Though they have a benign histologic appearance, lacking the nuclear and cytoplasmic features of a malignancy and a metastatic potential, DT may cause debilitating symptoms such as pain, deformity and in some cases life-threatening organ damage because of their locally invasive nature. DT may range from small slow-growing masses to rapidly enlarging aggressive tumors. The clinical course of the disease is unpredictable but increasing information suggests that an initial phase of growth may be followed by a long period of growth arrest with tumor stabilization or even regression [4–6].

2.2 Incidence

Though the actual incidence is likely significantly higher due to misdiagnosis, multiple and confusing pathologic nomenclature and underreporting, the current estimate is an incidence of 2–4 per million per year. Desmoid tumors are undisputedly very rare, with only 900 new cases diagnosed each year in the US. These tumors constitute 0.03% of all biopsy-analyzed neoplasms and < 3% of all biopsy-analyzed soft-tissue tumors [7]. These tumors have been documented in patients between 3 and 67 years [8], with a peak incidence of 25–35. The female to male ratio ranges from 1.4 to 1.8 [9–12]. Reitamo et al. noted that in females under the age of 15 an

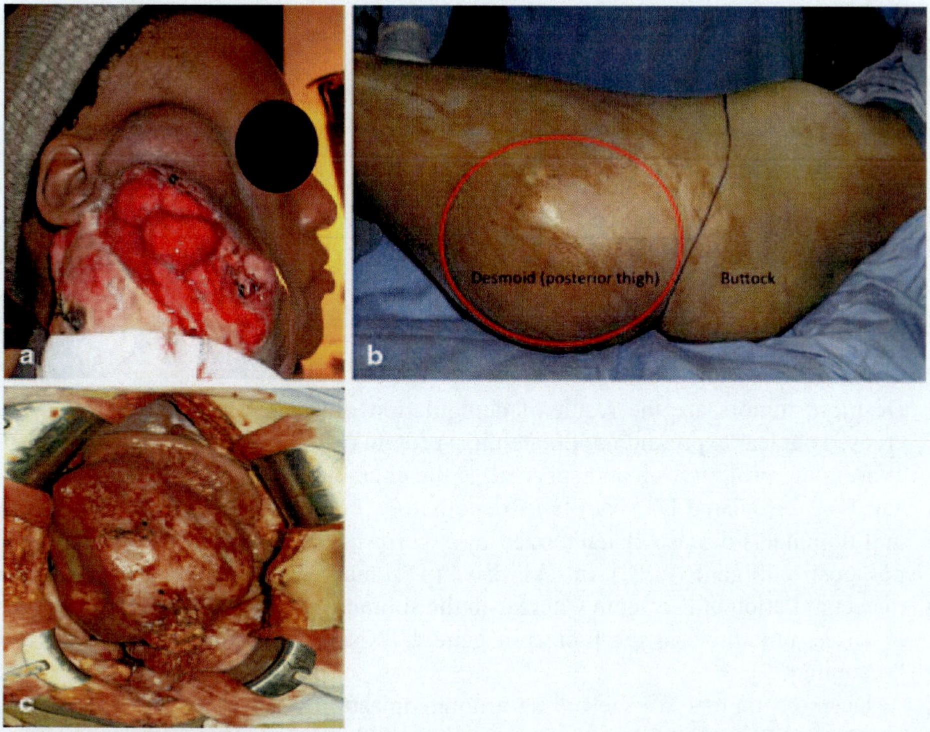

Fig. 2.1 Extra-abdominal and intra-abdominal tumors. **a** Head and neck **b** Lower extremity **c** Intra-abdominal (*mesenteric*) desmoid (Courtesy of Raphael E. Pollock, MD, PhD, University of Texas MD Anderson Cancer Center)

extra-abdominal location was more common while in females aged 18–36 an abdominal location was more common. DT occur in the abdominal wall with a female to male ratio of 7:1 [13]. There was no association with race [14]. In one study, 16% of primary tumors were < 5 cm, 28% were between 5 and 10 cm and 50% were greater than 10 cm [15]. While the majority of desmoid tumors are sporadic, approximately 5% are associated with Familial Adenomatous Polyposis (FAP).

2.3 FAP

Desmoid tumors may present sporadically or as a manifestation of a hereditary syndrome called Familial Adenomatous Polyposis (FAP). FAP is a familial cancer predisposition syndrome characterized by the development of hundreds to thousands of premalignant adenomatous polyps in the colon and rectum by the age of 40 years [16]. Unless treated at an early age, almost all patients with FAP will develop colorectal cancer [17]. In fact, FAP is responsible for 1% of all cases of colorectal cancer [18]. The treatment of choice is prophylactic surgery comprising colectomy with ileorectal anastomosis or restorative proctocolectomy [19].

A significant percentage (3.5–32%) of FAP patients will develop DT during their lifetime [20–22]. The risk of patients with FAP-developing DT is 800–1,000-fold higher compared to the general population [23]. The peak incidence of DT in FAP is between the second and the third decade [24]. In the majority of cases DT occur following prophylactic surgery for FAP [25, 26] with surgical trauma identified as a trigger for the development of DT in FAP. However, in some cases, DT may be the first manifestation of FAP with about 4% of cases of DT appearing as an incidental finding at the time of primary surgery [27]. Family history is a predisposing factor for DT formation in FAP patients [28, 29], with an observed increased risk of 2.5 times in first-degree relatives [29].

2.4 Etiology

Desmoid tumors are the result of deregulation of connective tissue growth. Increased nuclear expression of β-catenin, a protein responsible for regulation of gene expression, proliferation and survival, is the characteristic feature in both sporadic and FAP-associated DT. Familial Adenomatous Polyposis is a hereditary (autosomal dominant) disease characterized by a germ-line mutation in the adenomatous polyposis coli gene (APC). In FAP-driven DT, inactivation of the APC gene leads to accumulation of β-catenin whereas in the sporadic setting, in approximately 85% of cases, mutations in the β-catenin gene CTNNBi lead to increased activity of β-catenin [30].

Desmoid tumors are viewed as a nonneoplastic process by some authors and as a well-differentiated low-grade sarcoma by others [31]. The characterization of desmoid tumors as a neoplastic process rather than as an inflammatory fibrous reaction has been bolstered by the molecular studies of X-chromosome inactivation that confirmed that DT are the result of a clonal process [31, 32]. Nonrandom X-chromosome inactivation, trisomy 8 and/or 20 was demonstrated in greater than 30% of sporadic DT [33]. DT behave aggressively as locally infiltrating mesenchymal monoclonal proliferations that lack metastatic potential [34].

2.5 Clinical Presentation

In sporadic desmoids, between 37 and 50% of DT arise in the abdominal region [35–37]. The most common extra-abdominal sites are the shoulder girdle, chest wall and inguinal regions [38] (see Fig. 2.2).

Patients with intra-abdominal desmoids may have asymptomatic masses which silently enlarge and infiltrate into adjacent structures [2] or may have symptoms of weight loss, cachexia, malaise, compression of ureters, renal failure, small bowel compression, perforation and peritonitis [35, 41, 42]. In sporadic DT, infiltration of intestinal or visceral structures is less common but muscle, nerve and vessel involvement may result in debilitating symptoms such as pain, restricted mobility or deformity. A characteristic example of such presentation is the infiltration of the brachial plexus by a shoulder girdle tumor which may result in pain in

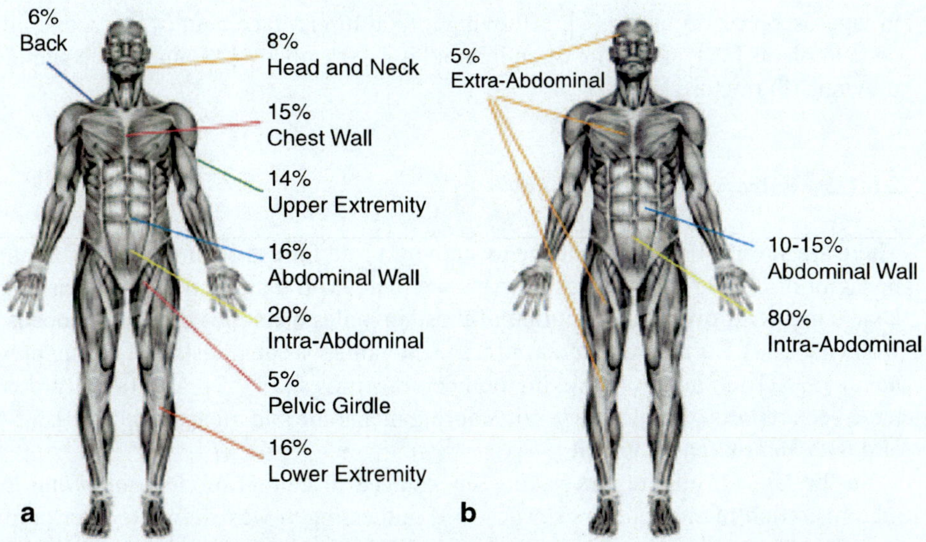

Fig. 2.2 **a** Locations of all desmoid tumors [39]. **b** FAP-associated desmoid tumors [40]

the shoulder and arm and weakness of the upper limb. The management of such cases is challenging as surgical excision is often not a feasible option. Due to their aggressive infiltrating nature DT may cause impairment or loss of function of vital organs. DT of the upper chest wall may engulf organs in the mediastinum including the trachea or the esophagus. As a result patients may suffer from dyspnoea/asphyxiation and dysphagia, respectively. Weiss et al. reported a patient with quadriceps paralysis and neurogenic bladder from focal invasion of the lumbosacral plexus [43].

2.6 Clinical Considerations

2.6.1 Risk Factors

2.6.1.1 Trauma

Trauma has been theorized to increase the risk of DT occurrence. Antecedent trauma, often surgical, has been reported at the site of the DT in approximately 25% of cases [10, 29, 44]. Moreover, 68–86% of abdominal wall and intra-abdominal wall DT are noted after abdominal surgery, the majority within the first 5 postoperative years [21]. FAP patients appear to be at even greater risk for DT development following surgical trauma with a reported 84% of cases of FAP-associated desmoids occurring within 5 years of abdominal surgery [45]. There have been reports of DT in laparoscopic port sites [46], following a total hip replacement [47], around silicone implants [48], at the site of an internal jugular catheter [49] and at the site of a previous rib fracture [50].

2.6.1.2 Estrogen and Pregnancy

There are several lines of evidence to support a role for estrogen in modulating the behavior of DT. Several studies have shown that DT in females of childbearing age have a greater growth rate than that of those in males or in pre- or postmenopausal women [3, 51]. Further, an increased frequency rate was demonstrated during pregnancy [9, 51] and in females taking oral contraceptives [28, 52]. Additionally, there have been reports of tumor regression during menarche and menopause [51, 53, 54] and with Tamoxifen treatment [55].

In the lab, fibrous tumors have been induced in animal models following the administration of exogenous estrogen [53] and estrogen was shown to exert a mitogenic influence on many cell types, including fibroblasts [56]. Additionally, in a study of human DT, estrogen receptors (ER) were observed in 33% of all DT examined, with an equal incidence in males and females and with antiestrogen binding sites found in 79% of samples, including some which were ER negative [57].

In pregnancy-associated DT, the mass is most frequently located within one of the two rectus muscles of the abdominal wall without involving the midline [58, 59]. Pregnancy-associated DT may develop during any trimester or postpartum.

While the history of antecedent trauma is 28% of sporadic DT [60], such a history is ostensibly missing in pregnant DT patients. It has been theorized that the combination of an altered hormonal milieu and the trauma of stretching of the abdominal aponeurosis during the advancement of pregnancy are contributing factors [61]. There has been one report of a DT that developed at the site of a prior caesarean section scar during a subsequent pregnancy [16].

A study of FAP patients revealed no association between the female gender or pregnancy and the risk of the development of DT [62]. After examining the divergent natural histories and behaviors of pregnancy-associated DT and FAP-associated DT, one group of investigators concluded that these two types of DT are separate entities [61].

2.6.2 Unique Tumor Locations

2.6.2.1 Head and Neck DT

Head and neck DT are a more aggressive disorders that affect a younger population. Twelve percent of extra-abdominal DT arise in the head and neck [63]. The mean age is 16.87 years, with 57.32% of cases under 11 years. Children with DT of the head and neck are younger at the time of diagnosis than children with DT at other sites [64–66]. There is a 30% local recurrence (LR) with a male to female ratio of 1:1 [67]. One explanation for the often difficult clinical course is the restricted anatomy containing crucial neural and vascular structures [67].

2.6.2.2 Breast

Desmoid tumors are rarely seen in the breast and can simulate breast carcinoma [68].

2.6.3 FAP vs. Non-FAP

Anatomic locations differ between FAP and sporadic DT, with more intra-abdominal or abdominal than extra-abdominal wall tumors. In a Mayo clinic review from 1976 to 1999, 67% of FAP-associated DT were abdominal as compared to 11% sporadic. Limb DT accounted for 1.4% in FAP patients and 34.7% in non-FAP patients [69]. While one large study reported a female to male ratio of 3.0 in FAP patients with DT [28], some studies failed to show the female predominance in FAP-associated DT that has been shown in sporadic DT [29, 44]. Additionally, desmoid development occurred an average of 6 years earlier in FAP patients [22]. Eighty to 90% of FAP individuals will carry an alteration in the APC gene on chromosome number 5. The majority will have a family history of colorectal cancer and polyposis. But, up to 33% of FAP patients with DT will have a de novo mutation within the APC gene and therefore no family history of DT [69].

2.6.4 Multicentricity

There have been 10–20 reports of multicentric extra-abdominal DT, mostly in FAP patients [70–73]. These usually recur in the same limb in proximity to the site of the primary tumor. They do not grow simultaneously, with the second growth generally occurring years later [74].

2.7 Clinical Course

DT remains an enigmatic disease with a variable course that can range from an incidental small tumor that can remain small and stable or become large and grow rapidly, causing death in a matter of months or years. The morbidity and mortality is largely determined by the location of the tumor and therefore the adjacent structures the tumor may infiltrate or compress. According to Church, 10% of DT will resolve spontaneously, 30% will undergo cycles of progression and resolution, 50% will remain stable after diagnosis and 10% will progress rapidly [75].

Some of the local recurrence (LR) rates are determined by tumor location. For example, extremity tumors are considered locally aggressive and have LR ranging from 24 to 77% [76–80]. LR rates for intra-abdominal tumors are higher than for extra-abdominal tumors, reported to be 57–86% [28, 81, 82]. One review found LR to be 24% for abdominal wall, 43% for extra-abdominal and 77% for intra-abdominal tumors [2]. In a study of 78 FAP patients that studied progression-free survival rates after surgery versus conservative care, it was determined that extra-abdominal and abdominal wall DT had better outcomes and more benefit overall from surgical intervention than intra-abdominal tumors [22].

Gender has been shown not to be a prognostic factor for LR [4, 83]. There is disagreement about whether age may play a role in recurrence. Some studies have shown that younger age was associated with increased local treatment failure [39, 84] while others did not [75, 85]. One study found the recurrence rate in children to be 88%, twice that of adults (38%) [10]. Also controversial is the role of age in LR risk. Some studies show increased risk of LR in female patients older than 30 [88] while others show increased risk in patients under 30 [9]. One larger study of 103 patients over 26 years found no correlation with recurrence to age, gender, or site [83]. There is some suggestion that size of the primary tumor is an important predictor for recurrence [40] but that a single recurrence did not significantly increase the likelihood of a subsequent recurrence [10].

There is ongoing controversy over the significance of margin status in predicting LR. In one series, response rates of 72% and 41% were reported for tumor-free and tumor-positive margins, respectively [86]. Other studies show no correlation with margin status. The MSKCC (Memorial Sloan-Kettering Cancer Center) and Istituto Nazionale Tumori experiences showed no significant difference (22% negative vs. 24% positive [76] and 21% positive vs. 18% negative) [87].

The limitations in the studies stem from the small subject numbers and the mix of intra- and extra-abdominal tumors as well as primary and recurrent lesions, leading to conflicting results about the biology of these elusive tumors [9, 70, 76–81, 88–90]. The difficulties of interpretation of the data are compounded by the unpredictable natural course of this tumor that can apparently regress even without treatment [75].

2.8 Conclusions

Desmoid tumors are an enigmatic, elusive disease that continue to defy definition. Due to their rarity and the practical limitations in their study, these tumors often evade accurate characterization. As they can arise in many locations throughout the body, thereby presenting unique challenges to physicians in many different fields, the most appropriate and fruitful approach to caring for any individual desmoid tumor patient is a multidisciplinary one.

References

1. Goldblum J, Fletcher JA (2002) Desmoid-type fibromatoses. In: Fletcher CDM, Unni KK, Mertens F (Eds) World Health Organization classification of tumours. Pathology and Genetics of Tumours of Soft Tissue and Bone. IARC Press, Lyon, pp 83–84
2. Easter DW, Halasz NA (2010) Recent trends in the management of desmoid tumors. Summary of 19 cases and review of the literature. Ann Surg 210:765–769
3. Hayry P, Reitamo JJ, Totterman S et al (1982) The desmoid tumor. II. Analysis of factors possibly contributing to the etiology and growth behavior. Am J Clin Pathol 77:674–680
4. Phillips SR, A'Hern R, Thomas JM (2004) Aggressive fibromatosis of the abdominal wall, limbs and limb girdles. Br J Surg 91(12):1624–1629
5. Bonvalot S, Eldweny H, Haddad V et al (2008) Extra-abdominal primary fibromatosis: aggressive management could be avoided in a subgroup of patients. Eur J Surg Oncol 34(4):462–468
6. Stoeckle E, Coindre JM, Longy M et al (2009) A critical analysis of treatment strategies in desmoid tumours: a review of a series of 106 cases. Eur J Surg Oncol 35:129–134
7. Micke O, Seegenschmiedt MH (2005) Radiation therapy for aggressive fibromatosis (desmoid tumors): results of a national Patterns of Care Study. Int J Radiat Oncol Biol Phys 61:882–891
8. Brodsky IT, Gordan MS, Hajdu SI, Burt M (1992) Desmoid tumors of the chest wall. A locally recurrent problem. J Thorac Cardiovasc Surg 104:900–903
9. Posner MC, Shiu MH, Newsome JL, Hajdu SI, Gaynor JJ, Brennan MF (1989) The desmoid tumor. Not a benign disease. Arch Surg 124:191–196
10. Lopez R, Kemalyan N, Moseley HS, Dennis D, Vetto RM (1990) Problems in diagnosis and management of desmoid tumors. Am J Surg 159:450–453
11. Jarvinen HJ (1987) Desmoid disease as a part of familial adenomatous polyposis coli. Acat Chir Scand 153:379–383
12. Klemmer S, Pascoe L, DeCosse J (1987) Occurrence of desmoids in patients with familial adenomatous polyposis of the colon. Am J Med Genet 28:385–392
13. Pack GT, Ehrlich HE (1944) Neoplasms of the anterior abdominal wall with special consideration to desmoid tumours. Int Abstr Surg 79:177–198
14. Wong SL (2008) Diagnosis and management of desmoid tumors and fibrosarcoma. J Surg Onc 97:554–558
15. De Camargo VP, Keohan ML, D'Adamo DR, Antonescu CR, Brennan MF, Singer S, Ahn LS, Maki RG (2010) Clinical outcomes of systemic therapy for patients with deep fibromatosis (desmoid tumor). Cancer 116:2258–2265
16. De Cian F, Delay E, Rudigoz RC, Rachere D, Rivoire M (1999) Desmoid tumor arising in a cesarean section scar during pregnancy: monitoring and management. Gynecol Oncol 75:145–148
17. Herman K, Marcinek A (1996) Abdominal desmoid in a 28 year-old pregnant woman. Ginekol Pol 67:374–375
18. Burke AP, Sobin LH, Shekitka KM et al (1990) Intra-abdominal fibromatosis: a pathologic analysis of 130 tumors with comparison of clinical subgroups. Am J Surg Pathol 14:335–341
19. Suarez V, Hall C (1985) Mesenteric fibromatosis. Br J Surg 72:976–978
20. Bertario L, Russo A, Sala P et al (2003) Multiple approach to the exploration of genotype-phenotype correlations in familial adenomatous polyposis. J Clin Oncol 21:1698–1707
21. Clark SK, Phillips RK (1996) Desmoids in familial adenomatous polyposis. Br J Surg 83:1494–1504
22. Nieuwenhuis MH, Casparie M, Mathus-Vliegen LM, Dekkers OM, Hogendoorn PC, Vasen HF (2010) A nation-wide study comparing sporadic and familial adenomatous polyposis-related desmoid-type fibromatoses. Int J Cancer 129(1):256–261
23. Fong Y, Rosen PP, Brennan MF (1999) Multifocal desmoids. Surgery 114:902–906

24. Godwin Y, McCulloch TA, Scully L (2001) Extra-abdominal desmoid tumour of the breast: review of the primary management and the implications for breast reconstruction. Br J Plast Surg 54:268–271
25. Corsten M, Donald P, Boggan J et al (1998) Extra-abdominal fibromatosis (desmoid tumor) arising in the infratemporal fossa: a case report. Skull Base Surg 8(4):237–241
26. Heinimann K, Mullhaupt B, Weber W et al (1998) Phenotypic differences in familial adenomatous polyposis based on APC germline mutation status. Gut 43:675–679
27. Sleijfer S (2009) Management of aggressive fibromatosis: can we unravel the maze of treatment options? Eur J Cancer 45(17):2928–2929
28. Jones IT, Jagelman DG, Fazio VW, Lavery IC, Weakley FL, McGannon E (1986) Desmoid tumors in familial polyposis coli. Ann Surg 204:94–97
29. Gurbuz AK, Giardiello FM, Petersen GM, Krush AJ, Offerhaus GJ, Booker SV, Kerr MC, Hamilton SR (1994) Desmoid tumours in familial adenomatous polyposis. Gut 35:377–381
30. De Bree E, Keus R, Melissas J, Tsiftsis D, van Coevorden F (2009) Desmoid tumors: need for an individualized approach. Expert Rev Anticancer Ther 9:525–535
31. Li M, Cordon-Cardo C, Gerald WL, Rosai J (1996) Desmoid fibromatosis is a clonal process. Hum Pathol 27:939–943
32. De Wever I, Dal Cin P, Fletcher CD et al (2000) Cytogenetic, clinical and morphologic correlations in 78 cases of fibromatosis: a report from the CHAMP Study Group. Chromosomes and morphology. Mod Pathol 13:1080–1085
33. Fletcher JA, Naeem R, Xiao S, Corson JM (1995) Chromosome aberrations in desmoid tumors: trisomy 8 may be a predictor of recurrence. Cancer Genet Cytogenet 63:527–529
34. Alman BA, Pajerski ME, Diaz-Cano S et al (1997) Aggressive fibromatosis (desmoid tumor) is a monoclonal disorder. Diagn Mol Pathol 6:98–101
35. Lewis JJ, Boland PJ, Leung DH, Woodruff JM, Brennan MF (1999) The enigma of desmoid tumor. Ann Surg 229:866–873
36. Weiss S, Goldblum JR (Eds) (2001) Enzinger and Weiss's soft tissue tumors, 4th edn. Mobis, St Louis, pp 641–693
37. Bruce JM, Bradley EL 3rd, Satchidanand SK (1996) A desmoid tumor of the pancreas. Sporadic intra-abdominal desmoid revisited. Int J Pancreatol 19:197–203
38. Khorsand J, Karakousis CP (1985) Desmoid tumours and their management. Am J Surg 149:215–218
39. Lev D, Kotilingam D, Wei C, Ballo MT, Zagars GK, Pisters PW, Lazar AA, Patel SR, Benjamin RS, Pollock RE (2007) Optimizing treatment of desmoid tumors. J Clin Oncol 25(13):1785–1791
40. Sturt JNH, Clark SK (2006) Current ideas in desmoid tumors. Familial Cancer 5:275–285
41. Corbel L, Souissi M, Chretien Y, Dufour B (1992) Desmoid tumor of the mesentery. An uncommon cause of ureteral obstruction. J Radiol 73:669–672
42. Anthony T, Rodriquez-Bigas MA, Weber TK, Petrelli NJ (1996) Desmoid tumor. J Am Coll Surg 182:369–377
43. Weiss AJ, Lackman RD (1989) Low-dose chemotherapy of desmoid tumors. Cancer 64:1192–1194
44. McAdams WA, Goligher JC (1970) The occurrence of desmoids in patients with familial polyposis coli. Cr J Surg 57:618–631
45. Bertario L, Russo A, Sala P et al (2001) Genotype and phenotype factor as determinant of desmoid tumors in patients with familial adenomatous polyposis. Int J Cancer 95:102–107
46. Lynch HT, Fitzgibbons R Jr (1996) Surgery, desmoid tumors and familial adenomatous polyposis: case report and literature review. Am J Gastroenterol 91:2598–2601
47. Gebhart M, Fourmarier M, Heymans O, Alexiou J, Yengue P, De Saint-Aubain N (1999) Development of a desmoid tumor at the site of a total hip replacement. Acta Orthop Belg 65:230–234
48. Reitamo JJ, Hayry P, Nykyri E, Saxen E (1982) The desmoid tumor. I. Incidence, sex, age, and anatomical distribution in the Finnish population. Am J Clin Pathol 77:665–673

49. Skhiri H, Zellama D, Ameur FM, Moussa A, Gmar BS, Achour A, Ben Dhia N, Zakhama A, Elmay M (2004) Desmoid cervical tumor following the placing of an internal jugular catheter. Presse Med 33:95–97 (French)
50. Wiel Marin A, Romagnoli A, Carlucci I, Veneziani A, Mercui M, Destito C (1995) Thoracic desmoid tumors: a rare evolution of rib fracture. Etiopathogenesis and therapeutic considerations. G Chir 16:341–344
51. Reitamo JJ, Scheinin TM, Hayry P (1986) The desmoid syndrome. New aspects in the cause, pathogenesis and treatment of the desmoid tumor. Am J Surg 151:230–237
52. Waddell WR (1975) Treatment of intra-abdominal and abdominal wall desmoid tumors with drugs that affect the metabolism of cyclic 3″.5″-adenosine monophosphate. Ann Surg 181:299–302
53. Dahn I, Johnsson N, Lundh G (1963) Desmoid tumors. A series of 33 cases. Acta Chir Scand 126:305–314
54. Lofti AM, Dozois RR, Gordon H, Hruska LS, Weiland LH, Carryer PW, Hurt RD (1989) Mesenteric fibromatosis complicating familial adenomatous polyposis: predisposing factors and results of treatment. Int J Colorectal Dis 4:30–36
55. Wilcken N, Tattersall MH (1991) Endocrine therapy for desmoid tumors. Cancer 68:1384–1388
56. Dhingra K (1999) Antiestrogens-tamoxifen, SERMS and beyond. Invest New Drugs 17:285–311
57. Lim CL, Walker MJ, Mehta RR et al (1986) Estrogen and antiestrogen binding sites in desmoid tumors. Eur J Cancer Clin Oncol 22:583
58. Gansar GF, Markowitz IP, Cerise EJ (1987) Thirty years of experience with desmoid tumors at Charity Hospital. Surg 53(6):318–319
59. Galetotti F, Facci E, Bianchin E (2006) Desmoid tumour involving the abdominal rectus muscle: report of a case. Hernia 10:278–281
60. Enzinger FM, Weiss SW (1995) Soft tissue tumors, 3rd Edn. Mosby Year Book Inc., Saint Louis.
61. Johner A, Tiwari P, Zetler P, Wiseman SM (2009) Abdominal wall desmoid tumors associated with pregnancy: current concepts. Expert Rev Anticancer Ther 9(11):1675–1682
62. Nieuwenhuis MH, De Vos tos Nederveen Cappel W, Botma A et al (2008) Desmoid tumors in a Dutch cohort of patients with familial adenomatous polyposis. Clin Gastroenterol Hepatol 6:215–219
63. Conley J, Healey WV, Stout AP (1966) Fibromatosis of the head and neck. Am J Surg 112(4):609–614
64. Ayala AG, Ro JY, Goepfert H, Cangir A Khorsand J, Flake G (1986) Desmoid fibromatosis: a clinicopathologic study of 25 children. Semin Diagn Pathol 3:138–150
65. Scougall P, Staheli LT, Chew DE, Taylor TKF, Almquist EE (1987) Desmoid tumors in childhood. Orthop Rev 16:481–488
66. Spiegel DA, Dormans JP, Meyer JS et al (1999) Aggressive fibromatosis from infancy to adolescence. J Pediatr Oprthop 19:776–784
67. Kruse AL, Luebber HT, Gratz KW, Obwegeser JA (2010) Aggressive fibromatosis of the head and neck: a new classification based on a literature review over 40 years (1968–2008). Oral Maxillofac Surg 14(40):227–232
68. Greenberg D, McIntyre H, Ramsaroop R, Artyr J, Harman J (2002) Aggressive fibromatosis of the breast: a case report and literature review. Breast J 8:55–57
69. Fallen T, Wilson M, Morlan B, Lindor NL (2006) Desmoid tumors-a characterization of patients seen at Mayor Clinic 1976–1999. Fam Cancer 5:191–194
70. Rock MG, Pritchard DJ, Reiman HM et al (1984) Extra-abdominal desmoid tumors. J Bone Joint Surg 66A:1369–1373
71. Wagstaff MJD, Raurell A, Perks AGB (2004) Multicentric extra-abdominal desmoid tumours. Br Assoc of Plastic Surgeons 57:362–365
72. Antal I, Szendroi M, Kovacs G et al (1994) Multicentric extra-abdominal desmoid tumour: a case report. J Cancer Res Clin Oncol 120:490–494

73. Maurer F, Horst F, Pfannenberg C et al (1996) Multifocal extra-abdominal desmoid tumour-diagnostic and therapeutic problems. Arch Orthop Trauma Surg 115:359–362
74. Barber HM, Galasko CSB, Woods CG (1973) Multicentric extra-abdominal desmoid tumours. Report of two cases. J Bone Joint Surg 55:858–863
75. Church JM (1995) Desmoid tumours in patients with familial adenomatous polyposis. Semin Colon Rectal Surg 6:29–32
76. Merchant NP, Lewis JJ, Leung DH, Woodruff JM, Brennan MF (1999) Extremity and trunk desmoid tumors: a multifactorial analysis of outcome. Cancer 86:2045–2052
77. Wold LE, Weiland LH (1983) Tumefactive fibro-inflammatory lesions of the head and neck. Am J Surg Pathol 7:477–482
78. Exelby PR (1981) Surgery of soft tissue sarcomas in children. Natl Cancer Inst Monogr 153–157
79. Scott RJ, Taeschner W, Heinimann K et al (1997) Association of extracolonic manifestations of familial adenomatous polyposis with acetylation phenotype in a large FAP kindred. Eur J Hum Genet 5:43–49
80. Thomas JA, Kothare SN (1972) Desmoid tumors of the abdominal wall. Indian J Cancer 9:66–69
81. Rodriguez-Bigas MA, Mahoney MC, Karakousis CP, Petrelli NJ (1994) Desmoid tumors in patients with familial adenomatous polyposis. Cancer 74:1270–1274
82. Penna C, Tiret E, Parc R et al (1993) Operation and abdominal desmoid tumors in familial adenomatous polyposis. Surg Gyencol Obstet 177:263–268
83. Pignatti G, Barbanti-Brodano G, Ferrari D, Gherlinzoni F, Bertoni F, Bacchini P, Barbieri E, Giunti A, Campanacci M (2000) Extraabdominal desmoid tumor: a study of 83 cases. Clinical Orthop and Related Research 375:207–213
84. Sorensen A, Keller J, Nielsen OS, Jensen OM (2002) Treatment of aggressive fibromatosis. A retrospective study of 72 patients followed for 1–27 years. Acta Orthop Scan 73:213–219
85. De Bree E, van Coevorden F, Keus RB, Tsiftsis DD (2004) Treatment of extremity desmoid tumours. Eur J Surg Oncol 30:1141–1142
86. Nuyttens JJ, Rust PF, Thomas CR, Turrisi III (2000) Surgery versus radiation therapy for patients with aggressive fibromatosis or desmoid tumors. A comparative review of 22 articles. Cancer 88:1517–1523
87. Gronchi A, Casali PG, Mariani L et al (2003) Quality of surgery and outcome in extra-abdominal aggressive fibromatosis: a series of patients surgically treated at a single institution. J Clin Oncol 21:190–197
88. Pritchard DJ, Nascimento AG, Petersen IA (1996) Local control of extra-abdominal desmoid tumors. J Bone Joint Surg 78:848–854
89. Miralbell R, Suit HD, Mankin HJ, Zuckerberg LR, Stracher MA, Rosenberg AE (1990) Fibromatoses: from postsurgical surveillance to combined surgery and radiation therapy. Int J Radiat Oncol BIol Phys 18:535–540
90. Anthony T, Rodriguez-Bigas MA, Weer TK, Petrelli NJ (1996) Desmoid tumors. J Am Coll Surg 182:369–377

Chapter 3
Pathology of Desmoid Tumors

Wai Chin Foo and Alexander J. Lazar

Contents

Abstract Desmoid fibromatosis is an uncommon locally aggressive fibroblastic/myofibroblastic neoplasm with no metastatic ability. The pathologic diagnosis is usually straightforward but can be difficult in small biopsies and in recurrences associated with scars from a prior procedure. Immunohistochemistry, specifically β-catenin, and more recently, molecular diagnostics can play an important role in its diagnosis. This chapter reviews the clinical and pathological features, highlights the role of immunohistochemistry and molecular studies in distinguishing desmoids from potential mimics, and briefly discusses the clinical behavior with reference to possible predictors of recurrence.

Keywords Desmoid fibromatosis • Differential diagnosis • Histology • Immunohistochemistry • Molecular • Recurrence • β-Catenin • *CTNNB1* • *APC*

W. C. Foo (✉)
Department of Pathology, University of Texas; MD Anderson Cancer Center, Houston, Texas 77030, USA
e-mail: wfoo@mdanderson.org

C. Litchman (ed.), *Desmoid Tumors*,
DOI 10.1007/978-94-007-1685-8_3, © Springer Science+Business Media B.V. 2012

3.1 Introduction

Desmoid fibromatosis, also termed desmoid tumor, deep fibromatosis, and aggressive fibromatosis, is a locally aggressive mesenchymal neoplasm that arises from deep muscle fascia, aponeurosis, and tendons. It is uncommon, representing less than 2% of all soft tissue sarcomas and a much smaller percentage of mesenchymal tumors in general. It has an incidence of two to four patients per million of the population per year. John MacFarlane, who noticed tumors in the abdominal walls of women who had recently given birth, first recognized and described desmoid fibromatosis in 1832. Arthur Purdy Stout later recognized similar tumors occurring at other anatomic sites. Since then, there has been advancements in the diagnosis and pathogenetic understanding of desmoid tumors, including recognition of its distinct clinical associations, and more recently, its unique genetic aberrations.

3.2 Pathological Description

The presentation of desmoid tumors is characterized by where they arise. The potential anatomic locations can be divided into three groups: extra-abdominal, abdominal wall, and intra-abdominal. Regardless of anatomic location, desmoid fibromatoses share a common macroscopic and microscopic appearance (Fig. 3.1). They are frequently large tumors with infiltrative borders. There is considerable size variability ranging from less than 5 cm to greater than 20 cm in greatest dimension. As expected, those arising in the mesentery (intra-abdominal) are generally larger than those arising in the abdominal wall or in extra-abdominal sites given the usual delay in presentation of the former. Gross surfaces appear fibrous, being white or tan with coarse trabeculations. In recurrent lesions, macroscopic distinction from scar tissue is generally not possible.

Microscopically, the tumor is composed of uniform, palely eosinophilic spindle cells with tapering, vesicular nuclei. Nucleoli are inconspicuous, and atypia and nuclear hyperchromasia are not seen. The overall cellularity and mitotic activity is variable, but mitoses are generally sparse and do not appear to be predictive of outcome. Cellularity can range from very sparse and fibrotic (perhaps best exemplified by Gardner-type fibromas, but also seen in sporadic cases) to relatively cellular, appearing almost storiform in areas. Generally, though, the overall pattern is mostly enlongated fascicles. Ultrastructural studies indicate that the spindle cells have features of both fibroblasts and myofibroblasts, but this is not useful in making diagnostic distinctions. Architecturally, the tumor cells are typically arranged in long, sweeping fascicles, and vague whorls in a background of eosinophilic, collagenized stroma with prominent thin-walled vessels. The stroma can also show myxoid features, reportedly more common in the breast and the mesentery, but can be seen in other more common sites. Keloidal-type hyalinization of collagen has been described, predominantly in mesenteric desmoids [9], and is also seen in a small subset of cases at other sites (Fig. 3.1f). Other histological features that have been recognized include

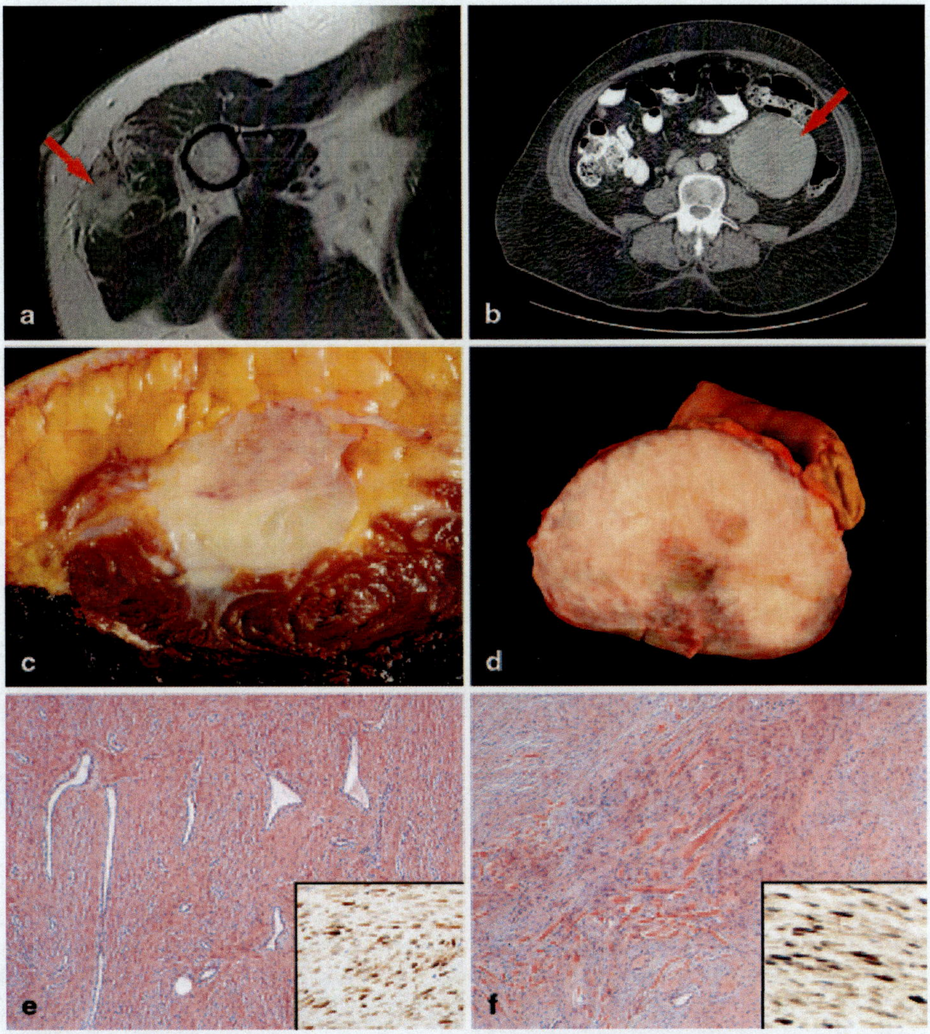

Fig. 3.1 **a** Magnetic Resonance Imaging (MRI) shows a desmoid (*red arrow*) with infiltrative borders in the shoulder. **b** Computed Tomography (CT) image reveals a large intra-abdominal desmoid (*red arrow*) associated with the mesentery of the small bowel. **c** The resected shoulder tumor shows infiltration of the adipose tissue and skeletal muscle. **d** The mesenteric desmoid is better circumscribed in this case and reveals some central degeneration and hemorrhage at the periphery. **e** Characteristic spindle cell morphology is seen with prominent vessels. **f** Sclerotic or hyalinized collagen (red-colored fibers in the *central* and *left* portions of the image) similar to those seen in cutaneous keloid-type scars is sometimes seen. Insets in panels e and f demonstrate nuclear accumulation of β-catenin on immunohistochemistry

scattered lymphocytes, nodular lymphoid aggregates, and atypical multinucleated cells which represent degenerating skeletal muscle at the periphery of extra-abdominal and abdominal wall tumors (Fig. 3.2e). The presence of atypical multinucleated cells can often be demonstrated by immunohistochemistry for smooth muscle actin (SMA), desmin, and sometimes myoD1 and myogenin are expressed in these distressed cells. Often more recognizable skeletal muscle is in the vicinity.

3.3 Immunohistochemistry

β-Catenin is a protein important in the Wnt signaling pathway and functions with E-cadherin as a constituent of adherens junctions. It is primarily present in the cell membrane and cytoplasm and colocalizes to a large extent with E-cadherin in adherens junctions in most nonneoplastic (normal) and neoplastic tissues (see Chap. 4). Epithelial-type tissues tend to show a membranous distribution of β-catenin with cytoplasmic reactivity while mesenchymal tissues usually show only cytoplasmic reactivity. Tissues with an activated Wnt pathway can show nuclear reactivity for β-catenin (such as germinative cells in the hair follicle). Point mutations in exon 3 of the gene β-catenin (*CTNNB1*) or inactivating mutations in the *APC* gene result in distinct nuclear accumulation and localization of β-catenin [5, 17, 20, 21] (Fig. 3.1e,f, insets). As such, antibody to β-catenin is useful in distinguishing desmoids from its histologic mimics, which generally lack this feature. Nuclear reactivity shows relatively high specificity, up to 70%, for desmoids regardless of site. Nuclear reactivity can also be seen in synovial sarcomas, solitary fibrous tumors, and endometrial stromal sarcomas albeit with a lower sensitivity. Active scar tissue can also show nuclear accumulation of β-catenin, though it is usually considerably less intense and scattered than seen in desmoids. This is expected as the Wnt pathway is activated and necessary for efficient wound healing. It should be noted that both membranous and cytoplasmic reactivity can be seen in other neoplastic and nonneoplastic tissues [5, 17, 20, 21].

Other antibodies that have been examined in desmoids include antibodies to smooth muscle actin, desmin, and KIT. Cytoplasmic reactivity with antibodies to smooth muscle actin is frequently positive. Desmin antibody may also show focal cytoplasmic reactivity in a small subset of cases. Neither desmin nor smooth muscle actin are specific for desmoids fibromatosis [30]. Yantiss et al. originally reported weak immunoreactivity to KIT antibody in up to 75% of intra-abdominal fibromatoses [31]. However, more recent evaluations with KIT antibody have shown only minimal, if any, immunoreactivity in desmoids [18].

3.4 Differential Diagnosis

The differential diagnosis of desmoid fibromatosis includes reactive conditions, such as scar and nodular fasciitis, and other mesenchymal neoplasms, including low-grade fibromyxoid sarcoma, malignant peripheral nerve sheath tumor, non-

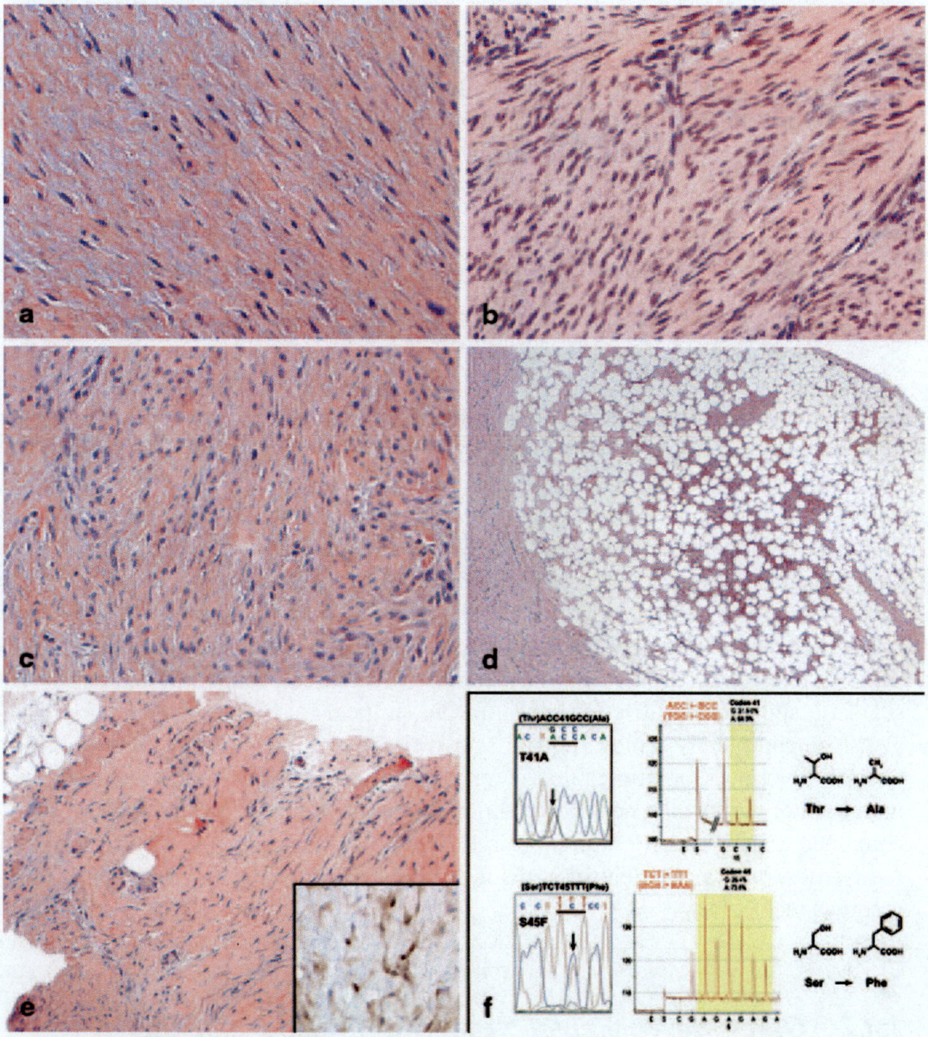

Fig. 3.2 **a** Desmoids can be relatively hypocellular and will sometimes show myxoid change. **b** Other cases can be more cellular. **c** Cases can also show more plump nuclei and the degree of collagen deposition is variable. Multiple cellular patterns can be seen in the same case. **d** Significant infiltration of adipose or other tissues is often a feature. **e** Needle biopsies can be difficult to distinguish from scar. Correlation with clinical and radiologic features can be helpful in making this distinction. This case shows infiltration of skeletal muscle. Immunohistochemistry to evaluate nuclear accumulation of β-catenin can show only focal results and be difficult to interpret in needle biopsies. **f** The two most common *CTNNB1* mutation in desmoids, T41A and S45F, are depicted by Sanger- and pyro-type DNA sequencing tracing (*left* and *right*, respectively) while the amino acid changes encoded by these two events is shown at the far *right*

lipogenic well-differentiated liposarcoma, inflammatory myofibroblastic tumor, schwannoma, and gastrointestinal stromal tumor (Table 3.1). The superficial fibromatoses such as palmar (Dupuytren), plantar and penile (Peyronie) types occur in distinct anatomic locations and usually do not enter the differential diagnosis if appropriate clinical history is known.

3.4.1 Reactive Fibroblastic/Myofibroblastic Proliferations

Scars and other benign proliferations or neoplasms, such as nodular fasciitis, can sometimes be misconstrued for fibromatoses. Scar can be especially vexing in assessing a biopsy from, or surgical margins of, excisions in recurrent lesions. Generally, the spindle cells in these reactive proliferations are arranged more haphazardly and in shorter fascicles. The cytomorphology of the lesional cells in nodular fasciitis is often more stellate and strongly and diffusely express SMA. Intra-lesional hemorrhage is also less commonly seen in desmoid fibromatosis. Immunohistochemistry has limited utility in distinguishing scar and desmoid as the former can show some nuclear reactivity for β-catenin as activation of the Wnt pathway is critical for wound healing. Desmoid fibromatosis will often show more intense and uniform nuclear accumulation of β-catenin. The degree of reactivity overlaps with scar in a significant subset of cases. In the surgical management of desmoid, the goal is to completely remove a prior scar while minimizing morbidity, such as loss of limb function. Sometimes this is not possible and fibrotic tissue extending to a margin may suggest the need for additional treatment. If the initial desmoid sample contained a characteristic mutation in *CTNNB1*, as do approximately 80% of sporadic cases, this can be helpful in distinguishing recurrence from scar by molecular methods (see below).

3.4.2 Other Mesenchymal Neoplasms that are Potential Mimics of Desmoid

Low-grade fibromyxoid sarcoma is a spindle cell sarcoma characterized by alternating zones of collagenous and myxoidstroma, by only mildly atypical spindle cells, and by a rich vascular network. They harbor t(7; 16) or t(11; 16) translocations, which result in joining *FUS* with *CREB3L2* or *CREB3L1*, respectively. Despite its bland appearance, and unlike desmoid tumors, they have the ability to metastasize. Immunohistochemistry for β-catenin may be useful in separating the two tumors; however, nuclear immunoreactivity in low-grade fibromyxoid sarcomas has been reported in the literature [22]. Fluorescence in situ hybridization (FISH) for the *FUS* (16p11) gene rearrangement or reverse transcriptase-polymerase chain reaction (RT-PCR) to demonstrate the characteristic fusion transcript can also be used to definitively distinguish the two tumors [15].

Table 3.1 Immunohistochemistry and molecular features in desmoid tumors and its differential diagnosis

Tumor type	β-Catenin	SMA	Desmin	Caldesmon	CD34	S-100	KIT	Other IHC	Molecular features
Desmoid fibromatosis	+	+	rare	–	–	–	–		β-Catenin (*CTNNB1*) mutations; germline mutations in *APC* gene
Low-grade fibromyxoid sarcoma (LGFMS)	rare	–	–	–	+	–	–		*FUS* (16p11) gene rearrangement
Malignant peripheral nerve sheath tumor (MPNST)	–	–	–	–	–	+	–	GFAP	
Well-differentiated liposarcoma, non-lipogenic	–	+	+	–	–	–	–		Amplification 12q13–15
Inflammatory myofibroblastic tumor (IMT)	–	+	+	–	–	–	–	ALK-1 (mostly in children and young adults)	2p23 and ALK gene rearrangement
Schwannoma	–	–	–	–	–	+	–		
Gastrointestinal stromal tumor (GIST)	–	–	+	+	+	rare	+		KIT and *PDGFRA* genotyping

Most malignant peripheral nerve sheath tumors (MPNST) are easily distinguishable from desmoid fibromatoses. However, the distinction between histologically "low-grade" MPNST and desmoid fibromatoses can be more challenging in small biopsies. Generally, there is a greater degree of atypia and nuclear hyperchromasia as well as more consistently wavy, elongated nuclei in MPNST compared to fibromatoses. Immunoreactivity for S-100 protein (patchy) and glial fibrillary acidic protein (GFAP) may also be useful as it is absent in desmoid tumors. Conversely, β-catenin immunoreactivity in MPNST has not been reported in the literature [22].

Non-lipogenic well-differentiated liposarcomas, as their name implies, are predominantly relatively bland to mildly atypical spindle cell neoplasms without an adipocytic component. These liposarcomas and desmoids can occur in similar anatomic locations. Though both tumors are locally aggressive, unlike desmoids, the liposarcomas have the potential to dedifferentiate as a form of tumor progression that confers the ability for very aggressive local behavior and distant metastasis. Thus pathologic distinction from desmoid fibromatoses is important in treatment planning. The degree of atypia and nuclear hyperchromasia may help in separating liposarcoma from fibromatoses. Ancillary FISH studies to demonstrate 12q15 amplification can be used as such amplification has not been found in fibromatoses.

Inflammatory myofibroblastic tumor (IMT) is a cellular spindle cell neoplasm commonly seen to arise in the mesentery. The degree of cytological atypia is greater than in desmoids, and there is a more extensive inflammatory infiltrate, typically lymphocytes and plasma cells, in IMT. Analogous to the spindle cells in fibromatosis, the IMT cells are arranged in long fascicles. As their name implies, the tumor cells appear to be myofibroblastic in origin. As such, inflammatory myofibroblastic tumors show immunoreactivity to smooth muscle actin and desmin. ALK-1 immunoreactivity can also be seen in a subset of these lesions but not in fibromatoses. Many cases with ALK reactivity will show *ALK* (2p23) gene rearrangement by FISH, but this is more common in pediatric cases [1, 10]. β-Catenin nuclear immunoreactivity is not seen in IMT.

Schwannomas show variable cellularity with a combination of Antoni A (cellular) and B (less cellular) areas. The underlying architecture of the spindle cells is often more storiform and shows nuclear palisading. Fascicles can also be seen. In older cases, thickened and hyalinized vessel walls can be encountered. These lesions will show diffuse and strong reactivity for S-100 protein and lack nuclear accumulation of β-catenin on immunohistochemistry.

Finally, the spindle cell variant of gastrointestinal stromal tumors (GIST) is also in the differential diagnosis. These spindle cells have eosinophilic, syncytial cytoplasm and, frequently, intra-cytoplasmic vacuoles. Skenoid fibers, which are globular extracellular collagen deposits, can also be seen. None of these features have been described in fibromatoses. Furthermore, the long, sweeping fascicles and pink, collagenous stroma common in fibromatosis are notably absent in gastrointestinal stromal tumors. Immunohistochemistry for β-catenin and KIT may also be useful, the former a marker for desmoids and the latter for GIST. While KIT immunoreactivity has been described in fibromatoses [31], more recent studies have shown that false positivity was due to cross reactivity due to overly aggressive antigen retrieval [18, 19]. CD34 reactivity is present in around 70% of GIST and is not commonly encountered in desmoids [30]. KIT or *PDGFRA* genotyping can also be helpful in distinguishing GISTs.

3.4.3 Molecular Diagnosis in Desmoid Tumors

Approximately 85% of sporadic desmoids will show one of three characteristic mutations involving codons 41 (threonine to alanine) and 45 (serine to phenylalanine or proline) of exon 3 in *CTNNB1* (Fig. 3.2f). This test is extremely robust as it involves amplification of a small region of tumor genomic DNA which is readily obtainable from formalin-fixed, paraffin-embedded tissue blocks, including core needle biopsies. In our hands, β-catenin immunohistochemistry in needle biopsy specimens is often disappointing, perhaps due to distortion during fixation (Fig. 3.2e). Demonstration of a characteristic *CTNNB1* mutation is often a definitive diagnostic finding and is particularly valuable for initial biopsies that are equivocal or cases arising in unusual clinical settings such as a second neoplasm in a cancer patient.

3.5 Clinical Behavior

Desmoids are locally aggressive tumors but have no capacity to metastasize. They frequently recur within 2 years after the initial excision [3, 24, 26, 28]. Recurrence rates vary depending on their location with higher rates reported in those arising in extra-abdominal locations [14, 23] and in patients with FAP syndrome [8, 29]. Despite their aggressive behavior and propensity to recur, they rarely lead to death with overall survival rates at 10 years exceeding 90% [14]. More recently, a watch and wait approach has been advocated for desmoid fibromatosis, with excision for cases that progress under observation [4, 6, 12, 16, 27].

3.5.1 Predicting Recurrence

Because of their propensity to recur locally, there is interest in determining which tumors are more likely to behave aggressively and recur. Epidemiologic variables associated with an increased risk of recurrence is discussed in detail in Chap. 2. Genetic predisposition (germline APC mutations) probably increase the likelihood of recurrence. Trisomy 8 is found in desmoids as well as other fibrous/fibrosing lesions, such as Dupuytren contracture and Peyronie disease [7, 11, 13], though these lack *CTNNB1* mutations. In two small studies, the abnormality was notably present in a majority of recurrent desmoids, suggesting it may indicate a higher risk of recurrence [11, 13]. Subsequent studies have found conflicting results. Bridge et al. found that none of the recurrences had gain of chromosome 8 [7]. Its use as a potential prognosticator requires further evaluation.

As discussed above, mutations in the *CTNNB1* gene have been found to be prevalent (up to 87%) in sporadic desmoid tumors. Two large series demonstrated that the specific types of mutations discovered were only three different point mutations [2, 17]. Of these, the more common mutation in codon 45 (serine to phenylalanine; S45F) was found to correlate with increased likelihood of recurrence [17]. However, this correlation was not clearly demonstrated in a subsequent series [25]. Its use as a predictor of recurrence require further studies which are currently ongoing.

3.6 Conclusions

Desmoid fibromatosis is a rare but recognizable mesenchymal neoplasm. Its deceptively bland appearance belies its locally aggressive nature and tendency to recur. Although the diagnosis is usually straightforward, it can be confused for both reactive conditions and other mesenchymal neoplasms. In this regard, immunohistochemistry, specifically β-catenin, and more recently, molecular diagnostics have proven exceedingly useful. Despite advancements in our understanding of this disease, the ability to predict recurrence remains difficult. Looking forward, it is likely that molecular analysis will increasingly impact the diagnosis and our understanding of this disease.

References

1. Alaggio R, Cecchetto G et al (2010) Inflammatory myofibroblastic tumors in childhood: a report from the Italian Cooperative Group studies. Cancer 116(1):216–226
2. Amary MF, Pauwels P et al (2007) Detection of beta-catenin mutations in paraffin-embedded sporadic desmoid-type fibromatosis by mutation-specific restriction enzyme digestion (MSRED): an ancillary diagnostic tool. Am J Surg Pathol 31(9):1299–1309
3. Ballo MT, Zagars GK et al (1999) Desmoid tumor: prognostic factors and outcome after surgery, radiation therapy, or combined surgery and radiation therapy. J Clin Oncol 17(1):158–167
4. Bertagnolli MM, Morgan JA et al (2008) Multimodality treatment of mesenteric desmoid tumours. Eur J Cancer 44(16):2404–2410
5. Bhattacharya B, Dilworth HP et al (2005) Nuclear beta-catenin expression distinguishes deep fibromatosis from other benign and malignant fibroblastic and myofibroblastic lesions. Am J Surg Pathol 29(5):653–659
6. Bonvalot S, Eldweny H et al (2008) Extra-abdominal primary fibromatosis: aggressive management could be avoided in a subgroup of patients. Eur J Surg Oncol 34(4):462–468
7. Bridge JA, Sreekantaiah C et al (1992) Clonal chromosomal abnormalities in desmoid tumors. Implications for histopathogenesis. Cancer 69(2):430–436

8. Burke AP, Sobin LH, Shekitka KM (1990) Mesenteric fibromatosis. A follow-up study. Arch Pathol Lab Med 114(8):832–835
9. Burke AP, Sobin LH et al (1990) Intra-abdominal fibromatosis. A pathologic analysis of 130 tumors with comparison of clinical subgroups. Am J Surg Pathol 14(4):335–341
10. Coffin CM, Hornick JL, Fletcher CD (2007) Inflammatory myofibroblastic tumor: comparison of clinicopathologic, histologic, and immunohistochemical features including ALK expression in atypical and aggressive cases. Am J Surg Pathol 31(4):509–520
11. Dal Cin P, Sciot R et al (1994) Some desmoid tumors are characterized by trisomy 8. Genes Chromosomes Cancer 10(2):131–135
12. de Bree E, Keus R et al (2009) Desmoid tumors: need for an individualized approach. Expert Rev Anticancer Ther 9(4):525–535
13. Fletcher JA, Naeem R et al (1995) Chromosome aberrations in desmoid tumors. Trisomy 8 may be a predictor of recurrence. Cancer Genet Cytogenet 79(2):139–143
14. Gronchi A, Casali PG et al (2003) Quality of surgery and outcome in extra-abdominal aggressive fibromatosis: a series of patients surgically treated at a single institution. J Clin Oncol 21(7):1390–1397
15. Guillou L, Benhattar J et al (2007) Translocation-positive low-grade fibromyxoid sarcoma: clinicopathologic and molecular analysis of a series expanding the morphologic spectrum and suggesting potential relationship to sclerosing epithelioid fibrosarcoma: a study from the French Sarcoma Group. Am J Surg Pathol 31(9):1387–1402
16. Lazar AJ, Hajibashi S, Lev D (2009) Desmoid tumor: from surgical extirpation to molecular dissection. Curr Opin Oncol 21(4):352–359
17. Lazar AJ, Tuvin D et al (2008) Specific mutations in the beta-catenin gene (CTNNB1) correlate with local recurrence in sporadic desmoid tumors. Am J Pathol 173(5):1518–1527
18. Lucas DR, al-Abbadi M et al (2003) c-Kit expression in desmoid fibromatosis. Comparative immunohistochemical evaluation of two commercial antibodies. Am J Clin Pathol 119(3):339–345
19. Miettinen M, Sobin LH, Sarlomo-Rikala M (2000) Immunohistochemical spectrum of GISTs at different sites and their differential diagnosis with a reference to CD117 (KIT). Mod Pathol 13(10):1134–1142
20. Montgomery E, Folpe AL (2005) The diagnostic value of beta-catenin immunohistochemistry. Adv Anat Pathol 12(6):350–356
21. Montgomery E, Torbenson MS et al (2002) Beta-catenin immunohistochemistry separates mesenteric fibromatosis from gastrointestinal stromal tumor and sclerosing mesenteritis. Am J Surg Pathol 26(10):1296–1301
22. Ng TL, Gown AM et al (2005) Nuclear beta-catenin in mesenchymal tumors. Mod Pathol 18(1):68–74
23. Pignatti G, Barbanti-Brodano G et al (2000) Extraabdominal desmoid tumor. A study of 83 cases. Clin Orthop Relat Res 375:207–213
24. Rock MG, Pritchard DJ et al (1984) Extra-abdominal desmoid tumors. J Bone Joint Surg Am 66(9):1369–1374
25. Salas S, Chibon F et al (2010) Molecular characterization by array comparative genomic hybridization and DNA sequencing of 194 desmoid tumors. Genes Chromosomes Cancer 49(6):560–568
26. Sorensen A, Keller J et al (2002) Treatment of aggressive fibromatosis: a retrospective study of 72 patients followed for 1–27 years. Acta Orthop Scand 73(2):213–219
27. Stoeckle E, Coindre JM et al (2009) A critical analysis of treatment strategies in desmoid tumours: a review of a series of 106 cases. Eur J Surg Oncol 35(2), 129–134
28. Stojadinovic A, Hoos A et al (2001) Soft tissue tumors of the abdominal wall: analysis of disease patterns and treatment. Arch Surg 136(1):70–79
29. Sturt NJ, Gallagher MC et al (2004) Evidence for genetic predisposition to desmoid tumours in familial adenomatous polyposis independent of the germline APC mutation. Gut 53(12):1832–1836

30. Yamaguchi U, Hasegawa T et al (2004) Differential diagnosis of gastrointestinal stromal tumor and other spindle cell tumors in the gastrointestinal tract based on immunohistochemical analysis. Virchows Arch 445(2):142–150
31. Yantiss RK, Spiro IJ et al (2000) Gastrointestinal stromal tumor versus intra-abdominal fibromatosis of the bowel wall: a clinically important differential diagnosis. Am J Surg Pathol 24(7):947–957

Chapter 4
APC/β-Catenin Deregulation in Desmoid Tumors: Important Implications for Diagnosis, Prognosis, and Therapy

Chiara Colombo and Dina Lev

Contents

Abstract Understanding the molecular aberrations driving the inception and progression of desmoid tumors (DTs) is crucial to devising an effective management for these neoplasms. The APC/β-catenin pathway is known to be deregulated in DT. This chapter illuminates the molecular mechanisms of APC/β-catenin pathway signaling, elucidates the potential deregulations and mutations at play in DTs, and most importantly evaluates the possible implications of this pathway on DT diagnosis, prognosis, and therapy.

Keywords APC • β-Catenin • Mutations • Sequencing • Prognostic biomarkers • Targeted therapy

C. Colombo (✉)
Department of Surgical Oncology and the Sarcoma Research Center, University of Texas; MD Anderson Cancer Center, Houston, Texas 77030, USA
e-mail: ccolombo@mdanderson.org

C. Litchman (ed.), *Desmoid Tumors*,
DOI 10.1007/978-94-007-1685-8_4, © Springer Science+Business Media B.V. 2012

4.1 Introduction

Elucidating the molecular aberrations driving the inception and progression of desmoid tumors (DTs) is of crucial importance in developing treatment strategies for the management of these neoplasms. Insights from studies of familial adenomatosis polyposis (FAP)-associated DTs provided initial insight into the potential role of the APC/β-catenin pathway in this disease [1, 2]. These observations were followed by the identification of somatic APC mutations in a small subset of sporadic DTs and, most importantly, a high prevalence (~85%) of *CTNNB1* (the gene coding for β-catenin) mutations in this cohort of tumors [3]. Whatever the underlying genetic alteration, in DT these mutations are translated into enhanced β-catenin signaling [4]. This deregulation of the β-catenin pathway against the backdrop of relative genomic stability suggests that this pathway might possibly be an "Achilles heel" of DT and a major driver of this neoplastic process. This chapter illuminates the molecular mechanisms of β-catenin pathway signaling, elucidates the potential deregulations at play in DTs, and most importantly evaluates the possible implications of this pathway on DT diagnosis, prognosis, and therapy.

4.2 APC/β-Catenin Signaling: Molecular Considerations

APC and β-catenin are both important components of the canonical Wnt pathway [5]. The term Wnt is derived from the combination of the Drosophila segment polarity gene Wingless and the mouse protooncogene Int-1. These are both secreted glycoproteins with at least 16 different members that are involved in cell growth regulation [6]. This physiologically important pathway plays a major role in the development of diverse organisms including Dictyostelium, Drosophila, Xenopus, and humans and is essential for embryologic development as well as growth and control of homeostatic tissues [7]. Although the components of this pathway differ between organisms, the end point of Wnt signaling is gene transcription regulation mediated by β-catenin [8]. In brief (see below for further information and depiction in Fig. 4.1), the Wnt/β-catenin signaling pathway starts with binding of the secreted Wnt ligand to its cell surface receptors which include seven transmembrane Fz-Frizzled receptors and the low-density lipoprotein receptor-related protein (LRP) coreceptors LRP5 and LRP6; such binding results in phosphorylation of the cytoplasmic dishevelled (dvl) protein [6, 9]. Phosphorylated dvl prevents phosphorylation of β-catenin by the APC/axin/CK1/GSK-3β. β-Catenin phosphorylation allows recognition by ubiquitin ligase, thereby ultimately targeting the protein for destruction in the proteosome. Unphosphorylated β-catenin is stable and can translocate to the nucleus to interact with the TCF family of transcription factors to activate downstream genes [10–15]. Normally, the Wnt pathway is tightly regulated; mutations or imbalance in its components can promote tumorigenesis [16]. Specific details of the structure, function, and regulation of APC and β-catenin molecules most pertinent to DT are provided below.

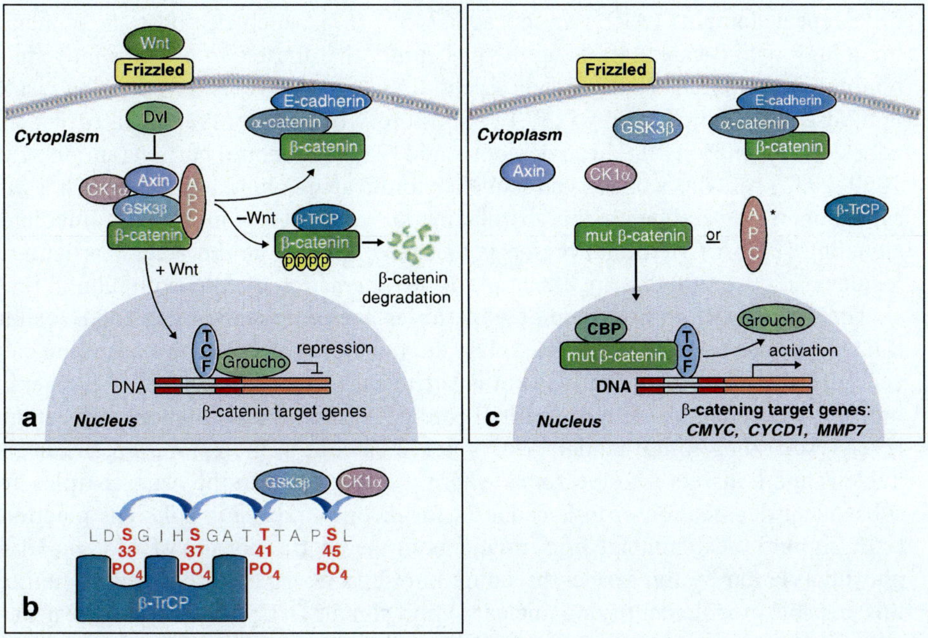

Fig. 4.1 The Wnt/β-catenin signaling pathway. **a** β-Catenin has dual roles in the cell. It has a structural component at the membrane as part of the adherens junction complex. It also has a signaling role in the cytoplasm and nucleus. The relationship between these pools is not fully understood. In the absence of extracellular Wnt ligand, β-catenin in the cytoplasm is phosphorylated by the APC destruction complex and marked for degradation in the proteosome. If Wnt ligand is present, the APC complex is inhibited and unphosphorylated β-catenin is stable and can accumulate in the nucleus and affect gene expression. **b** In the APC complex, phosphorylation is primed by CK1α at serine 45 and then completed sequential by GSK-3β at 41, 37, and 33. This sequence must follow this order. Any interruption and β-catenin is not marked for destruction and will instead have access to the nucleus. **c** When *CTNNB1* is mutated (usually at position 45 or 41 in DTs), the phosphorylation sequence cannot be performed and stabilized β-catenin can translocate to the nucleus to interact with cotrascriptional factors belonging to the TCF family to activate downstream genes (c-MYC, Cyclin D1, etc.). While *CTNNB1* mutation is more common in sporadic desmoids, APC mutations (*) prevent the APC complex formation and β-catenin phosphorylation. This is the major mechanism seen in desmoids associated with familial adenomatous polyposis (FAP). See text for additional details

4.2.1 APC

The APC gene was first identified by several groups who simultaneously localized it to chromosome 5q21 [17, 18]. This gene is composed of 21 exons, the largest one being exon 15, comprising more than 75% of the entire coding sequence [19]. The main protein product is a 2843 amino acid protein; several isoforms are known to exist expressed in a tissue-specific pattern, but their exact function is not yet known [20, 21]. Three distinct regions of APC are of major functional importance. These include the highly conserved proximal N-terminal region containing seven Armadillo repeat domains (ARD; amino acids 453–767) which demonstrate sequence homology with β-catenin, raising the possibility that these two proteins may share binding partners [22]. This region is essential for cell survival and its deletion results in mouse embryonic lethality [23]. Furthermore, a role in cytoskeletal integrity, cell adhesion, and motility has been demonstrated [24]. The central portion (amino acids 1020–2033) contains a conserved sequence implicated in binding Axin which is disrupted upon Wnt activation, thereby playing an essential role in β-catenin-mediated signaling [22]. A C-terminal region is enriched in basic amino acids, particularly residues 2,200–2,400 that are essential for the interaction of APC with tubulin [25].

The role of APC in β-catenin degradation is not completely understood. A shuttling model has been proposed to explain the function of APC. In mutant colon cancer cells, the overexpression of Axin is sufficient to reduce the level of β-catenin, indicating a potential but not essential role of APC in the regulation of β-catenin levels. According to the model, APC binds β-catenin in the cytoplasm and in the nucleus and transfers it to the zones where it either binds to the Axin complex for subsequent degradation or to E-cadherin for incorporation into adherens junctions [26]. To bind β-catenin, specific fragments in the central portion of APC mandate phosphorylation by the serine–threonine kinase GSK-3 [19]. Recent data support this possible model, identifying nuclear export signals (NES) in APC that are necessary for its exit from the nucleus; in almost all APC truncations found in sporadic colorectal tumors, NES are deleted, indicating that APC is contained in the nucleus. These cells also express high levels of nuclear β-catenin indicating that APC could enhance β-catenin nuclear localization [26].

4.2.2 β-Catenin

Human β-catenin, a homolog of the Drosophila Armadillo protein, is a multifunctional protein that plays essential roles in development and tissue maintenance [27]. This 92 kDa protein is encoded by the *CTNNB1* gene mapping to chromosome 3p21 [28]. β-Catenin is composed of 781 amino acids and it contains three major domains: first, a 150-amino acid N-terminal domain which contains the binding site for α-catenin and the phosphorylation sites for GSK-3β [8], second, a 550-amino acid central armadillo repeat domain (present also in APC protein), highly conserved between species and containing binding sites for TCF/LEF, APC, Axin, and E-cadherin [8, 29], and, third, a 100-amino acid C-terminus that also plays a major role in transcriptional coactivation with TCF/LEF [30]. Functionally, β-catenin is involved in two crucial developmental processes: first, specific cell–cell interactions through adherens junctions (mainly in epithelial origin cells) via binding to E-cadherin and α-catenin on the cell surface [31] and, second, regulation of gene expression through Wnt signaling activation, resulting in β-catenin nuclear translocation and interaction with transcription regulators of the TCF/LEF family [31].

β-Catenin signaling is tightly regulated in normal cells [27]. Generally, cytoplasmic β-catenin levels are kept low via continuous ubiquitin–proteasome-mediated degradation of this protein, a process which is regulated by a multiprotein complex-containing axin, APC, GSK-3β, and CK1α [24]. CK1α and GSK-3β mediate the degradation of β-catenin molecules by phosphorylating specific amino N-terminal residues (Ser45 by CK1α, and Thr41, Ser 37, and Ser33 by GSK-3β in this sequential order), thereby marking the protein and rendering it as recognizable by β-transducin repeat-containing protein (β-TrCP), a component of the E3 ubiquitin ligase. This results in degradation of β-catenin by the 26S proteasome complex [32]. Physiological Wnt pathway activation as well as aberrant signaling (e.g., mutations in Wnt pathway component including direct β-catenin mutations) results in accumulation of nonphosphorylated β-catenin in the cytoplasm. Nonphosphorylated β-catenin escapes recognition by β-TrCP, thereby avoiding degradation. It is translocated into the nucleus where β-catenin forms transcriptional-permissive protein complexes (described below) that act as coregulators to induce transcription of target genes such as *c-MYC*, *c-JUN*, MMP7, Nr-CAM, and *cyclin D1* [10–14]. Earlier studies have demonstrated that β-catenin harbors two transactivation domains, N-terminal activation domain (NTAD) and C-terminal activation domain (CTAD) [33–35]; each of these domains is capable of potently stimulating gene expression. In particular, the CTAD has been shown to be sufficient both for signaling and for oncogenic transformation [36].

4.2.3 TCF/LEF Family of Transcription Factors

The vertebrate genome encodes for four transcription factor (TCF)/Lymphoid Enhancing Factor (LEF) proteins (TCF1, TCF3, TCF4, and LEF1), containing a highly conserved high-mobility group (HMG) box as a DNA-binding domain [37]. These proteins bind and bend DNA and act as adaptors to allow other factors to bind and modify the transcription of target genes. In principle TCF/LEF proteins are thought to act as constitutive transcriptional inhibitors; i.e., in the absence of nuclear β-catenin, TCF/LEF proteins are bound to the corepressors Gro/TLE and CtBP, and actively suppress target gene transcription. Both Gro/TLE and CtBP interact with histone deacetylases to silence transcription by altering local chromatin structure [38]. Once in the nucleus, β-catenin binds to TCF/LEF family members to form a stable complex by displacing Gro/TLE [39]; this allows β-catenin to recruit a variety of coactivators necessary for its protranscriptional activity. Of major relevance to this issue is the finding that in DTs β-catenin specifically binds to TCF-3 [40]. This is in contrast to other neoplastic contexts such as colorectal cancer or pilomatricoma, in which β-catenin acts primarily through TCF-4 and LEF-1, respectively [41]. This ability of β-catenin to bind to a specific transcription factor like TCF-3 may be cell lineage dependent in that the TCF family of transcription factors appears to be differentially expressed in various tissues and cell types. Selectivity of β-catenin for a certain member of the TCF family is also possible, but the mechanisms for such specificity are not known and could involve additional protein(s) in the nuclear transcription factor complex. Thus, while β-catenin mutations occur in a variety of cancers (described below), the downstream effects may not be equivalent as the TCF family member involved may differentially modulate the function of β-catenin in different tumors.

4.3 APC/β-Catenin Deregulation in Desmoid Tumors

As commonly occurs with other major cellular and molecular pathways, Wnt signaling is frequently subverted by neoplasia to provide advantages in growth and survival [7]. Among the various molecules involved in the Wnt pathway, β-catenin, APC, and Axin are frequently mutated in human cancer, suggesting a possible role in tumorigenesis [42, 43]. Presented below are data describing the prevalence and distribution of APC/β-catenin mutations in DTs. Desmoids are demonstrably monoclonal neoplasms; in some salient regards they mimic an "uncontrolled" wound healing process. Several lines of evidence establish a role for β-catenin in wound healing. For example, Cheon et al. demonstrated that β-catenin is transiently elevated in fibroblasts during tissue repair and that forced β-catenin overexpression results in the formation of hypertrophic scars in mice [4]. A large number of growth factors and cytokines such as PDGF and TGF are secreted from platelets at the site of injury and induce β-catenin signaling in fibroblast in a paracrine manner [44]. Decreased β-catenin signaling is observed at the late stages of scaring [4]. Taken together, the reality that β-catenin plays a physiological role in wound healing is consistent with the possibility that deregulation of this pathway is of functional relevance in DT.

4.3.1 APC Mutations

In accord with the role of APC as a tumor suppressor, deactivating APC mutations are relatively common cancer-related alterations and are present in the vast majority of colorectal polyps and sporadic colorectal carcinomas [45, 46]. More than 1,600 mutations, both germline and somatic, have been described. The majority lead to an early stop codon and a truncated protein that can no longer facilitate the phosphorylation and degradation of β-catenin [19]. While germline mutations have been found throughout the span of this gene, sporadic mutations tend to be clustered in a small region at the 5′ end between codons 1280 and 1500 of APC, designated a mutation cluster region (MCR) [45]; this region is essential for APC interaction with β-catenin and Axin [22, 47].

Familial adenomatosis polyposis (FAP) is a hereditary genetic syndrome where germline APC mutations drive the formation of thousands of colonic polyps and eventually colorectal cancer [48]. Several extra-intestinal manifestations commonly occur in the context of FAP including a high incidence of DTs (described in 10–15% of FAP patients) [48]. Interestingly APC genotype correlates with disease phenotype and clinical manifestations: APC mutations between codon 1249 and 1330 correlate with a severe form of FAP exhibiting an early onset of colon cancer and a large number of colonic polyps (>5,000) [19], whereas those mutations occurring in codons 1445–1578 are associated with a less severe polyposis phenotype but an increased frequency of DTs and upper gastrointestinal polyposis [49]. Mutations at the extreme 5′ or 3′ ends of APC, or involving an alternatively spliced exon 9, correlate with an attenuated polyposis phenotype (AAPC) which is characterized either by a late age of onset and/or <100 colorectal adenomas [50, 51]. As suggested by the Knudsen model, most FAP patients develop a second-hit mutation leading to biallelic APC inactivation, enhanced β-catenin signaling, and tumorigenesis [45, 52–54]. When APC mutation-containing cells were transiently or stably transfected with full-length wild-type APC gene, the β-catenin protein levels and cell proliferation were shown to be significantly decreased [55].

Gardner syndrome is the acronym used to describe FAP patients harboring DT. Most desmoids in this context occur within the intestinal mesentery although extra-abdominal desmoids can also develop [48]. As is with FAP in general, the site of APC mutation may also be a factor in determining the severity of desmoids. For example, a germline mutation at the extreme 3′ end of the APC gene (codons 2643–2644) has been identified in a French-Canadian kindred as resulting in a very severe desmoid phenotype characterized by the presence of multiple DTs in the trunk and extremities with a 100% penetrance but the virtual absence of colon or upper gastrointestinal polyps [1]. Interestingly, it has been hypothesized that the second-hit APC mutations in some FAP desmoid patients may be caused by misalignment of DNA strands during wound healing subsequent to abdominal surgery [56]. In FAP-associated DTs, second-hit somatic mutations were found to occur distal to codon 1400 when the germline mutation is proximal to codon 1400, while allelic loss (LOH) occurs when the germline mutation is distal to codon 1449 [57]. Although both colonic adenomas and DTs in the background of FAP harbor APC mutation as the initiating molecular event, it is intriguing that the former can progress into a highly aggressive malignant cancer whereas the latter does not have this capacity [58]. This finding might be explainable by the difference in the cell of origin of these two tumors and/or differential β-catenin downstream targets.

APC mutations (either biallelic mutation or more commonly loss of heterozygosity) also occur in 5–10% of sporadic DTs, developing in patients without a germline mutation. Consistent with this finding, cytogenetic studies have demonstrated that partial deletions in the long arm of chromosome 5 (the location of the APC gene) occur in some DTs [59, 60]. The absence of a complete APC protein or gain of function/dominant negative function of a truncated mutated APC protein in the initiation of desmoid tumors merits further study and could shed light on the role of APC in this tumor.

4.3.2 β-Catenin Mutations

The observation that β-catenin nuclear protein level is elevated in virtually all sporadic DTs despite the fact that >90% exhibit a wild type and functional APC

Table 4.1 *CTNNB1* mutation prevalence documented in various neoplasms

Neoplasm	N	*n*	%
Liver carcinoma	3,029	516	17
Hepatoblastoma	541	231	43
Endometrial carcinoma	851	183	22
Wilm's tumor	707	151	21
Colon adenocarcinoma	2,779	161	5
Ovarian carcinoma	753	84	11
Pancreatic carcinoma	285	82	29
Gastric adenoma	262	83	32
Craniopharyngioma	181	73	40
Gastric carcinoma	1,252	60	5
Pilomatrical carcinoma (skin)	197	61	31
Thyroid carcinoma	157	30	19
Melanoma	456	26	6
Biliary tract neoplasms	67	28	42
Colangiocarcinoma	341	13	4

The online Catalog of Somatic Mutations in Cancer (COSMIC) site of Wellcome Trust, Sanger Institute (http://www.sanger.ac.uk/perl/genetics/CGP/cosmic), was utilized to acquire the frequency of APC and β-catenin somatic mutation in a variety of tumor types

gene led to the search for other possible Wnt pathway deregulations [61]. These investigations highlighted the propensity of direct *CTNBB1* (the gene coding for β-catenin) mutations in sporadic DTs. *CTNBB1* and APC mutations are mutually exclusive [62]. Mutations in *CTNNB1* have been found in many human cancers at various prevalence levels; e.g., colon carcinoma, hepatocellular carcinoma, pancreatic cancer, gastric cancer, melanoma, hepatoblastoma, and Wilm's tumors (Table 4.1) [3, 61, 63–66]. *CTNBB1* mutations almost exclusively occur in exon 3 of gene in the region encoding the phosphorylation domain of β-catenin. Mutations at these sites do not affect β-catenin mRNA expression. Instead they prevent proper, sequential phosphorylation of β-catenin, thereby rendering it refractory to regulation by the axin–APC complex and eventually leading to stabilization and nuclear accumulation of β-catenin [67, 68]. Interestingly, a high incidence of stabilizing *CTNBB1* mutations tends to occur in *less* aggressive types of cancer that have minimal metastatic capacity, e.g., endometrioid ovarian cancer [69] in which *CTNNB1* are particularly common, albeit with variability in reported prevalence ranges (16–54%) [70]. Endometrioid ovarian cancers harboring *CTNNB1* mutations are more frequently identified as low-grade, highly differentiated lesions [71] that have better prognosis and decreased metastatic capacity [72]. Comparable findings are also seen in colon cancer, where *CTNNB1* mutations are identified in more benign tumor subsets associated with microsatellite instability (MSI+) such as hereditary nonpolyposis colorectal cancer (HNPCC) [73, 74]. The biological implications of this finding are yet to be determined.

Initial reports evaluating small-sample cohorts suggested that *CTNNB1* mutations occur in approximately 50% of sporadic DTs [63]. However, subsequent stud-

Table 4.2 *CTNNB1* mutational spectrum in relatively large studies of desmoid tumors

Study	*n*/total	T41A	S45F	S45P	%
Miyoshi et al. [63]	7/13	4	3	–	54
Tejpar et al. [61]	22/42	10	12	–	52
Abraham et al. [64]	15/33	11	3	–	45
Amary et al. [3]	66/76	27	34	5	87
Lazar et al. [65]	117/138	69	39	9	85
Domont et al. [66]	129/155	64	53	9	83

ies utilizing larger numbers of samples have identified a mutational prevalence of 85–88% (Table 4.2) [65]. Together, these investigations establish sporadic DTs as the tumor type that bears one of the highest rates of *CTNNB1* mutation yet described. Interestingly, only three different point mutations in two different codons (41 and 45) are almost invariably identified in mutated samples: ACC to GCC in codon 41 (41A; replacement of threonine by alanine); TCT to TTT in codon 45 (45F; replacement of serine by phenylalanine), and TCT to CCT in codon 45 (45P; replacement of serine with proline) [65]; these two residues are target to phosphorylation by GSK-3β and CK1, respectively. Indeed, among solid tumors it is unusual and fortuitous to demonstrate only three specific mutations; i.e., two involving codon 45 and one involving codon 41. In contrast, most other neoplasms harboring exon 3 *CTNNB1* mutations exhibit a much wider variety of mutations at multiple critical codons [68, 27]. This finding could imply that these specific *CTNNB1* mutations may be critical in desmoid development. Moreover, it may suggest that the *type* of mutation observed in the *CTNNB1* gene could affect or even alter the signaling properties of β-catenin in ways that are conducive to desmoid formation.

Considered together, APC and *CTNBB1* mutations can be identified in the vast majority of DTs. However, it is important to note that in 5–10% of DTs where increased nuclear β-catenin expression is observed, neither of these mutations can be identified, suggesting yet to be identified alterations driving Wnt pathway signaling. Further studies are needed to determine the exact aberrations operative in wild-type DT.

4.4 β-Catenin Downstream Effectors in Desmoid Tumors

Loss of APC function and gain-of-function mutations in exon 3 of *CTNBB1* result in the consequent nuclear accumulation of this nascent transcription factor. Many proteins encoded by β-catenin/TCF transcriptional targets presumably affect neoplastic transformation, thereby ultimately impacting on subsequent tumor cell proliferation, differentiation, survival, migration, and invasion. Much of the data regarding cancer-related deregulated β-catenin signaling effects stem from colon cancer studies where a multitude of potential overexpressed downstream transcriptional targets such as *CCND1*, c-*MYC*, *MMP-7*, fascin, *CX43*, *ITF2*, *PPAR-delta*, and others have been identified. These targets are thought to contribute to tumorigenesis and progression [24]. The high prevalence of APC/CTNBB1 mutations in DTs suggests that aberrant β-catenin signaling is an important contributor to the pathophysiology of this disease and may potentially serve as the substrate of their "oncogenic addiction." This hypothesis is strengthened by the previously published finding that transgenic mice in which mutated, stabilized β-catenin is conditionally expressed in mesenchymal cells develop desmoid tumors after transgene induction [4]. Furthermore, fibroblasts from these mice exhibit increased proliferation, motility, and invasiveness. However, the molecular mechanisms resulting in these potential stabilized β-catenin-induced effects and the altered gene expression affecting the finely tuned equilibrium between proliferation and differentiation that lead to desmoid tumorigenesis and growth are not well characterized. It is quite likely that the effects of β-catenin stabilization vary between tumor types as reflected by their significantly varied biological behaviors. Some β-catenin target genes identified in colon cancer such as *PPAR-delta*, *c-Myc*, and *c-jun* have been evaluated in desmoids and have not been found to be upregulated [40, 44]. One possibility explaining this difference is that β-catenin binds different transcription factors in a tumor type-dependent manner, thereby inducing different downstream effects. The finding that desmoids express TCF3 rather than TCF4 or LEF1 and that β-catenin binds TCF3 in these tumors supports this possibility [40]. Target genes of β-catenin/TCF3 in desmoid tumors are largely unknown; only limited studies have evaluated potential desmoid-associated gene expression deregulation [14, 15, 75–79]. Several candidate genes, including IGFBP6 and WT1, were found to be repressed and induced respectively in DTs compared to normal fibroblasts and were shown to potentially constitute β-catenin downstream targets [15, 78]. In addition to β-catenin/TCF3 target genes, high-throughput expression arrays have identified expression of molecules that regulate cell cycle, tissue remodeling, and growth in several small-desmoid cohort series [80]. While limited, these studies suggest that comprehensive gene expression analysis of desmoid tumors harboring different β-catenin mutations could be useful as a robust strategy to identify heretofore not determined β-catenin/TCF3 target genes that have roles in the pathogenesis of desmoids and possibly other types of human cancers that possess β-catenin pathway defects.

4.5 β-Catenin as a Desmoid Tumor Diagnostic and Prognostic Biomarker

DT diagnosis is commonly made on the basis of clinical, radiological, and histological parameters and is highly dependent on pathologist expertise. As a hallmark of DT, determining β-catenin expression levels and mutational status can be clinically meaningful (Fig. 4.2). Immunohistochemical detection of nuclear β-catenin has been shown to be helpful in DT differential diagnosis [3] and is commonly included as part of the diagnostic armamentarium. While not entirely specific for DT, in the differential diagnosis of spindle cell lesions with fibrous differentiation, nuclear accumulation of β-catenin is highly suggestive of a desmoid diagnosis [81, 82].

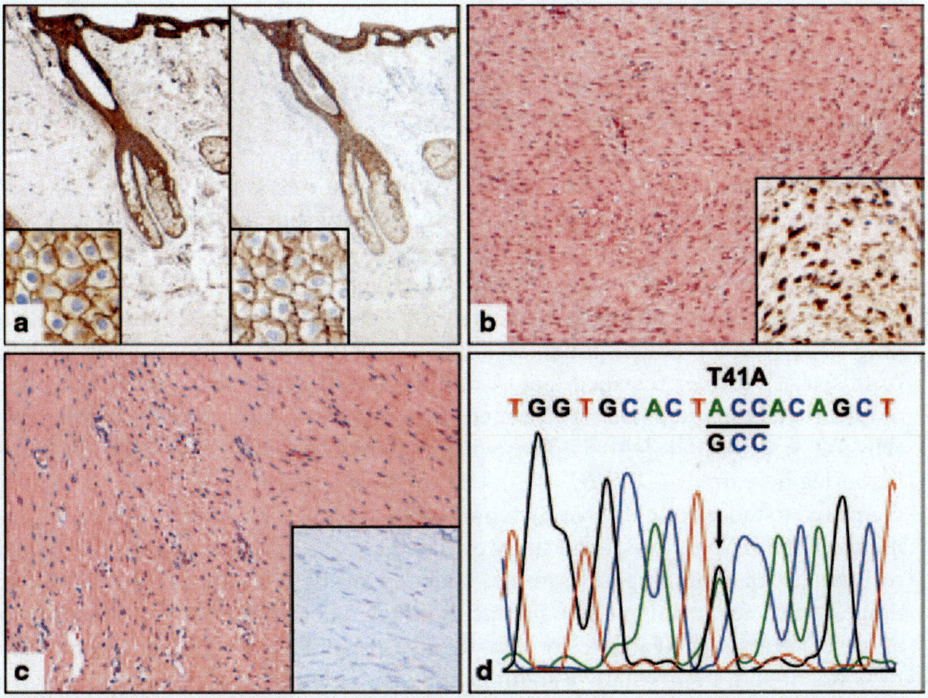

Fig. 4.2 *CTNNB1* mutations and β-catenin protein expression in desmoid tumors. **a** β-Catenin (*left*) and E-cadherin (*right*) immunostaining of a hair follicle of normal skin. Both are present and concentrated in adherens junctions at the cell membrane of the epithelial cells as the insets show. **b** Desmoid tumors have distinct nuclear accumulation of β-catenin as seen in the inset. **c** While scars have a similar histologic appearance, they generally lack distinct nuclear accumulation. **d** Mutations in exon 3 of *CTNNB1*, the gene encoding β-catenin, can often be demonstrated with PCR amplification of tumor DNA and Sanger sequencing (T41A mutation in this case, causing the normally phosphorylated threonine to be substituted by alanine which cannot be phosphorylated)

The percentage of nuclear β-catenin staining in various larger studies ranges from 33–100%, depending on the number of samples and type of antibody used, although most studies indicate that the vast majority of cases are reactive [61, 64, 82–85]. Additional information regarding β-catenin immunostaining can be found in other sections of this book.

However, it is important to note that with all diagnostic investigations there are definite assay limitations, and nuclear β-catenin expression has been reported in several other desmoid differential diagnosis pathologic entities [82–84]. Moreover, tumor cells within desmoids may only be focally positive for β-catenin [86]. Finally, IHC analysis is antibody-, specific technical algorithm-, observer-, and interpretation-dependent and as such may therefore yield equivocal results [82]. It has been suggested that β-catenin immunohistochemistry is a more sensitive assay when applied in excisional biopsies or surgical specimens than in small-core needle biopsies. This concern is particularly evident during follow-up surveillance where differentiating between normal postsurgical scarring and recurrent DT is of major (yet challenging) clinical importance. Current studies are evaluating the role of *CTNNB1* mutational analysis as a potential tool for "difficult to diagnose" DTs. Initial results (unpublished data) suggest the usefulness of this diagnostic approach.

A potential role for *CTNBB1* type-specific mutational status as a disease prognosticator has also been suggested [65]. In an initial study evaluating a cohort of 89 primary sporadic DTs treated at a single institution, the estimated 5-year recurrence-free survival rate for *CTNNB1* gene 41A mutation-harboring tumors was 83%, and the median time to recurrence has not been achieved; tumors lacking a mutation followed an equivalent course [65]. In remarkable contrast, 45F *CTNNB1* gene mutation-harboring tumors demonstrated a 5-year recurrence-free survival rate of only 47%, with a median time to recurrence of 3.16 years. A multivariate analysis of this series further revealed that of all the tumor and clinical factors evaluated, only 45F mutation retained significance as a marker for increased risk of recurrence (HR 4.279; 95% CI 1.7–10.5). These data possibly suggest that sporadic desmoids harboring an exon 3 *CTNNB1* 45F mutation have a markedly inferior outcome as compared to those patients bearing tumors with a 41A *CTNNB1* gene mutation or no mutation in *CTNNB1*. A second study evaluated 101 surgically excised primary and recurrent extra-abdominal DT samples obtained through Conticanet (the connective tissue cancer network including France, Belgium, and Switzerland); a follow-up of at least 5 years was available for all patients [66] and a *CTNNB1* mutation rate of 83% was found. In this study a significantly shorter 5-year recurrence-free survival was found for mutated tumors compared to wild-type *CTNNB1* harboring DTs. Only a nonsignificant trend for enhanced recurrence was found for DTs harboring 45F mutations as compared to 41A. The discrepancy between these two series can possibly be explained by the difference in tumor cohorts studied: in the former study only *primary* intra- and extra-abdominal tumors were evaluated whereas in the latter both *primary and recurrent* lesions were included but only those located extra-abdominally. It is apparent that additional studies evaluating a larger number of patients are needed to resolve this discrepancy and confirm or refute the predictive utility of *CTNNB1* mutational status.

4.6 Potential Therapeutic Strategies Targeting β-Catenin Signaling Pathway

The typically indolent growth of desmoids and their lack of metastatic capacity suggest a possible suitability as candidates for molecular-targeted therapies. If used in conjunction with surgical resection, such focused interventions could potentially forestall recurrence and might possibly even serve as efficacious induction therapy, thereby potentially mitigating surgical morbidity. Based on the findings above, β-catenin signaling blockade might be an attractive therapeutic approach for desmoid treatment. Switching off crucial β-catenin signaling upon which desmoid cells may be dependent could potentially elicit significant antidesmoid effects; of necessity, such targeting must spare normal cells. However, agents directly down-

Table 4.3 Potential drugs targeting β-catenin signaling pathway

	Name	Function	Reference
Existing drugs	NSAIDs	Suppression of Tcf gene expression	Wang [88]
	COX2 inhibitors	Suppression of Tcf gene expression	Steinbach [98]
	Imatinib	PDGFRB/KIT inhibitor	Dufresne 2010 [99]
Small molecules			
	PKF118–310	TCF/β-catenin inhibitor	Barker 2006 [100]
	PFK115–744	TCF/β-catenin inhibitor	Barker 2006 [100]
	PKF115–584	TCF/β-catenin inhibitor	Lepourcelet et al. [87]
	PFK222–815	TCF/β-catenin inhibitor	Barker 2006 [100]
	ZTM000990	TCF/β-catenin inhibitor	Barker 2006 [100]
	CGPO49090	TCF/β-catenin inhibitor	Lepourcelet et al. [87]
	ICG-001	CREB binding protein inhibitor	Emami [89]
Others molecules			
	Quercetin	TCF inhibitor	Park [90]
	2,4 diamino-quinazoline	TCF/β-catenin inhibitor	Chen [91]
	XAV939	Tankyrase 1/Axin inhibitor	Huang [92]

regulating β-catenin are not yet available, and such agents, when developed, may not be clinically useful if they compromise normal β-catenin physiological functioning due to nonselective blockade [87]. For these reasons, approaches that target specific β-catenin protumorigenic downstream effects rather than directly downregulate β-catenin per se may be more applicable. Inhibitors of the β-catenin signaling pathway have recently received attention as plausible candidates for anticancer drug development (Table 4.3) [88–92]. Many compounds, i.e., antiinflammatory drugs, vitamins, and recently the tyrosine kinase inhibitor imatinib, have been identified as potentially inhibiting β-catenin signaling, perhaps offering an explanation for the favorable responses to these agents observed in some desmoid patients [44, 93, 94]. However, these compounds principally attenuate the cytoplasmic expression and enhance the degradation of wild-type β-catenin; in that most desmoids harbor stabilized mutated β-catenin, therapies to block molecular events downstream of β-catenin stabilization, such as nuclear localization, protein–protein interaction, transcriptional activity, and/or inhibition of specific β-catenin deregulated target genes might be more appealing.

Stabilized β-catenin nuclear localization and function is tightly regulated via dynamic interaction with a multitude of proteins. Among these binding partners, some function to enhance β-catenin/TCF-induced transcription while others act as naturally expressed inhibitors [95]. One potential novel therapeutic approach to indirectly inhibit β-catenin signaling is to target applicable β-catenin activating binding-partners and/or block these enhancing protein–protein interactions. A recent search for small molecule antagonists targeting TCF/β-catenin interaction used high-throughput screening to identify agents that disrupt the TCF4/β-catenin complex [96]. For example, PKF115-584 and CGPO49090 are two small molecule compounds that share a common core chemical structure, a similar mechanism of action (including the ability to disrupt the Tcf-/β-catenin complex), and have shown promise in preclinical colon cancer models [87]. Similarly, reconstitution and/or mimicry of β-catenin inhibitory binding-proteins are another current area of intensive research. For example, a recent study using a recombinant adenovirus encoding ICAT (a β-catenin negative regulator) inhibited the growth of colorectal tumor cells harboring β-catenin mutations in vitro and in vivo [97]. In contrast, ICAT did not inhibit growth of normal or tumor cells containing wild-type β-catenin. Alternatively, identification of β-catenin target genes expressed in a variety of cancers might offer novel opportunities for developing therapeutics against targets that have critical roles in tumor progression; such an approach might be anticipated to generate therapeutics having fewer side effects. Taken together approaches such as those described above might be highly relevant for desmoid therapy. However, little is currently known about either β-catenin binding partners and/or target genes in the desmoid microenvironment, and future studies bridging this knowledge gap are crucially needed.

4.7 Conclusions

β-Catenin pathway deregulation is the most common molecular event attributed to DT occurring through mutations in the APC or *CTNBB1* genes as well as other yet to be identified mechanisms. Initial insights suggest that this pathway contributes to DT growth and progression. Additional studies are needed to further unravel the possible implications of this pathway on DT diagnosis, prognosis, and most importantly therapy.

References

1. Couture J, Mitri A, Lagace R et al (2000) A germline mutation at the extreme 3′ end of the APC gene results in a severe desmoid phenotype and is associated with overexpression of beta-catenin in the desmoid tumor. Clin Genet 57:205–212
2. Bertario L, Russo A, Sala P et al (2001) Genotype and phenotype factors as determinants of desmoid tumors in patients with familial adenomatous polyposis. Int J Cancer 95:102–107
3. Amary MFC, Pauwels P, Meulemans E et al (2007) Detection of beta-catenin mutations in paraffin-embedded sporadic desmoid-type fibromatosis by mutation-specific restriction enzyme digestion (MSRED): an ancillary diagnostic tool. Am J Surg Pathol 31:1299–1309
4. Cheon SS, Cheah AYL, Turley S et al (2002) β-Catenin stabilization dysregulates mesenchymal cell proliferation, motility, and invasiveness and causes aggressive fibromatosis and hyperplastic cutaneous wounds. PNAS 99(10):6973–6978
5. Logan CY, Nusse R (2004) The Wnt signaling pathway in development and disease. Annu Rev Cell Dev Biol 20:781–810

6. Kikuchi A, Yamamoto H, Kishida S (2007) Multiplicity of the interactions of Wnt proteins and their receptors. Cell Signal 19:659–671
7. Polakis P (2000) Wnt signaling and cancer. Genes Dev 14:1837–1851
8. Kotiligam D, Lazar AJ, Pollock RE et al (2008) Desmoid tumor: a disease opportune for molecular insights. Histol Histopathol 23(1):117–126
9. Tolwinski NS, Wieschaus E (2004) Rethinking WNT signaling. Trends Genet 20(4):177–181
10. He TC, Sparks AB, Rago C et al (1998) Identification of c-MYC as a target of the APC pathway. Science 281(5382):1509–1512
11. Tetsu O, McCormick F (1999) Beta-catenin regulates expression of cyclin D1 in colon carcinoma cells. (javascript:AL_get(this, 'jour', 'Nature.')) Nature 398(6726):422–426
12. Crawford HC, Fingleton BM, Rudolph-Owen LA et al (1999) The metalloproteinase matrilysin is a target of beta-catenin transactivation in intestinal tumors. Oncogene 18(18):2883–2891
13. Conacci-Sorrell ME, Ben-Yedidia T, Shtutman M et al (2002) Nr-CAM is a target gene of the beta-catenin/LEF-1 pathway in melanoma and colon cancer and its expression enhances motility and confers tumorigenesis. Genes Dev 16(16):2058–2072
14. Denys H, De Wever O, Nusgens B et al (2004) Invasion and MMP expression profile in desmoid tumours. Br J Cancer 90(7):1443–1449
15. Denys H, Jadidizadeh A, Amini Nik S et al (2004) Identification of IGFBP-6 as a significantly downregulated gene by beta-catenin in desmoid tumors. Oncogene 23(3):654–664
16. Lucero OM, Dawson DW, Moon RT et al (2010) A re-evaluation of the "oncogenic" nature of Wnt/beta-catenin signaling in melanoma and other cancers. Curr Oncol Rep 12(5):314–318
17. Bodmer WF, Bailey CJ, Bodmer J et al (1987) Localization of the gene for familial adenomatous polyposis on chromosome 5. Nature 328(6131):614–616
18. Leppert M, Dobbs M, Scambler P et al (1987) The gene for familial polyposis coli maps to the long arm of chromosome 5. Science 238(4832):1411–1413
19. Goss KH, Groden J (2000) Biology of the adenomatous polyposis coli tumor suppressor. J Clin Oncol 18(9):1967–1979
20. Horii A, Nakatsuru S, Ichii S et al (1993) Multiple forms of the APC gene transcripts and their tissue-specific expression. Hum Mol Genet 2(3):283–287
21. Pyles RB, Santoro IM, Groden J et al (1998) Novel protein isoforms of the APC tumor suppressor in neural tissue. Oncogene 16(1):77–82
22. Rubinfeld B, Souza B, Albert I et al (1995) The APC protein and E-cadherin form similar but independent complexes with alpha catenin, beta-catenin, and plakoglobin. J Biol Chem 270(10):5549–5555
23. Smits R, Kielman MF, Breukel C et al (1999) Apc1638T: a mouse model delineating critical domains of the adenomatous polyposis coli protein involved in tumorigenesis and development. Genes Dev 13:1309–1321
24. Morin PJ, Weeraratna AT (2003) The APC tumor suppressor pathway. In: El-Deiry WS (ed) Methods in molecular biology, vol 222: tumor suppressor genes: pathways and isolation strategies. Wafik S. El-Deiry Humana Press, Totowa
25. Munemitsu S, Souza B, Müller O et al (1994) The APC gene product associates with microtubules in vivo and promotes their assembly in vitro. Cancer Res 54(14):3676–3681
26. Bienz M, Clevers H (2000) Linking colorectal cancer to Wnt signaling. Cell 103:311–320
27. Clevers H (2006) Wnt/beta-catenin signaling in development and disease. Cell 127(3):469–480
28. Kraus C, Liehr T, Hülsken J et al (1994) Localization of the human β-catenin gene (CTNNB1) to 3p21: a region implicated in tumor development. Genomics 23:273–274
29. Lazar AJ, Hajibashi S, Lev D (2009) Desmoid tumor: from surgical extirpation to molecular dissection. Curr Opin Oncol 21(4):352–359
30. Gottardi CJ, Gumbiner BM (2004) Distinct molecular forms of beta-catenin are targeted to adhesive or transcriptional complexes. J Cell Biol 167(2):339–349
31. Barker N (2008) The canonical Wnt/beta-catenin signalling pathway. Methods Mol Biol 468:5–15

32. Patton EE, Willems AR, Tyers M (1998) Combinatorial control in ubiquitin-dependent proteolysis: don't Skp the F-box hypothesis. Trends Genet 14(6):236–243
33. Hecht A, Litterst CM, Huber O et al (1999) Functional characterization of multiple transactivating elements in beta-catenin, some of which interact with the TATA-binding protein in vitro. J Biol Chem 274(25):18017–18025
34. Hsu SC, Galceran J, Grosschedl R (1998) Modulation of transcriptional regulation by LEF-1 in response to Wnt-1 signaling and association with beta-catenin. Mol Cell Biol 18(8):4807–4818
35. Willert K, Jones KA (2006) Wnt signaling: is the party in the nucleus? Genes Dev 20(11):1394–1404
36. Aoki M, Hecht A, Kruse U et al (1999) Nuclear endpoint of Wnt signaling: neoplastic transformation induced by transactivating lymphoid-enhancing factor 1. Proc Natl Acad Sci 96:139–144
37. Hoppler S, Kavanagh CL (2007) Wnt signalling: variety at the core. J Cell Sci 120:385–393
38. Courey AJ, Jia S (2001) Transcriptional repression: the long and the short of it. Genes Dev 15(21):2786–2796
39. Daniels DL, Weis WI (2005) Beta-catenin directly displaces Groucho/TLE repressors from Tcf/Lef in Wnt-mediated transcription activation. Nat Struct Mol Biol 12(4):364–371
40. Tejpar S, Li C, Yu C et al (2001) Tcf-3 expression and beta-catenin mediated transcriptional activation in aggressive fibromatosis (desmoid tumour). Br J Cancer 85:98–101
41. Morin PJ, Sparks AB, Korinek V et al (1997) Activation of beta-catenin-Tcf signaling in colon cancer by mutations in beta-catenin or APC. Science 275(5307):1787–1790
42. Kikuchi A (2003) Tumor formation by genetic mutations in the components of the Wnt signaling pathway. Cancer Sci 94(3):225–229
43. Polakis P (2007) The many ways of Wnt in cancer. Curr Opin Genet Dev 17(1):45–51
44. Poon R, Smits R, Li C et al (2001) Cyclooxygenase-two (COX-2) modulates proliferation in aggressive fibromatosis (desmoid tumor). Oncogene 20(4):451–460
45. Miyoshi Y, Nagase H, Ando H et al (1992) Somatic mutations of the APC gene in colorectal tumors: mutation cluster region in the APC gene. Hum Mol Genet 1(4):229–233
46. Jen J, Powell SM, Papadopoulos N et al (1994) Molecular determinants of dysplasia in colorectal lesions. Cancer Res 54(21):5523–5526
47. Kishida S, Yamamoto H, Ikeda S et al (1998) Axin, a negative regulator of the wnt signaling pathway, directly interacts with adenomatous polyposis coli and regulates the stabilization of beta-catenin. J Biol Chem 273(18):10823–10826
48. Groen EJ, Roos A, Muntinghe FL et al (2008) Extra-intestinal manifestations of familial adenomatous polyposis. Ann Surg Oncol 15(9):2439–2450
49. Caspari R, Olschwang S, Friedl W et al (1995) Familial adenomatous polyposis: desmoid tumours and lack of ophthalmic lesions (CHRPE) associated with APC mutations beyond codon 1444. Hum Mol Genet 4(3):337–340
50. Spirio LN, Samowitz W, Robertson J et al (1998) Alleles of APC modulate the frequency and classes of mutations that lead to colon polyps. Nat Genet 20(4):385–388
51. Brensinger JD, Laken SJ, Luce MC et al (1998) Variable phenotype of familial adenomatous polyposis in pedigrees with 3′ mutation in the APC gene. Gut 43(4):548–552
52. Knudson AG (1996) Hereditary cancer: two hits revisited. J Cancer Res Clin Oncol 122(3):135–140
53. Powell SM, Zilz N, Beazer-Barclay Y et al (1992) APC mutations occur early during colorectal tumorigenesis. Nature 359(6392):235–237
54. Miyaki M, Konishi M, Kikuchi-Yanoshita R et al (1994) Characteristics of somatic mutation of the adenomatous polyposis coli gene in colorectal tumors. Cancer Res 54(11):3011–3020
55. Li C, Bapat B, Alman BA (1998) Adenomatous polyposis coli gene mutation alters proliferation through its beta-catenin-regulatory function in aggressive fibromatosis (desmoid tumor). Am J Pathol 153(3):709–714
56. Miyaki M, Konishi M, Kikuchi-Yanoshita R et al (1993) Coexistence of somatic and germline mutations of APC gene in desmoid tumors from patients with familial adenomatous polyposis. Cancer Res 53(21):5079–5082

57. Latchford A, Volikos E, Johnson V et al (2007) APC mutations in FAP-associated desmoid tumours are non-random but not 'just right'. Hum Mol Genet 16(1):78–82
58. Miyaki M, Yamaguchi T, Iijima T et al (2008) Difference in characteristics of APC mutations between colonic and extracolonic tumors of FAP patients: variations with phenotype. Int J Cancer 122(11):2491–2497
59. Fletcher JA, Naeem R, Xiao S et al (1995) Chromosome aberrations in desmoid tumors. Trisomy 8 may be a predictor of recurrence. Cancer Genet Cytogenet 79(2):139–143
60. Bridge JA, Sreekantaiah C, Mouron B et al (1992) Clonal chromosomal abnormalities in desmoid tumors. Implications for histopathogenesis. Cancer 69(2):430–436
61. Tejpar S, Nollet F, Li C et al (1999) Predominance of beta-catenin mutations and beta-catenin dysregulation in sporadic aggressive fibromatosis (desmoid tumor). Oncogene 18(47):6615–6620
62. Sparks AB, Morin PJ, Vogelstein B et al (1998) Mutational analysis of the APC/beta-catenin/Tcf pathway in colorectal cancer. Cancer Res 58(6):1130–1134
63. Miyoshi Y, Iwao K, Nawa G et al (1998) Frequent mutations in the beta-catenin gene in desmoid tumors from patients without familial adenomatous polyposis. Oncol Res 10(11–12):591–594
64. Abraham SC, Reynolds C, Lee JH et al (2002) Fibromatosis of the breast and mutations involving the APC/beta-catenin pathway. Hum Pathol 33(1):39–46
65. Lazar AJ, Tuvin D, Hajibashi S et al (2008) Specific mutations in the beta-catenin gene (CTNNB1) correlate with local recurrence in sporadic desmoid tumors. Am J Pathol 173(5):1518–1527
66. Dômont J, Salas S, Lacroix L et al (2010) High frequency of beta-catenin heterozygous mutations in extra-abdominal fibromatosis: a potential molecular tool for disease management. Br J Cancer 102(6):1032–1036
67. Polakis P, Hart M, Rubinfeld B (1999) Defects in the regulation of beta-catenin in colorectal cancer. Adv Exp Med Biol 470:23–32
68. Willert K, Nusse R (1998) Beta-Catenin: a key mediator of Wnt signaling. Curr Opin Genet Dev 8:95–102
69. Fukuchi T, Sakamoto M, Tsuda H et al (1998) Beta-catenin mutation in carcinoma of the uterine endometrium. Cancer Res 58(16):3526–3528
70. Bell DA (2005) Origins and molecular pathology of ovarian cancer. Mod Pathol 18(Suppl 2):S19–S32
71. Oliva E, Sarrió D, Brachtel EF et al (2006) High frequency of beta-catenin mutations in borderline endometrioid tumours of the ovary. J Pathol 208(5):708–713
72. Irving JA, Catasús L, Gallardo A et al (2005) Synchronous endometrioid carcinomas of the uterine corpus and ovary: alterations in the beta-catenin (CTNNB1) pathway are associated with independent primary tumors and favorable prognosis. Hum Pathol 36(6):605–619
73. Johnson V, Lipton LR, Cummings C et al (2005) Analysis of somatic molecular changes, clinicopathological features, family history, and germline mutations in colorectal cancer families: evidence for efficient diagnosis of HNPCC and for the existence of distinct groups of non-HNPCC families. J Med Genet 42(10):756–762
74. Rowley PT (2005) Inherited susceptibility to colorectal cancer. Annu Rev Med 56:539–554
75. Alman BA, Naber SP, Terek RM et al (1995) Platelet-derived growth factor in fibrous musculoskeletal disorders: a study of pathologic tissue sections and in vitro primary cell cultures. J Orthop Res 13:67–77
76. Locci P, Bellocchio S, Lilli C et al (2001) Synthesis and secretion of transforming growth factor-b1 by human desmoid fibroblast cell line and its modulation by toremifene. J Interferon Cytokine Res 21:961–970
77. Saito T, Oda Y, Tanaka K et al (2001) Beta-catenin nuclear expression correlates with cyclin D1 overexpression in sporadic desmoid tumours. J Pathol 195(2):222–228
78. Amini Nik S, Hohenstein P, Jadidizadeh A et al (2005) Upregulation of wilms' tumor gene 1 (WT1) in desmoid tumors. Int J Cancer 114:202–208

79. Fen Li C, Kandel C, Baliko F et al (2005) Plasminogen activator inhibitor-1 (PAI-1) modifies the formation of aggressive fibromatosis (desmoid tumor). Oncogene 24:1615–1624
80. Bacac M, Migliavacca E, Stehle JC et al (2006) A gene expression signature that distinguishes desmoid tumours from nodular fasciitis. J Pathol 208:543–553
81. Carlson JW, Fletcher CD (2007) Immunohistochemistry for beta-catenin in the differential diagnosis of spindle cell lesions: analysis of a series and review of the literature. Histopathology 51:509–514
82. Bhattacharya B, Dilworth HP, Iacobuzio-Donahue C et al (2005) Nuclear Beta-catenin expression distinguishes deep fibromatosis from other benign and malignant fibroblastic and myofibroblastic lesions. Am J Surg Pathol 29:653–659
83. Montgomery E, Torbenson MS, Kaushal M et al (2002) Beta-catenin immunohistochemistry separates mesenteric fibromatosis from gastrointestinal stromal tumor and sclerosing mesenteritis. Am J Surg Pathol 26:1296–1301
84. Ng TL, Gown AM, Barry TS et al (2005) Nuclear beta-catenin in mesenchymal tumors. Mod Pathol 18:68–74
85. Rakheja D, Molberg KH, Roberts CA et al (2005) Immunohistochemical expression of beta-catenin in solitary fibrous tumors. Arch Pathol Lab Med 129(6):776–779
86. Montgomery E, Folpe AL (2005) The diagnostic value of beta-catenin immunohistochemistry. Adv Anat Pathol 12:350–356
87. Lepourcelet M, Chen YN, France DS et al (2004) Small-molecule antagonists of the oncogenic Tcf/beta-catenin protein complex. Cancer Cell 5(1):91–102
88. Wang D, DuBois RN (2010) The role of COX-2 in intestinal inflammation and colorectal cancer. Oncogene 29:781–788
89. Emami KH, Nguyen C, Ma H et al (2004) A small molecule inhibitor of beta-catenin/CREB-binding protein transcription. Proc Natl Acad Sci 101(34):12682–12687
90. Park CH, Chang JY, Hahm ER et al (2005) Quercetin, a potent inhibitor against beta-catenin/Tcf signaling in SW480 colon cancer cells. Biochem Biophys Res Commun 328(1):227–234
91. Chen Z, Venkatesan AM, Dehnhardt CM et al (2009) 2,4-Diamino-quinazolines as inhibitors of beta-catenin/Tcf-4 pathway: potential treatment for colorectal cancer. Bior Med Chem Lett 19(17):4980–4983
92. Huang SM, Mishina YM, Liu S et al (2009) Tankyrase inhibition stabilizes axin and antagonizes Wnt signalling. Nature 461(7264):614–620
93. Signoroni S, Frattini M, Negri T et al (2007) Cyclooxygenase-2 and platelet-derived growth factor receptors as potential targets in treating aggressive fibromatosis. Clin Canc Res 13(17):5034–5040
94. Heinrich MC, McArthur GA, Demetri GD et al (2006) Clinical and molecular studies of the effect of Imatinib on advanced aggressive fibromatosis (desmoid tumor). J Clin Oncol 24(7):1195–1203
95. Takemaru KI, Ohmitsu M, Li FQ, Klussmann E, Scott J (eds) (2008) Protein–protein Iinteractions as new drug targets. 261 Handbook of experimental pharmacology 186. Springer, Berlin
96. Zhang Q, Major MB, Takanashi S et al (2007) Small-molecule synergist of the Wnt/beta-catenin signaling pathway. Proc Natl Acad Sci 104:7444–7448
97. Sekiya T, Nakamura T, Kazuki Y et al (2002) Overexpression of Icat induces G(2) arrest and cell death in tumor cell mutants for adenomatous polyposis coli, beta-catenin, or axin. Cancer Res 62(11):3322–3326
98. Steinbach G, Lynch PM, Phillips RK et al (2000) The effect of celecoxib, a cyclooxygenase-2 inhibitor, in familial adenomatous polyposis. N Engl J Med 342(26):1946–1952
99. Dufresne A, Bertucci F, Penel N et al (2010) Identification of biological factors predictive of response to imatinib mesylate in aggressive fibromatosis. Br J Cancer 103(4):482–485
100. Barker N, Clevers H (2006) Mining the Wnt pathway for cancer therapeutics. Nature Rev Drug Discovery 5:997–1014

Chapter 5
Imaging Techniques in Desmoid Tumors

Robert A. Lefkowitz, Sinchun Hwang and Jonathan Landa

Contents

Abstract From an imaging perspective, desmoid tumors are best classified as extra-abdominal, abdominal wall, and intra-abdominal. MRI is the imaging modality of choice for extra-abdominal desmoids, demonstrating a lesion that can be well-defined, has infiltrative margins, or a combination of both. The lesions are low in T1 signal, while T2 signal is variable, depending upon the stage of evolution. During their early growth stage, desmoid tumors are highly cellular with relatively less collagen. As a result, they are predominantly high in T2 signal with small foci of low T2 signal, and demonstrate avid contrast enhancement. As they evolve over time, the tumors become less cellular and more densely collagenous, with a resultant decrease in T2 signal intensity and

R. A. Lefkowitz (✉)
Department of Radiology, Memorial Sloan Kettering Cancer Center, 1275 York Avenue, New York, NY 10065, USA
e-mail: lefkowir@MSKCC.org

C. Litchman (ed.), *Desmoid Tumors*,
DOI 10.1007/978-94-007-1685-8_5, © Springer Science+Business Media B.V. 2012

enhancement, and often with a concomitant decrease in size. Radiation and medical therapy can also result in these signal changes, suggesting treatment response even in the absence of decreases in size. Abdominal wall desmoid tumors can best be imaged with MRI or CT, while intra-abdominal desmoid tumors are best imaged with CT. CT demonstrates a mass which is nearly isodense to muscle on noncontrast images and which demonstrates mild-to-moderate enhancement with intravenous contrast. CT is superior to MRI in distinguishing intra-abdominal desmoids from adjacent bowel loops, although vascular involvement can be accurately assessed with either CT or MRI. MRI is sometimes desirable to CT for imaging of intra-abdominal desmoids, particularly in patients who cannot receive iodinated contrast material, either because of allergies or impaired renal function, or in patients in whom radiation exposure is a major concern. In patients with severe renal dysfunction, intravenous contrast should not be used with MRI either because of the risk of developing nephrogenic systemic sclerosis.

Keywords Desmoid • Fibromatosis • Intra-abdominal • Extra-abdominal • MRI • CT • Ultrasound • PET • Imaging

5.1 Introduction

The indications for imaging and the imaging features of desmoid tumors vary, depending upon the location of the lesions and histologic composition. These lesions are best classified according to location as: (1) extra-abdominal, (2) abdominal wall, and (3) intra-abdominal desmoid tumors (the last category includes mesenteric, retroperitoneal, and pelvic desmoid tumors) [7].

5.2 Extra-abdominal Desmoid Tumor

5.2.1 Radiographs

Plain radiographs of extra-abdominal desmoid tumor are usually normal. Radiographs occasionally reveal a soft tissue mass (Fig. 5.1) when it is large or displaces adjacent soft tissue structures; calcifications are rare [14]. Bone involvement by desmoid tumors can manifest as pressure erosions, periosteal reaction, and cortical thickening. Skeletal dysplasias, including undertubulation of long bones, have been also reported [14]. Although these findings can be helpful for tumor detection, they are nonspecific for diagnostic purposes.

5.2.2 Ultrasound

Ultrasound is utilized at some institutions as a first-line screening tool to confirm the presence of a soft tissue mass and is an excellent imaging modality to distinguish

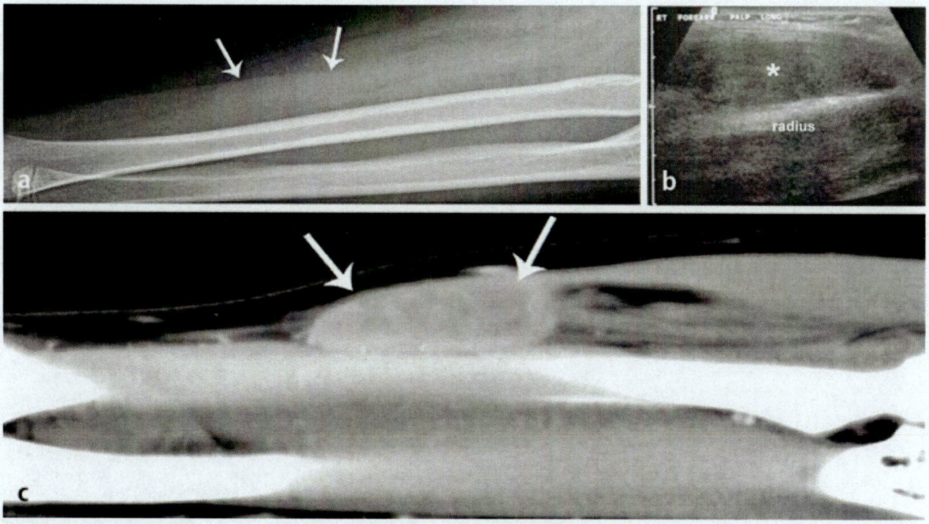

Fig. 5.1 Desmoid tumor in the forearm of a 15-year-old female. **a** Lateral radiograph of forearm shows a noncalcified soft tissue mass (*arrows*) without erosion of the adjacent radius. **b** Longitudinal ultrasound image shows a sharply bordered and diffusely hypoechoic soft tissue mass (*) adjacent to the radius. **c** Contrast-enhanced sagittal CT image shows a mildly enhancing well-circumscribed soft tissue mass (*arrows*) with a dense peripheral capsule

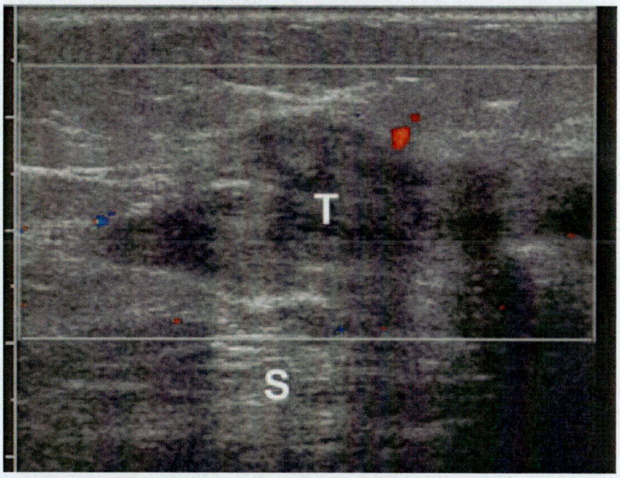

Fig. 5.2 Desmoid tumor in the popliteal fossa of a 27-year-old female. A longitudinal ultrasound image with color doppler shows a heterogeneously hypoechoic mass (*T*) with posterior acoustic enhancement in the adjacent soft tissues (*S*); the posterior acoustic enhancement is caused by the uniformity of the tumor which results in lack of impedance of the sound waves within the mass. The mass demonstrates poorly defined borders and is predominantly hypovascular

solid from cystic masses. However, for diagnosis and surveillance of desmoid tumors, ultrasound has a limited role compared to MRI, which is far superior in its ability to characterize the lesion, determine histologic stage, identify multifocal involvement, and assess involvement of adjacent bones and joints.

The sonographic appearance of desmoid tumors is variable depending on the amount of fibrous and collagenous content [16]. Desmoid tumors can be hypo-, iso- or hyperechoic with posterior acoustic shadowing; the borders can be sharply or poorly defined [14, 16] (Figs. 5.1 and 5.2). Because ultrasound provides real-time imaging, it is often employed to guide needle biopsies of the lesions.

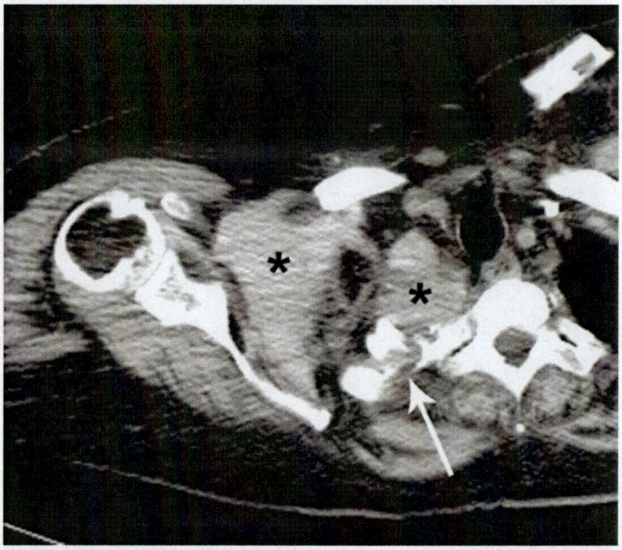

Fig. 5.3 Desmoid tumor in the right chest wall of a 55-year-old female. Noncontrast CT image demonstrates soft tissue masses (*) in the right axilla and extrapleural space adjacent to the right lung apex. The masses are higher in attenuation than adjacent muscle. Tumor erodes the adjacent ribs (*arrow*)

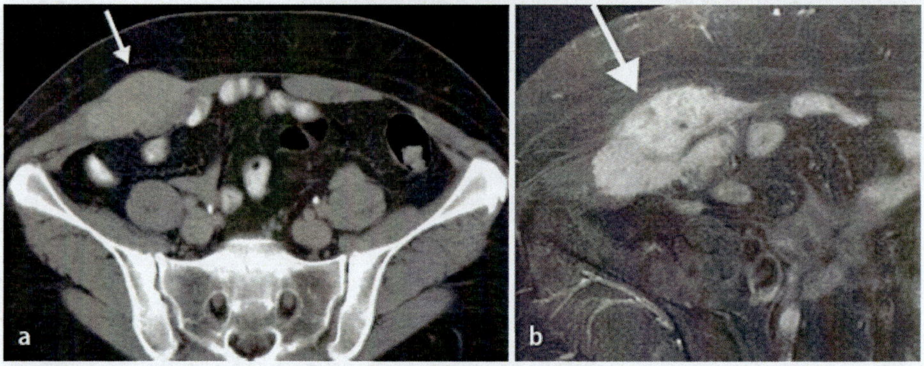

Fig. 5.4 Desmoid in abdominal wall of a 49-year-old female. **a** Contrast-enhanced CT image shows mild-diffuse enhancement of the soft tissue mass within the right rectus abdominis muscle (*arrow*). **b** Contrast-enhanced fat-suppressed T1-weighted image also demonstrates diffuse enhancement of the mass (*arrow*) due to the highly cellular composition of this particular tumor. MRI is generally more sensitive than CT in detecting contrast enhancement

5.2.3 Computed Tomography (CT)

CT scans usually reveal soft tissue masses with variable attenuation [31]. The lesion is usually iso- or hyperattenuating relative to that of skeletal muscle on noncontrast images, which is probably related to the collagen content of these tumors (Fig. 5.3). Contrast enhancement is variable, and occasionally quite prominent, probably related to the abundant capillary network present in these tumors [5, 14]. The pattern of enhancement may be diffuse or heterogenous (Fig. 5.4). Due to their infiltrative pattern of growth along fascial planes, desmoid tumors often have poorly defined margins unless the lesions are surrounded by a fat plane [31]. Bone erosion and cortical scalloping can occasionally be detected in long-standing cases without involvement of the medullary cavity [14]. CT is superior to MRI for evaluating cortical bone (Fig. 5.3).

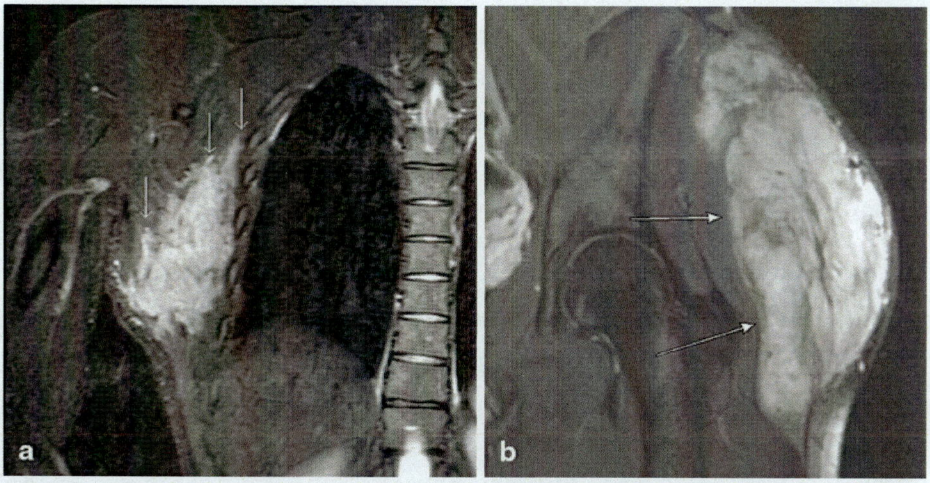

Fig. 5.5 **a** Desmoid tumor of chest wall in 18-year-old male demonstrating infiltrative margins. Coronal T2 WI shows very high T2 signal mass in the right lateral chest wall. Bands of high signal infiltrate along fascial planes (*arrows*). If attempting resection, the surgeon must be sure to include these linear extensions within the surgical margin. **b** Desmoid tumor in 20-year-old male demonstrating well-defined margins. Coronal T2 WI show predominantly high T2 signal desmoid tumor around the hip. Note that the interface (*arrows*) between the tumor and the surrounding muscles is smooth and sharply defined

5.2.4 Magnetic Resonance Imaging (MRI)

MRI is the modality of choice for imaging extra-abdominal desmoid tumors because of its superior soft tissue contrast, allowing easy delineation of these tumors from background muscle or fat [25]. A standard soft tissue tumor protocol should include spin echo T1-weighted images and fast-spin echo T2-weighted images with fat saturation with both sequences performed in two orthogonal planes (axial and sagittal or coronal) and spin echo T1-weighted fat-saturated images both before and after the intravenous administration of a gadolinium contrast agent, in at least one plane (usually the axial plane). When fat-suppression T2-weighted sequences cannot be obtained or are suboptimal due to factors causing inhomogeneous fat saturation (such as a large field of view or metallic hardware), short-tau inversion recovery (STIR) can be used. However, this sequence is more time consuming and has limited tissue contrast compared to spin echo T2-weighted sequences. An attempt should be made to image with the smallest possible field of view that covers the entire lesion using the appropriate imaging coil for the body part being scanned. However, for desmoids located in an extremity, some authors advocate imaging the entire extremity due a high incidence of multifocal disease in these patients.

Though most extra-abdominal desmoid tumors are solitary lesions, multifocal disease can occur within the same extremity in 10–15% of cases [31]. Multifocal disease can be synchronous or metachronous [4]. Approximately half of all extra-abdominal desmoid tumors have well-defined margins, while the remainder demonstrate infiltrative margins (Fig. 5.5) [7]. Extra-abdominal fibromatoses are typically 5–10 cm in greatest dimension, but can vary in size from very small lesions to

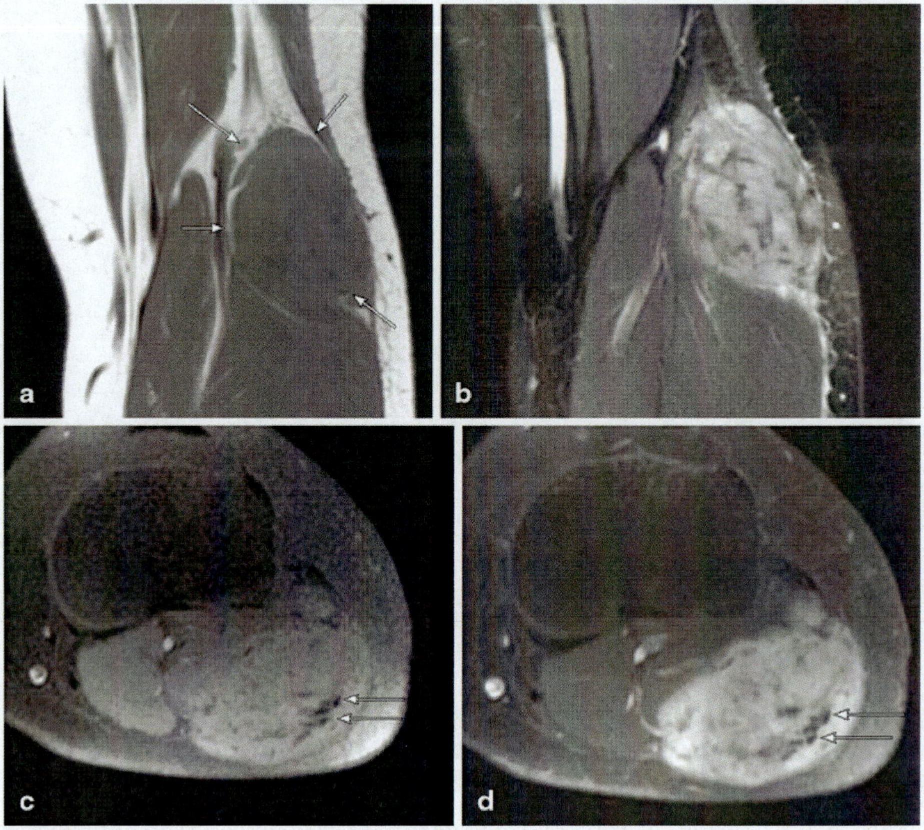

Fig. 5.6 16-year-old female with desmoid tumor in lateral popliteal region. **a** Coronal T1 WI demonstrating intermediate signal mass in an intermuscular location between the lateral head of the gastrocnemius and biceps femoris muscles. Note the rim of high signal fat (*arrows*) surrounding the mass illustrating the "split fat" sign. **b** On coronal T2 WI the mass is predominantly high in T2 signal with multiple curvilinear bands of low T2 signal representing areas of dense collagen, a characteristic appearance of desmoid tumors. These bands of collagen are also visible on the T1 WI (Fig. 5.6a). **c, d** T1-weighted fat saturated images obtained both before (Fig. 5.6c) and after (Fig. 5.6d) gadolinium-based contrast administration. The mass demonstrates avid enhancement. The bands of collagen seen on the T1- and T2-weighted sequences are hypovascular (*arrows* in Fig. 5.6d), thus appearing low in signal on the postcontrast images. Note the difference between this lesion and that in Fig. 5.4, which is intramuscular in location, confined within the rectus abdominus muscle

large, bulky masses that can exceed 15 cm [14]. They can be either intermuscular or intramuscular in origin. The intermuscular lesions are often surrounded by a rim of fat, which is high in T1 signal compared to the tumor; this finding is sometimes referred to as the "split fat" sign (Fig. 5.6) [14]. Murphy et al. describe a "fascial tail sign" which is present in 83% of extra-abdominal desmoid tumors, but is unusual in most other soft tissue tumors (Fig. 5.7). Desmoid tumor has a tendency to spread along fascial planes, and this mechanism of spread can manifest as a linear focus of signal abnormality extending a significant distance from the main mass, along the adjacent fascial planes. This sign has important diagnostic implications

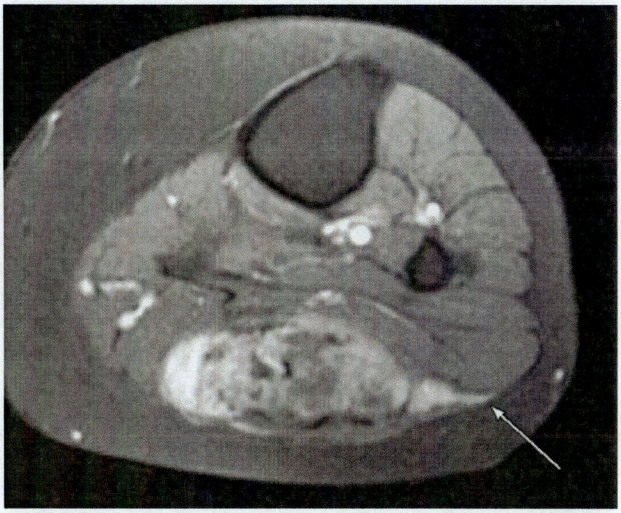

Fig. 5.7 Desmoid tumor of calf in 50-year-old female. Axial T1 postcontrast image with fat saturation demonstrating the "fascial tail" sign (*arrow*). This linear extension of high signal represents tumor spreading along the fascia which invests the lateral head of the gastrocnemius muscle. This "fascial tail" must be removed with the rest of the mass if this lesion is to be surgically excised in its entirety

for staging because complete surgical resection of these tumors requires inclusion of the "fascial tail" [14].

Desmoid tumors are typically intermediate signal on T1-weighted images, similar to that of muscle, but can have curvilinear bands or focal amorphous areas of low T1 signal signifying regions of dense fibrosis. Tumors that are diffusely acellular with dense collagen are markedly low in T1 signal [7].

Desmoids are usually heterogenous in T2 signal, with regions that vary from high to very low in signal depending on the relative amounts of collagen, cellular tissue, and myxoid tissue within the tumor [2, 8, 14]. According to Sundaram et al. areas that have a high percentage of collagen and low cellularity are low in T2 signal, while regions that are highly cellular, regardless of the collagen content, are high in T2 signal [8]. The presence of myxoid components also contributes high T2 signal intensity [14]. A number of soft tissue tumors, both benign and malignant, can demonstrate focal areas of low T2 signal within a predominantly high T2 signal mass, including synovial sarcoma and pigmented villonodular synovitis/giant cell tumor of tendon sheath (due to hemorrhage), fibrosarcoma, and malignant fibrous histiocytoma (due to fibrous tissue), and osteosarcoma, enchondroma, and chondrosarcoma (due to calcification) [11]. However, the pattern of low T2 signal in desmoid tumors is quite distinct from the aforementioned lesions, having discrete linear, curvilinear, or irregular bands of low T2 signal intensity on all pulse sequences. These bands of low signal are also hypovascular on postcontrast images and can be identified in 62–91% of all desmoid tumors [4, 7, 14]. Additional imaging features which suggest the diagnosis of desmoid tumor over sarcoma include an infiltrative growth pattern (sarcomas usually displace rather than infiltrate adjacent soft tissues), a tendency to cross fascial boundaries (sarcomas usually compress adjacent tissue forming a pseudocapsule and respect fascial boundaries until late in their course), and an absence of necrosis even with very large lesions (sarcomas, especially large ones, typically contain areas of necrosis) [7]. The necrotic areas in sarcomas are brighter than fat (closer to fluid) on standard (nonfat saturated) T2

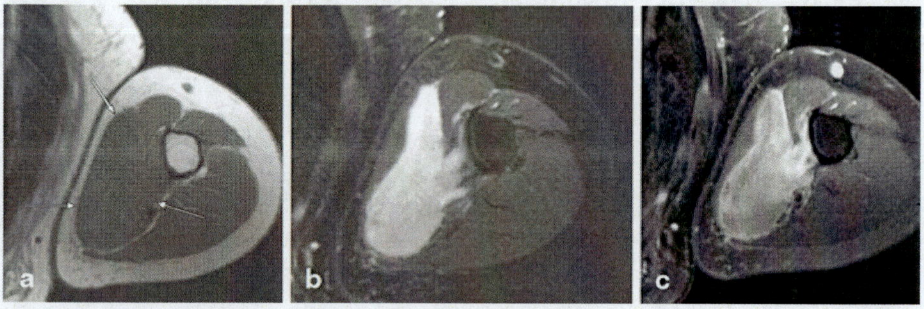

Fig. 5.8 32-year-old male with stage 1 desmoid tumor in medial aspect of upper arm. **a** T1 WI demonstrating mass (*arrows*) which is isointense to, and thus, difficult to distinguish from, adjacent skeletal muscle. **b** T2 WI with fat saturation demonstrates a mass which is uniformly high in signal consistent with a desmoid tumor that is highly cellular with little collagen. **c** T1 WI postgadolinium sequence with fat suppression demonstrates nearly uniform, avid enhancement consistent with a highly cellular desmoid. Note the convex borders of the tumor which are typical of stage 1 tumors

WI and do not enhance, whereas the highest signal intensity on T2 WI in desmoid tumors approximate that of fat [20].

The MR appearance of desmoid tumors changes with time as the lesion evolves or matures along three stages. During the first stage, the period of growth, desmoids are more cellular with relatively less collagen and contain large extracellular spaces. These features result in a lesion that is low in T1 signal and uniformly high in T2 signal. Foci of low T2 signal are generally absent during this stage of development. In this stage, the lesions tend to have convex borders and demonstrate moderate-to-strong, uniform enhancement with IV contrast (Fig. 5.8). The high cellularity during the first stage explains why desmoid tumors with high T2 signal are, statistically, more likely to grow, and to grow more rapidly than those with low or intermediate signal [14, 25]. During the second stage, there is an increased deposition of collagen centrally or peripherally within the lesion, resulting in a more heterogenous mass containing focal areas of low T2 signal. The cellular areas in the tumor which remain high in T2 signal continue to demonstrate moderate-to-strong enhancement, while the low T2 signal areas of dense collagen demonstrate minimal, if any, enhancement (Fig. 5.9). During the third and final stage, desmoid tumors become mostly fibrous in composition with a decrease in degree of cellularity. The volume of the extracelluar spaces within the tumor decreases with associated decrease in water content, and the overall size of the tumor decreases during this stage. As the size decreases, the tumor borders become less convex and more undulating. As a result of these histologic changes, tumors during this stage are low in T1 and T2 signal, reflecting the predominance of fibrous tissue and lack of cellularity. Enhancement during this stage is also dramatically less avid than earlier stages (Fig. 5.10) [4]. In cases of multifocal desmoid tumors within the same limb, the lesions are often asynchronous, with the more proximal lesions typically developing later than the distal ones and lagging behind the distal lesions in their evolution. Thus, subsequent development of a new lesion proximal to a resected lesion should not be construed

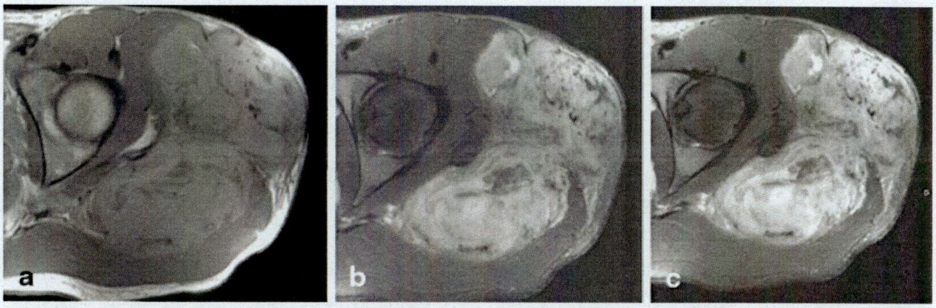

Fig. 5.9 20-year-old male with desmoid tumor of left buttock and hip regions which is probably in stage 2 of evolution. **a** Axial T1 WI demonstrating mass that is slightly hyperintense to adjacent skeletal muscle. Multiple bands of low signal collage are interspersed throughout the mass. **b** Axial T2 WI demonstrates a mass which is predominantly high in T2 signal, indicating regions of high cellularity. This lesion also contains focal areas of low T2 signal, which represents areas that are more collagenous and less cellular. The areas of collagen become more prominent as the desmoid matures. **c** Postgadolinium image of the identical region in **b**. Note that the cellular areas on the T2 WI correspond almost precisely to the enhancing regions on this sequence, while the low T2 signal regions are hypovascular (low signal) in **c**. The densely collagenous regions are low in signal on all pulse sequences and enhance very little, if at all

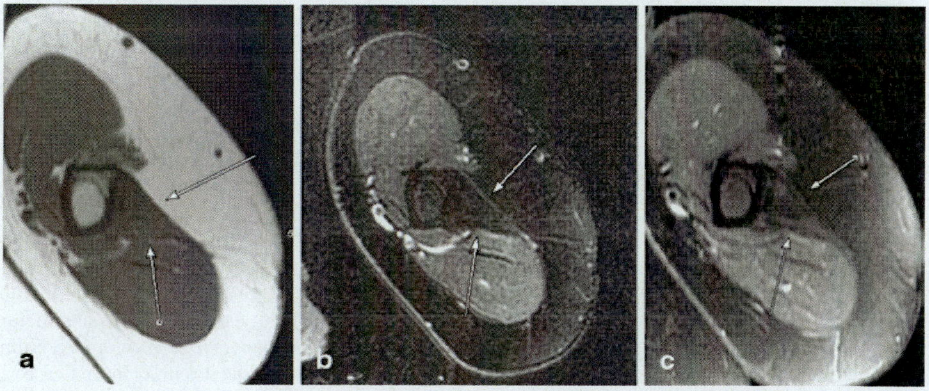

Fig. 5.10 45-year-old male with stage 3 desmoid tumor in lateral aspect of upper arm. **a** T1 WI demonstrates a mass (*arrows*) which is hypointense to muscle. **b** T2 WI with fat saturation demonstrates that the mass is very low in signal. The low signal on T1 and T2 WI signifies that the mass is predominantly collagenous in composition and is very low in cellularity. This represents the end stage in the evolution of desmoid tumors. Note that the borders are concave and slightly undulating (*posterior margin*) in contrast to the convex borders seen in earlier-stage tumors. **c** Postcontrast images demonstrate a hypovascular lesion, which is typical of this stage

as a recurrence if the new lesion is remote from the original one (Fig. 5.11) [4]. In contrast to the specific MR appearance of desmoid tumors, CT imaging features have not shown a good correlation with histologic findings, including its assessment of collagen and vascularity [20].

Primary desmoid tumors which demonstrate greater T2 signal intensity and enhancement before surgery—the ones that grow more rapidly—are believed to have

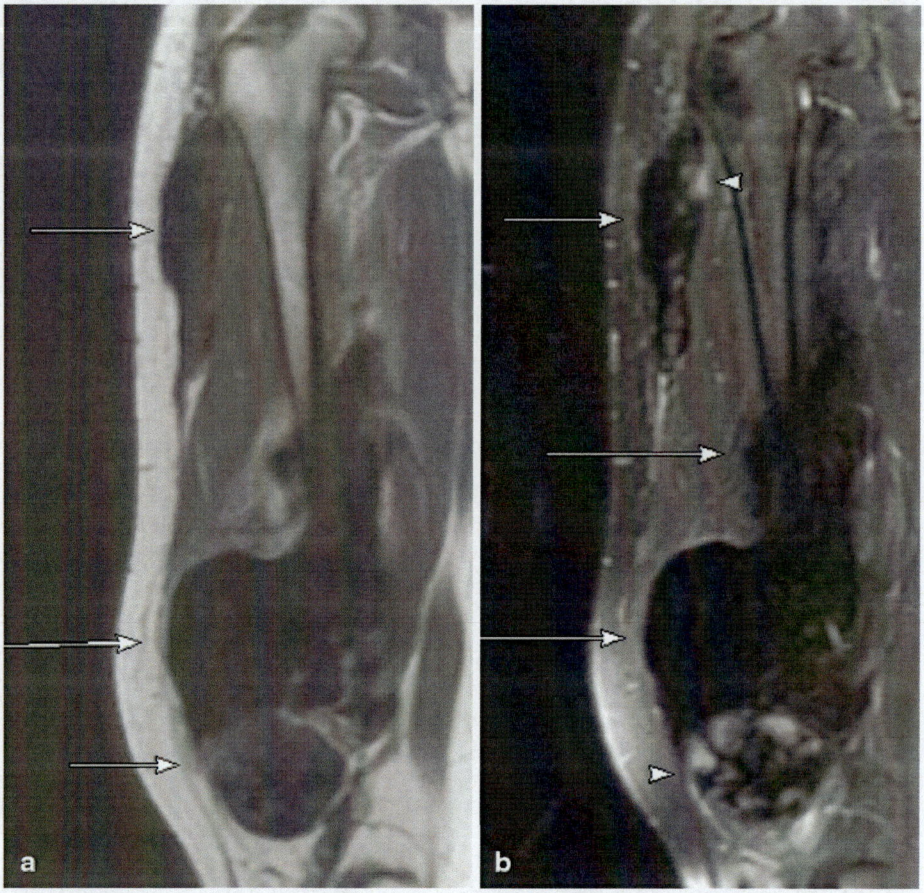

Fig. 5.11 26-year-old female with multifocal desmoid tumor of right thigh. **a** Coronal T1 and **b** T2-weighted images demonstrating multiple, predominantly low-signal soft tissue masses (*arrows*) of high collagen content with focal areas of high T2 signal (*arrowheads*) representing smaller cellular components. The masses extend from the hip to the distal femur. In this case, all the lesions are in approximately the same stage of evolution

an increased risk for recurrence postoperatively compared to their less cellular, lower T2 signal, and less avidly enhancing counterparts [14]. Thus, MR can help predict which patients are likely to have better outcomes postoperatively. MR imaging is also the preferred modality for monitoring patients after resection of desmoid tumors. Local recurrences most often occur near the resection margins, at sites where subtle, distant fascial spread was not appreciated preoperatively, and thus, left behind at surgery [31]. Recurrent desmoid tumors have identical histology, and, thus, the same imaging features as primary early-stage lesions, demonstrating uniformly high T2 signal, with or without interspersed low-signal collagenous bands, and moderate-to-strong enhancement (Fig. 5.12). On average, however, recurrent desmoid tumors tend to behave more aggressively than their primary counterparts,

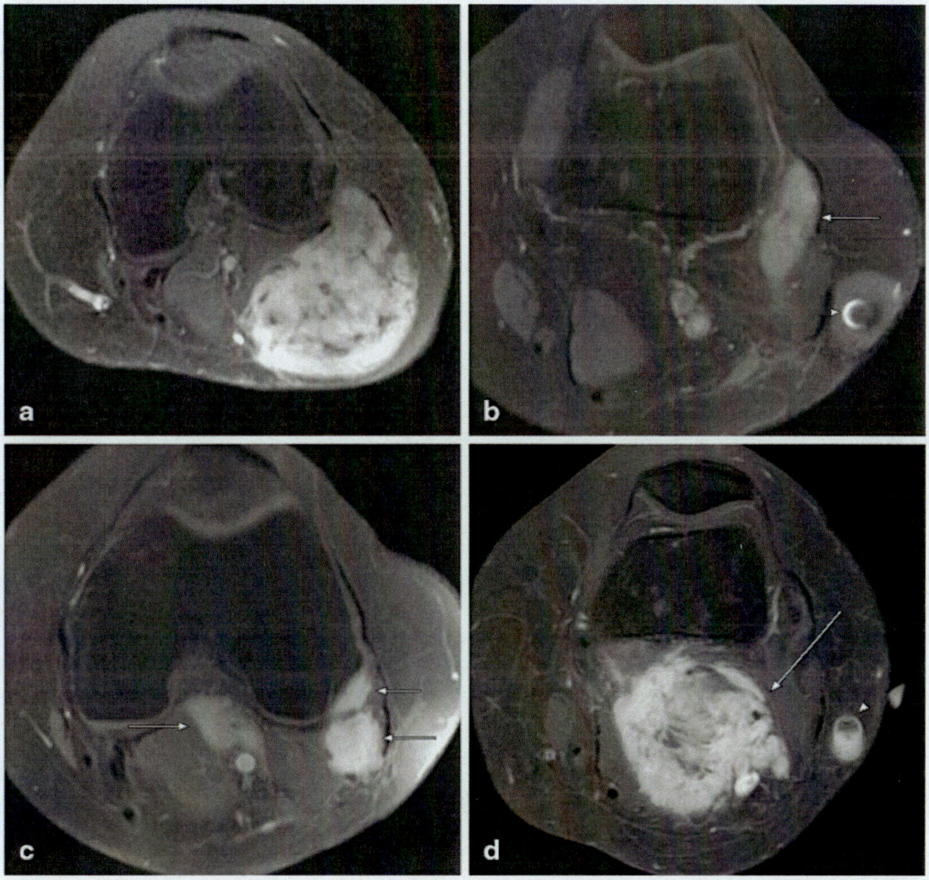

Fig. 5.12 Recurrent desmoid tumor of popliteal region in 17-year-old female. **a** Preoperative T1 WI with fat saturation demonstrating an 8 cm markedly enhancing mass consistent with a highly cellular desmoid tumor. Small foci of low signal within the mass are consistent with densely collagenous regions. It is believed that the highly cellular desmoids such as this one are more likely to recur after surgery. **b**, **c** Axial postcontrast images 10 months after surgical resection demonstrate four small hypervascular nodules (*arrows*) along the periphery of the operative bed (*resection margins*) consistent with locally recurrent cellular desmoid tumors. Note artifact from a surgical clip in **b** (*arrowhead*). **d** Axial postcontrast image 45 months after surgery demonstrating coalescence of the nodules into a single mass (*long arrow*). Note the resemblance of the recurrent tumor to the primary tumor in **a**. Clip artifact again seen (*arrowhead*)

with more rapid growth, an increased rate of extracompartmental spread, and an increased likelihood of bone invasion [4, 19]. Recurrences are also more likely to have infiltrative margins on imaging [7]. Recurrent desmoid tumors probably undergo the same evolutionary process as primary tumors, with growth arrest, some shrinkage, and eventual transformation into densely collagenous, dormant masses [4].

MR is also the imaging modality of choice to monitor the response of desmoid tumors to radiation or medical therapy. Tumors that respond to therapy not only demonstrate a decrease in size, but typically show a decrease in T2 signal as well, indicat-

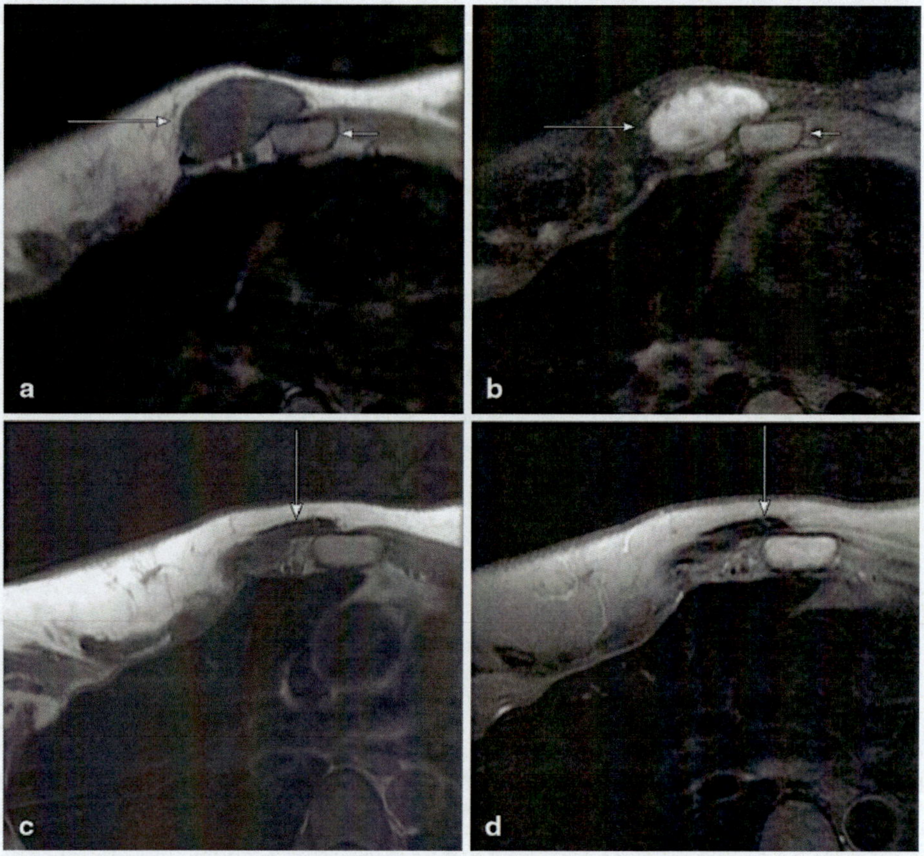

Fig. 5.13 27-year-old female with desmoid tumor of anterior chest wall. Patient was treated with Sorafenib. **a, b** show desmoid (*long arrow*) adjacent to sternum (*short arrow*) on T1 and T2 WI, respectively, prior to therapy. This is a cellular desmoid which is high in signal on T2 WI and intermediate in signal (isointense to muscle) on T1 WI. **c, d** are T1 and T2 WI images, respectively, 2 years after initiating Sorafenib therapy. The lesion (*arrows*) has decreased significantly in size and signal intensity on both sequences, consistent with treatment response (the tumor is now a collagen-predominant lesion)

ing the transformation to a less cellular, more collagenous state (Fig. 5.13) [31]. In a study by Castellazzi et al. desmoid tumors treated with chemotherapy had a higher rate of T2 signal loss than untreated lesions, suggesting the transformation into a more indolent phase. However, this loss of T2 signal was not always associated with a decrease in size, and thus, these tumors would not qualify as responders by standard Response Evaluation Criteria In Solid Tumors (RECIST) (Fig. 5.14) [19]. Further studies must be performed to determine whether or not the loss of T2 signal alone, even in the absence of response by traditional size criteria, results in improved clinical outcomes. If improved clinical outcomes are shown to be independently associated with T2 signal changes alone, then MR imaging would prove to be indispensable for determining desmoid tumor response rates for patients on medical therapy.

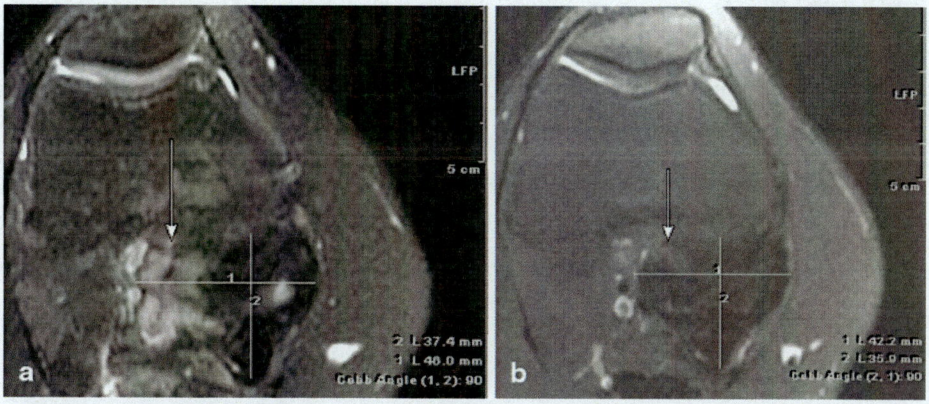

Fig. 5.14 29-year-old female with desmoid tumor of popliteal region, treated with Sorafenib. **a** Pretreatment scan, axial T2 WI, demonstrates a heterogenous mass with areas of both high and low signal, corresponding to areas of high and low cellularity, respectively. The mass measures 4.6 × 3.7. **b** Axial T2 WI 10 months after initiation of therapy. The tumor now measures 4.2 × 3.6 cm, which does not qualify as a response by RECIST or WHO criteria. However, the previously noted high T2 signal cellular areas (*arrow* in **a**) are now uniformly low in T2 signal (*arrow* in **b**), consistent with a change in composition to a more collagenous state. Some authors have suggested that change in signal alone is indicative of treatment response

5.2.5 *Fluorodeoxyglucose-Positron Emission Tomography (FDG-PET)*

FDG-PET has a well-known role in the evaluation of metastatic disease from soft tissue sarcomas [39]. However, its role in the evaluation of desmoid tumors is very limited at this time. It has been reported that PET scans demonstrate heterogeneous uptake of FDG related to the heterogenous histologic make-up of these tumors, which contain varying proportions of densely collagenous and more cellular components. Areas of dense collagen within desmoid tumor have low standardized uptake values (SUV) while more cellular areas have relatively higher SUVs [31]. Since the aggressiveness of these tumors is directly related to the degree of cellularity, FDG-PET may have a potential role in predicting the behavior of desmoid tumors.

FDG-PET has a well-established role in monitoring patients treated with chemotherapy for certain sarcomas. In fact, FDG-PET is considered the modality of choice for evaluating changes in metabolic activity of gastrointestinal stromal tumors, as it is the earliest indicator of treatment response, in patients treated with imatinib mesylate (Gleevac). Patients who respond to Gleevac may show dramatic decreases in FDG uptake within weeks, or even days [3]. The utility of FDG-PET is currently being investigated for desmoid tumors. In a pilot study, nine patients with desmoid tumors who were treated with imatinib were evaluated with serial PET scans and MRI. Following treatment, there was a decrease in median SUV_{max} of 29% on PET scans; however, by standard RECIST criteria, seven of nine (78%) patients demonstrated stable disease and two of nine (22%) demonstrated disease progression on MRI [7, 14]. A well-recognized pitfall of using standard RECIST and WHO criteria for assessing tumor response with patients on imatinib and other targeted therapies is that many lesions which demonstrate necrosis and fibrosis after treatment (histologic evidence of tumor response) will paradoxically show stable disease, or occasionally even progression, when using size criteria alone. It is for this reason that FDG-PET, which measures metabolic activity rather size, may also play a role in monitoring treatment response of desmoid tumors to targeted therapies.

5.3 Abdominal Wall Desmoid Tumor

Abdominal wall desmoids are histologically indistinguishable from extra-abdominal desmoid tumors. Their classification as a distinct entity relates not only to their location, but also to their unique epidemiology and lower recurrence rates as discussed in previous chapters. As a result of their identical histology, however, the imaging features of abdominal wall desmoid tumors are also identical to those of their extra-abdominal counterparts [14]. Since the abdominal wall tumors are relatively superficial in location, ultrasound can be used as a first-line screening tool to confirm the presence of a mass. As with extra-abdominal desmoid tumors, however, ultrasound has a limited role in diagnosis because the sonographic features are nonspecific. MRI and CT are the preferred imaging modalities.

In a study by Healy et al. CT and MRI were equally accurate in depicting the number, size, location, and margins of abdominal wall desmoid tumors [25]. CT typically demonstrates a mass which is isodense, and occasionally slightly hyperdense, to adjacent skeletal muscle on noncontrast images. The higher density lesions are probably those containing more prominent collagen. Hypodensity relative to muscle is the least common appearance, but can be seen in lesions with a prominent myxoid component [14]. The tumor margins are frequently indistinct due in part to the infiltrative growth pattern and in part to the similar attenuation of the tumor with adjacent muscle. Desmoid tumors usually demonstrate mild enhancement, but can enhance moderately. Those lesions which are more vascular than adjacent skeletal muscle are more likely to show well-defined or partially well-defined margins after contrast administration (Fig. 5.15) [14, 23, 31].

At our institution, MR is the imaging modality of choice for abdominal wall tumors due to the superior soft tissue contrast versus CT. Like their extra-abdominal counterparts, abdominal wall desmoid tumors are isointense to muscle on T1 WI and variable in signal on T2 WI depending on the degree of collagen, cellularity, and myxoid components. According to Murphey et al. the identification of a low to intermediate signal-intensity abdominal wall mass with linear extension along the superficial fascia (fascial tail sign) and containing low signal nonenhancing bands (collagen) is virtually diagnostic of abdominal wall desmoid tumor (Fig. 5.16) [14].

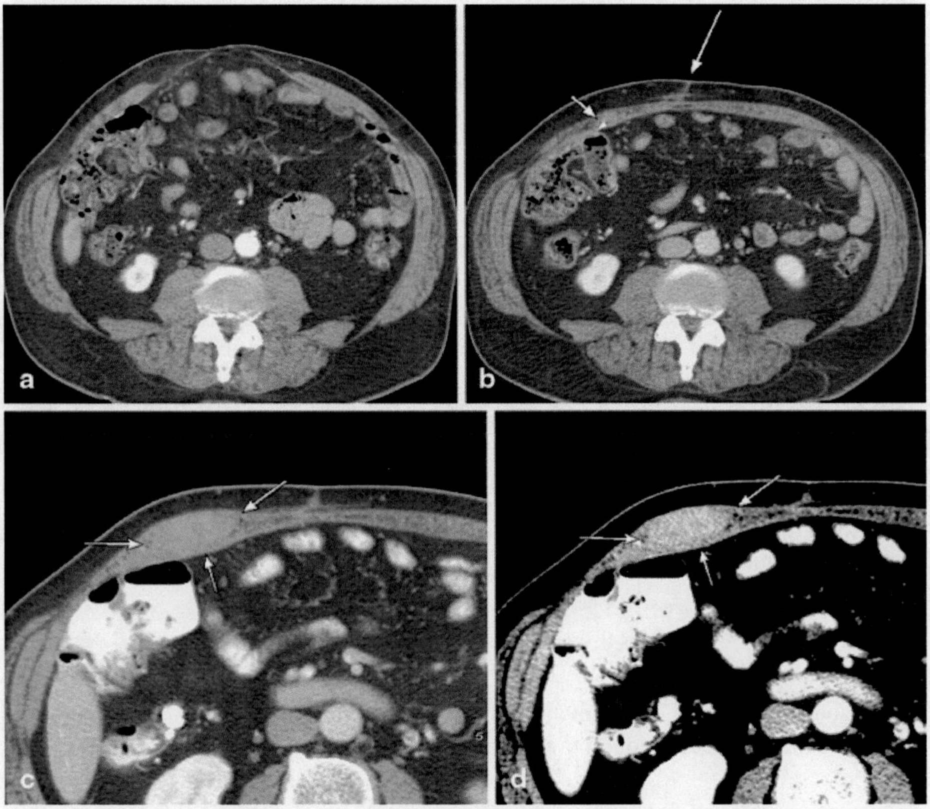

Fig. 5.15 CT scan of abdomen, axial images, with IV and oral contrast in 61-year-old male with a prior ventral hernia repair. **a** Contrast-enhanced CT scan demonstrating midline ventral hernia. **b** Follow-up CT scan at same location demonstrating new postoperative changes status post hernia repair (*long arrow*), including a surgical clip in the right rectus abdominus muscle (*short arrow*). **c** Contrast-enhanced CT performed approximately 1 year after surgery demonstrates a new 5 cm mass in the right rectus abdominus muscle (*arrows*) in the region of the hernia repair. The attenuation of the mass is only slightly greater than that of adjacent skeletal muscle, making it difficult to delineate the tumor margins. For this reason, intramuscular desmoids can be very subtle on CT. In this case the mass is large enough to expand the muscle, making the lesion more conspicuous—note, the asymmetry compared to opposite rectus muscle. **d** Same image with a "narrower window" which is created by adjusting the contrast of the image. The mass is now more obvious because a narrow window accentuates small differences in attenuation

5.4 Intra-abdominal Desmoid Tumor

5.4.1 Radiographs

Abdominal radiographs are often normal, but if the tumor is large enough, a nonspecific soft tissue mass may be evident. Other findings that can be seen on plain films include bowel obstruction and, infrequently, cavitation due to fistulization with bowel. Calcification is a distinctly unusual finding.

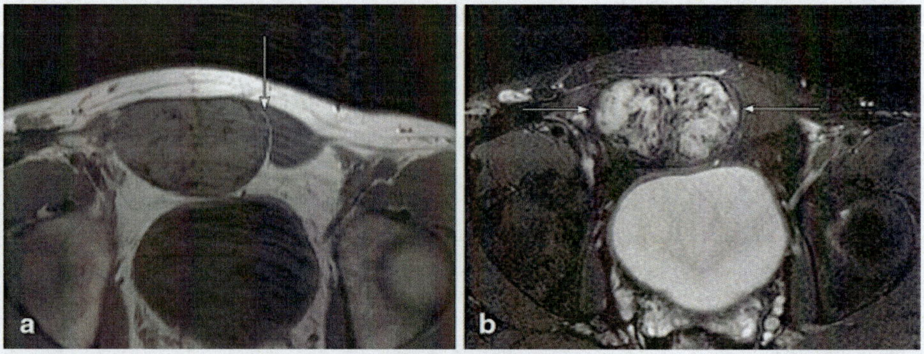

Fig. 5.16 MRI of lower abdominal wall in 32-year-old male with a 7 cm desmoid tumor in the right rectus abdominus muscle. **a** Axial T1 WI demonstrates an intermediate T1 signal mass with foci of low signal which represent bands of collagen. The mass expands the muscle and extends across the midline, but does not involve the contralateral rectus muscle. *Arrow* points to preserved fat plane between the mass and the left rectus muscle. **b** Axial T2 WI demonstrates a predominantly high signal mass with interspersed bands of low signal; this appearance is highly characteristic of a desmoid tumor

5.4.2 Ultrasound

Ultrasound is limited in the evaluation of intra-abdominal tumors because the images are markedly degraded by adjacent mesenteric fat and air within bowel.

5.4.3 Computed Tomography

Computed tomography is the imaging modality of choice for intra-abdominal desmoids (especially mesenteric and omental), both primarily and for follow-up [25, 36]. While MR images are frequently degraded by bowel peristalsis and respiratory motion, modern CT examinations performed with multidetector helical scans are acquired very rapidly, and thus, less susceptible to bowel and respiratory motion. In the study by Healy et al. which evaluated 22 intra-abdominal desmoid tumors, CT was more sensitive and specific than MRI for tumor detection, better able to determine the presence of bowel encasement or tethering, and more accurate for size estimation, in part related to CT's ability over MRI to distinguish tumor margins from adjacent bowel [25].

A positive oral contrast agent, such as barium or Gastrografin, is essential for CT since desmoid tumors are often in contact with bowel loops. Without an oral contrast agent, it can be extremely difficult to distinguish tumor from unopacified small bowel. The colon is less problematic since the presence of air and stool within the lumen allows easy distinction from solid masses even in the absence of oral contrast. Intravenous contrast should also be administered in patients with adequate renal function (generally a serum creatinine of less than 2.0 mg/dl) and without a

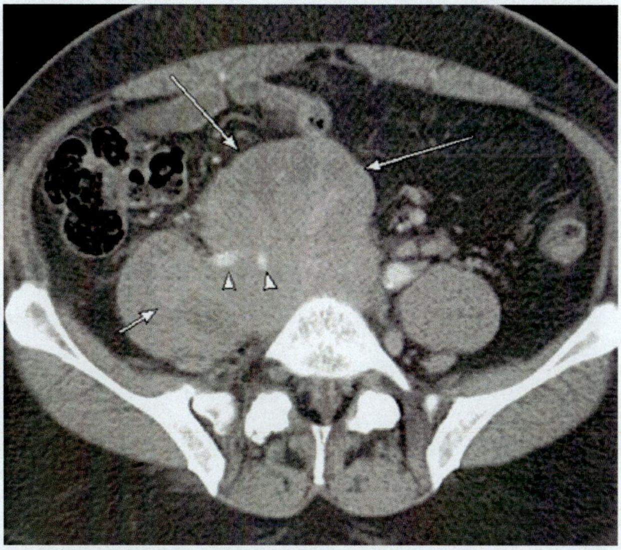

Fig. 5.17 52-year-old male with sporadic desmoid tumor located in retroperitoneum. The mass is solitary and has well-circumscribed margins (*long arrows*). At the interface with the right psoas muscle, the margin is more difficult to discern due to the similar attenuation of tumor to muscle, but is still well-circumscribed (*short arrow*). Note encasement of the right internal and external iliac arteries (*arrowheads*) by the tumor, rendering it unresectable

history of prior allergic reaction to contrast. Patients with an allergic history can be premedicated with steroids and antihistamines before the examination.

CT depicts intra-abdominal masses that are typically 5–10 cm in greatest dimension, but tumors can be as large as 25 cm [40]. They can be solitary or multiple [23]. Desmoid tumors that arise sporadically are most often located in the retroperitoneum or pelvis (Fig. 5.17). Those that occur in association with familial adenomatous polyposis/Gardner's syndrome typically occur in the mesentery or abdominal wall, most often within the rectus sheath. Pelvic desmoid tumor, a subtype of intra-abdominal desmoids, occurs in the iliac fossa or lower pelvis [16]. In patients with familial adenomatous polyposis, there is usually evidence of prior surgery (colectomy). Mesenteric desmoid tumors can vary from well-circumscribed to completely infiltrative with bands of fibrosis radiating into the mesenteric fat to a combination of well-circumscribed and infiltrative. The infiltrative and mixed morphologies are more often associated with desmoids arising in the mesentery than in the retroperitoneum or pelvis. Mesenteric tumors can also have a whorled, or coiled, appearance (Fig. 5.18) [36, 39]. Adenopathy or other evidence of metastatic disease is not seen with desmoid tumors, and an alternative diagnosis should be sought in the presence of these findings.

On noncontrast images, desmoid tumors are iso- to slightly hyperattenuating to adjacent muscle. Intra-abdominal desmoids typically enhance more than skeletal muscle, but the enhancement can be variable [16, 23, 36, 39]. They usually are relatively homogeneous throughout, but large lesions can occasionally contain focal low-attenuation areas which represent necrosis [23]. Less common causes of heterogeneity on CT include microhemorrhage, lymphocytic infiltration, calcification, cartilage formation, and osseous metaplasia.

Intra-abdominal desmoid tumors frequently involve the bowel; the mass-like forms displace or compress adjacent bowel loops, while the infiltrative forms cause

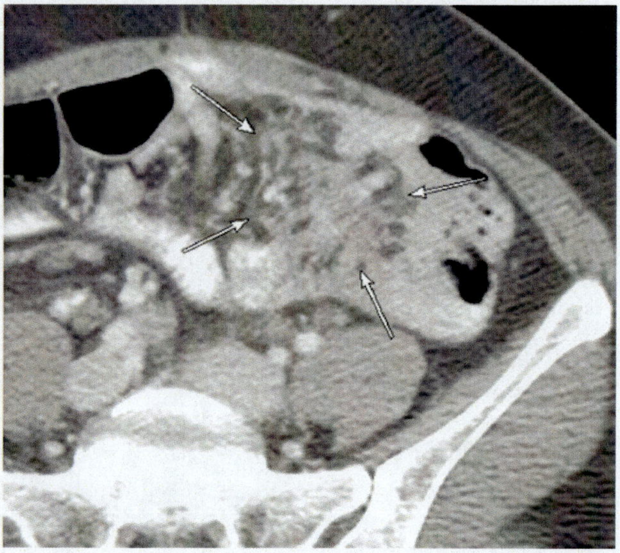

Fig. 5.18 46-year-old female with Gardner's syndrome and multifocal mesenteric desmoid tumor. Contrast-enhanced CT scan demonstrates an infiltrative desmoid tumor with multiple bands (*arrows*) radiating into the mesentery in a typical "whorled" configuration

angulation or spiculation of bowel loops (Fig. 5.19) [40]. The most common complication of bowel involvement is obstruction; less often, perforation, hemorrhage, or fistulous communication with bowel can result. Obstruction of the ureters can also occur with resultant hydroureteronephrosis (Figs. 5.20, 5.21). CT is useful for surgical planning and predicting prognosis [23]. Tumors that are large (> 10 cm), multiple, or infiltrative, and those that tether or encase small bowel loops or entrap the ureters are associated with a worse prognosis. Other findings that can be accurately assessed with CT for surgical planning include the relationship of tumor to major vascular structures, most commonly the superior mesenteric artery and vein, and involvement of adjacent organs.

5.4.4 Magnetic Resonance Imaging

MRI is preferable to CT for imaging of intra-abdominal desmoid tumors when patients are allergic to iodinated contrast or cannot receive IV contrast due to poor renal function (serum creatinine of 2.0 mg/dl or greater) or when the carcinogenic potential of radiation becomes a factor, specifically in young patients who must undergo multiple follow-up CT examinations. These issues are discussed in more detail later. Some authors argue that MRI is superior to CT in evaluating vascular involvement due to its superior soft tissue resolution and multiplanar capabilities [7]. However, this is not always the case, as the quality of MR examinations is quite variable. In addition, modern multidetector CT scanners can now produce high-quality sagittal and coronal reconstructions similar to MR.

On T1 WI, desmoid tumors are hypo- to isointense to muscle [39, 40]. Desmoid tumors have variable and often heterogeneous signal on T2 WI, but the most com-

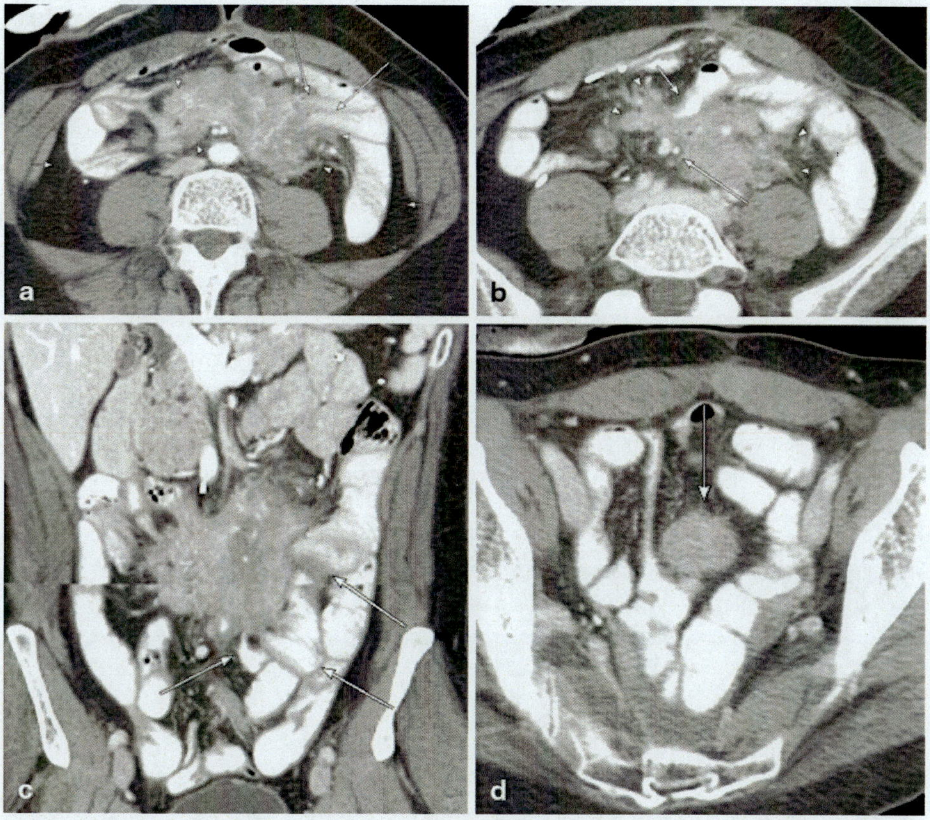

Fig. 5.19 40-year-old female with Gardner's syndrome. **a** Contrast-enhanced CT scan of abdomen and pelvis demonstrates a 9 cm mesenteric desmoid tumor with infiltrative margins and bands of fibrosis (*arrowheads*) radiating into mesenteric fat. The mass tethers adjacent small bowel loops, causing angulation and spiculation (*long arrows*). Note, absence of the ascending and descending colon from their normal locations (*short arrows*), consistent with prior total colectomy for colonic polyposis. **b** Section from same study from a slightly different location again demonstrates infiltrative margins (*arrowheads*), in addition to partial encasement of mesenteric vessels (*long arrow*) and small bowel loop (*short arrow*). **c** Coronal reformatted images of same patient again demonstrate tethering, angulation, and kinking of small bowel loops (*arrows*). **d** Images through pelvis demonstrate a separate focus of desmoid tumor (*arrow*) consistent with multifocal disease

mon appearance is that of a mass which is predominantly high in T2 signal [40]. This T2 hyperintensity reflects the high degree of cellularity which is present early in the course of the disease. As the lesion matures, the overall T2 signal intensity decreases as a consequence of increasing collagen and decreasing cellularity [39]. Some studies have shown that lesions with higher T2 signal are, statistically, more likely to grow, presumably related to the higher degree of cellularity [25]. Subsequent studies, however, have questioned this relationship by demonstrating no significant correlation between signal intensity and tumor behavior [19, 39]. These tumors typically show moderate to marked enhancement with gadolinium [39].

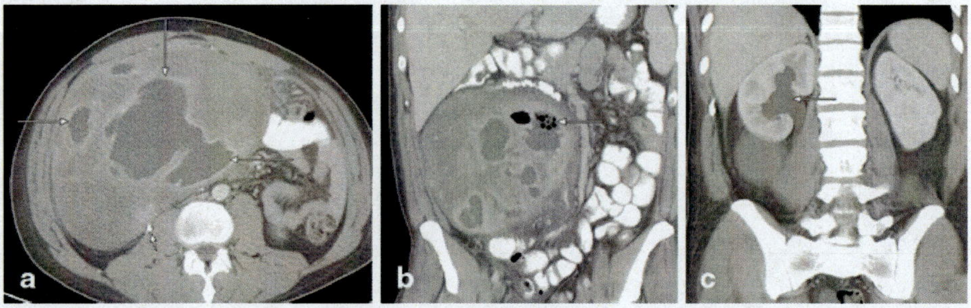

Fig. 5.20 32-year-old male with 23 cm sporadic desmoid tumor. **a** Axial contrast-enhanced CT image demonstrates large mass with several well-circumscribed areas of low attenuation (*long arrows*) consistent with necrosis. A right ureteral stent (*short arrow*) has been placed due to ureteral obstruction by the tumor. **b** Coronal reformatted image in same patient demonstrates foci of air (*arrow*) within the necrotic areas suggesting that the mass communicates with a bowel loop (*fistula*). **c** Same study showing dilated right renal collecting system (*arrow*) consistent with hydronephrosis due to ureteral obstruction

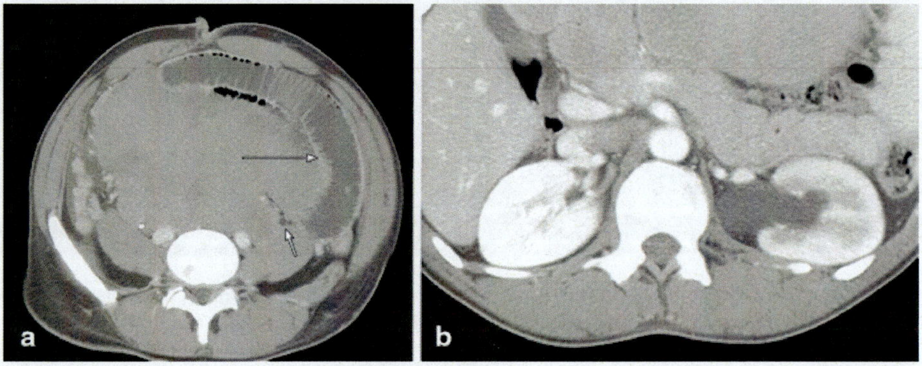

Fig. 5.21 Massive mesenteric desmoid tumor in 35-year-old male. **a** Contrast-enhanced CT demonstrates homogenous mass which encases the left ureter (*short arrow*). The image also shows a dilated loop of small bowel (*long arrow*) consistent with small bowel obstruction, also caused by the desmoid tumor. The actual site of obstruction is at a different level. **b** Same examination demonstrating left-sided hydronephrosis with a delayed nephrogram caused by obstruction of the ureter in **a**

Like their extra-abdominal counterparts, intra-abdominal desmoid tumors can also contain nonenhancing, low T1 and low T2 signal bands of dense collagen; these bands are highly characteristic of desmoid tumors (Fig. 5.22) [39].

5.4.5 Differential Diagnosis

The radiologic differential diagnosis for an intra-abdominal desmoid includes sarcoma (leiomyosarcoma, gastrointestinal stromal tumor, desmoplastic small-round-

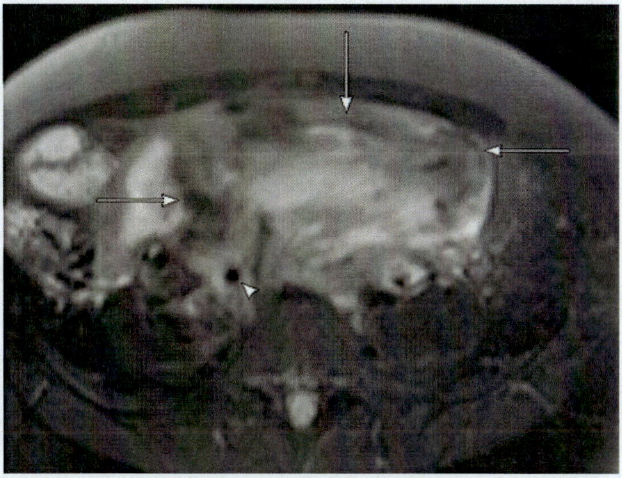

Fig. 5.22 MRI in 54-year-old male with desmoid tumor involving retroperitoneum and mesentery. Axial T2 WI demonstrates 17 cm high signal mass in midline containing multiple curvilinear bands of low T2 signal collagen (*arrows*), which are highly characteristic of desmoid tumors. Note that the mass encases the right common iliac artery (*arrowhead*)

cell tumor, and dedifferentiated liposarcoma), metastatic carcinoid, and other metastatic disease including carcinomatosis, lymphoma, schwannoma, mesenteric panniculitis, tuberculosis, and hematoma [36, 39]. Sarcomas typically appear more heterogenous than desmoid tumors on CT and MRI as a result of outstripping their blood supply with resultant necrosis, hemorrhage, and cystic change, particularly with large tumors [36]. Lymphomas can resemble desmoids with their homogenous, moderately enhancing appearance, but are usually associated with retroperitoneal or mesenteric adenopathy, and frequently, splenomegaly. Lymphadenopathy is not a feature of desmoid tumors. Further, lymphomas are also more pliable, and as a result, create less mass effect upon adjacent structures [36, 39]. The adenopathy from small bowel or appendiceal carcinoids can appear very similar to infiltrative desmoid tumor, presenting as a mesenteric soft tissue mass with bands of soft tissue radiating through the mesenteric fat with associated tethering of the bowel [39]. Unlike desmoid tumors, however, carcinoids usually present with a characteristic biochemical syndrome, often cause thickening of adjacent bowel loops and are more likely to calcify [36, 39]. Metastatic disease to the peritoneum is more likely to be multifocal and is usually associated with a history of a primary tumor (Fig. 5.23) [36].

5.5 Advantages MRI over CT

As discussed previously, MRI is the modality of choice for imaging extra-abdominal desmoid tumors, and probably abdominal wall tumors as well, because of its superior soft tissue contrast, allowing easy delineation of desmoids from background muscle and fat.

The ability to image in multiple planes has traditionally been an advantage of MRI over CT for imaging of both intra- and extra-abdominal tumors. However,

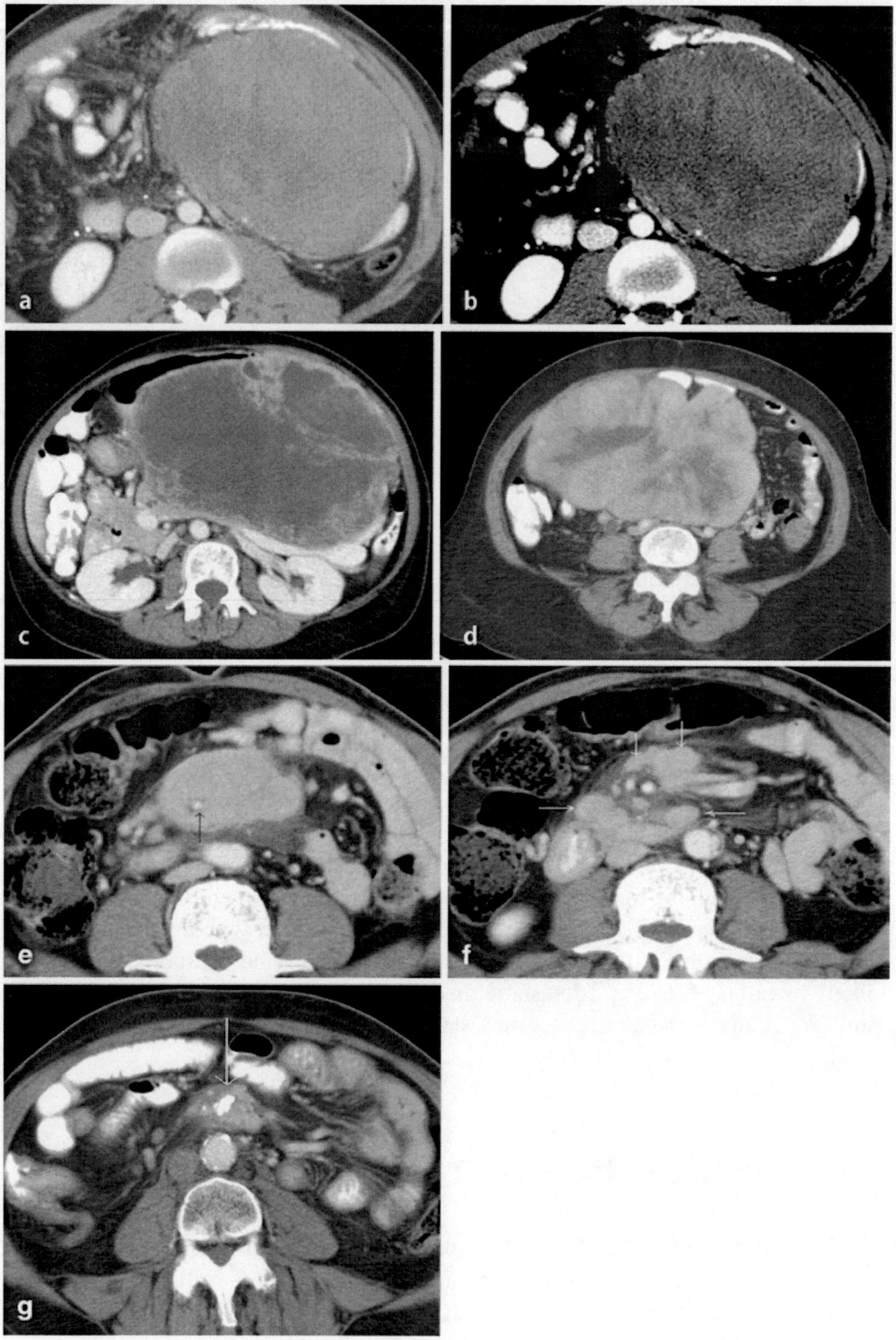

Fig. 5.23 Abdominal desmoid tumors compared with other retroperitoneal and peritoneal tumors. **a** 27-year-old male with a sporadic solitary mesenteric desmoid tumor with well-circumscribed margins. The tumor is very homogeneous and moderately enhancing, a common CT appearance

with the emergence of modern multidetector spiral scanners, high-quality sagittal and coronal reconstructions can now be created with CT as well. MRI has additional advantages over CT which favor its use even for abdominal imaging in the following situations: patients with moderate renal dysfunction or mild renal dysfunction with additional risk factors; patients with an allergic history to intravenous contrast; and patients in whom radiation dose is an important factor.

Contrast-induced nephropathy is most commonly defined as greater than 25%, or greater than 0.5 mg/dl, increase in serum creatinine level after administration of an iodinated contrast agent, most commonly for CT examinations or angiography, in the absence of an alternative cause [9, 43]. In hospitalized patients, it is the third leading cause of acute renal failure with mortality rates as high as 36% [1, 43]. In patients with serum creatinine ranging from 1.2–1.5 mg/dl and above, the risk for developing contrast-induced nephropathy increases dramatically [38, 43]. The pathogenesis appears to be the result of both a direct toxic effect on the renal tubular epithelial cells and to contrast-induced renal medullary ischemia, at least in part related to the increased osmotic load in the blood from the contrast injection in combination with other factors, including the viscosity and direct molecular toxicity of the contrast media [12]. The well-established risk factors for contrast nephropathy included preexisting renal insufficiency, especially in patients with diabetes, and the dose of IV contrast administered [18, 29, 43]. Other possible but less established risk factors include dehydration, advanced age, diabetes without preexisting renal insufficiency, renal transplantation, and multiple myeloma [29, 33, 43]. At our institution, iodinated intravenous contrast is contraindicated in patients with a serum creatinine of 2.0 mg/dl or greater. For patients with a serum creatinine between 1.4 and 1.9 mg/dl, a reduced dose of contrast can be administered (maximum dose of 100 cc of Omnipaque 300). Under special circumstances, patients with severe renal failure can receive IV contrast if they are on dialysis.

Gadolinium-based IV contrast agents (GBCAs) are much less nephrotoxic than iodinated contrast agents, and thus, can be administered in patients with mild-to-moderate renal dysfunction. This is in part due to the small volume of contrast re-

---

for abdominal desmoids. **b** Same image in **a** except with narrow windows. Some heterogeneity is now apparent within the tumor, although relatively mild given the large size of the mass. Abdominal desmoid tumors typically appear much more homogenous on CT than on MRI, probably due to the superior contrast resolution of the latter (compare with MRI in Fig. 5.22). **c** 48-year-old female with large gastrointestinal stromal tumor arising from greater curvature of stomach. Note dominant central area of necrosis, which is highly atypical of desmoid tumors, even very large ones. **d** 53-year-old female with primary leiomyosarcoma of pelvis extending into abdomen. The mass is somewhat more heterogenous on CT than a typical desmoid of this size. **e** 65-year-old male with lymphoma. Homogenous mesenteric mass encasing superior mesenteric artery (*arrow*) superficially resembling a desmoid tumor. However, on a lower section in the same exam **f**, multiple mesenteric lymph nodes (*arrows*) are associated with the dominant mass, strongly suggesting the diagnosis of lymphoma. **g** 69-year-old male with carcinoid tumor metastatic to mesenteric lymph node. The midline mesenteric mass has similarities to a desmoid tumor, including tethering of adjacent mesenteric vessels and small bowel loops. However, the presence of coarse calcifications favor the diagnosis of carcinoid tumor quired in MR imaging, resulting in a reduced osmotic load, which inflicts less stress upon the kidneys (MR is very sensitive to small concentrations of gadolinium; hence, the small volume required). Until recently, patients who could not receive iodinated contrast due to moderate-to-severe renal failure had been able to undergo contrast-enhanced MR examinations without concern for adverse affect. In recent years, however, the recognition of a disorder called nephrogenic systemic fibrosis (NSF) has resulted in new restrictions on the administration of GBCAs in patients with chronic renal insufficiency having a glomerular filtration rate (GFR) of less than 30 ml/min/1.73 m2 and in patients with acute renal insufficiency [24]. NSF is a debilitating and potentially life-threatening disorder characterized by widespread progressive fibrosis which initially affects the skin, with changes that mimic progressive systemic sclerosis. There is a predilection for peripheral extremity involvement that can subsequently involve the torso. Unlike scleroderma, however, NSF spares the face and lacks the serologic markers of scleroderma [24, 32]. Later in the course of the disease, this deposition of fibroblasts and collagen can extend beyond the skin to involve multiple organ systems, including muscle, bone, lungs, pleura, pericardium, myocardium, kidney, testes, and dura [32]. GBCAs are nontoxic when the gadolinium molecule remains in its chelated form; however, in patients with renal insufficiency, most of these agents, which are cleared by the kidneys, are not excreted from the body in a timely fashion and can destabilize over time, releasing toxic-free gadolinium into the bloodstream. It is this nonchelated form of gadolinium which is believed to incite the chain of events resulting in systemic fibrosis [28]. More recently, NSF has been shown to occur primarily in patients on dialysis, only rarely in patients with very limited renal function (GFR < 30 ml/min/1.73 m2) who are not on dialysis, and almost never in all other patients. Thus, the risk of developing NSF can be minimized in patients with renal insufficiency by avoiding the use of GBCAs in patients on dialysis, by reducing the administered dose as much as technically feasible, and by using only certain types of GBCAs (certain agents have a more stable chelation and, thus, are less likely to destabilize over time) [24, 28, 37]. For those patients who cannot receive any IV contrast agents, either iodinated or GBCAs, because of renal insufficiency, MR is usually preferred over CT, even for abdominal desmoids, because of its excellent soft tissue contrast resolution in the absence of IV contrast.

Another advantage of MRI is that allergic reactions to GBCAs are extremely rare. In one study by Li et al. which evaluated over 9,528 patients who received GBCAs, only 45 (0.48%) patients experienced contrast reactions, and a vast majority of these, 96%, were characterized as mild; only 2% of the reactions (less than 0.01% overall) were severe [35]. With the advent of low-osmolar nonionic contrast media for use with CT, angiography and other radiographic examinations, contrast reactions have decreased by 75% compared to the older high-osmolar agents; nonetheless, reaction rates for low-osmolar nonionic contrast media still remained higher than those of GBCAs (3.1% reaction rate for low-osmolar nonionic contrast, with an overall rate of 0.04% for severe reactions) [42]. In summary, patients are more likely to experience adverse reactions to IV contrast with CT than with MRI. Many patients who cannot undergo contrast-enhanced CT because of contrast allergy, can safely undergo MR examinations; the reverse is true much less frequently.

The risk of radiation exposure with repeated CT scans is another advantage of MRI over CT. Magnetic resonance imaging does not emit ionizing radiation. This can be of particular concern in patients with desmoid tumors, who are frequently young and often must undergo multiple imaging studies to monitor their condition. The typical radiation dose received by an adult during a routine CT examination of the abdomen and pelvis is 10 mSv. In comparison, the average person in the United States receives an effective dose of about 3 mSv per year from naturally occurring radioactive materials and cosmic radiation from outer space [22]. The carcinogenic effect of CT scan have been estimated by applying organ-specific cancer incidence or mortality data that were derived from studies of atomic-bomb survivors [17]. According to these data, the estimated lifetime attributable risk of death from cancer as a result of one standard abdominal CT varies from 0.14% for an infant to 0.06% for a 25-year-old, to approximately 0.01%, for a 65-year-old (children are most susceptible both because their tissues are inherently more radiosensitive and because they have more remaining years of life during which a radiation-induced cancer could develop) [17]. The exposure is cumulative in patients who have multiple CT examinations. At these doses, it is believed that each additional CT scan a patient receives during his/her lifetime results in an increased risk of cancer by incremental amounts—in other words, a linear dose response [44].

5.6 Advantages of CT over MRI

CT is the modality of choice for intra-abdominal desmoids because it is much less susceptible to motion artifact compared with MRI and because of its superior ability to distinguish tumor from adjacent bowel. With the advent of rapid multidetector helical CT scanners over the past decade, images through the entire abdomen can now be acquired within a single breath-hold, minimizing motion artifact. However, motion artifact from the bowel peristalsis remains a significant factor in abdominal MR examinations. A number of methods can be employed to minimize this MRI artifact, including the use of rapidly acquired sequences such as single-shot fast-spin echo (SSFSE) or the intravenous administration of certain drugs prior to the examination to suppress peristalsis, such as glucagon or hyoscine *N*-butylbromide (Buscopan) [41]. Abdominal wall and diaphragmatic motion due to respiration can also degrade MR images. When needed various techniques have been employed to minimize MR artifacts caused by this motion, including breath-hold imaging, respiratory-triggered imaging, breathing-averaged sequences, and very fast-gradient-echo sequences.

Abdominal desmoid tumors are readily distinguished from bowel on CT scans performed with oral contrast that is well-distributed throughout the small bowel. If the scan is acquired too early or late with respect to the ingestion of oral contrast, unopacified loops of small bowel can obscure small desmoid tumors. Distinguish-

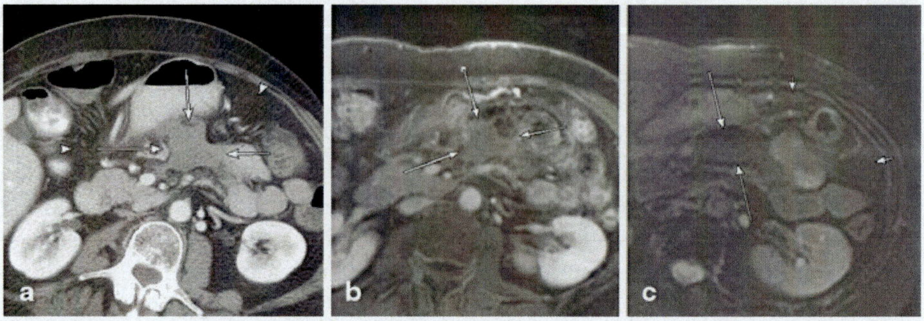

Fig. 5.24 61-year-old female with mesenteric desmoid tumor. **a** Contrast-enhanced CT demonstrates fairly well-defined mass (*arrows*) along the root of the mesentery. The lesion is easy to identify because it contrasts with the dark, low attenuation mesenteric fat (*arrowheads*). **b** Post-contrast T1 WI from MRI performed several months later. The lesion (*arrows*) is slightly less well-defined on MRI than CT. **c** T2 WI from same examination in **b**. The lesion (*long arrows*) is extremely difficult to appreciate on this sequence because it is low in signal due to the presence of abundant collagen. The low signal of the mass is nearly identical to that of the background mesenteric fat (*short arrows*), thus accounting for the lack of conspicuity

ing tumor from bowel is even more problematic with MR imaging. In addition to the motion artifact created by peristalsis, bowel that is fluid-filled is high in T2 signal, obscuring high T2 signal cellular desmoids. Bowel loops that are filled with air are low in signal on all MR sequences, potentially obscuring densely collagenous desmoids which are also low signal. These densely collagenous tumors are also hard to differentiate from mesenteric fat when fat-saturated sequences are utilized (Fig. 5.24). Desmoids that are heterogenous in signal can similarly mimic bowel that is partially filled with fluid and air. Various positive and negative oral contrast agents have been tested to improve conspicuity of abdominal tumors on MR with some promising results, although the technical feasibility of administering many of these agents discourages their routine use. Negative oral contrast agents, such as ferumoxsil, a superparamagnetic iron-based substance, cause marked signal loss within the lumen of bowel on both T1 and T2-weighted images, accentuating processes that are high in signal (such as the high T2 signal of cellular desmoids). Negative oral contrast agents also decrease the amount of noise created from bowel motion [15]. Positive oral contrast agents, including gadolinium-based formulas, are high in signal on certain sequences (gadolinium is high signal on T1 WI), accentuating tumors that are low in signal (most tumors, including desmoids, are low in T1 signal).

Another advantage of CT over MRI is that a number of implanted devices can become hazardous when exposed to the strong magnetic fields that are present within the bore of an MR machine. These powerful magnetic fields, which are as high as 3 Tesla in clinical scanners, can induce currents in the wires within devices such as pacemakers and cochlear implants, resulting in malfunction. The magnetic fields can also cause some insecure, magnetically susceptible objects to migrate within soft tissues (examples include iron-containing foreign bodies in the orbit and some older types of aneurysm clips). Strong magnetic fields can also cause burns by depositing energy in certain metallic objects [27]. To prevent these complications, many devices are now manufactured with MRI compatible materials.

Finally, patients who are claustrophobic or have severe pain may not be able to tolerate the long imaging times—which vary from one-half to one full hour—and confined spaces required for body MRI examinations. Medications, such as Valium, are occasionally successful in helping patients tolerate the exam. CT is more tolerable for these patients because it is much less constricting (shaped more like a donut rather than the long, narrow tube of a standard MR magnet) and much faster (total imaging times typically on the order of 5–10 min).

5.7 Conclusions

Desmoid tumors can appear as infiltrative or well-circumscribed masses on cross-sectional imaging that infiltrate or displace adjacent structures. Intra-abdominal tumors are best imaged with contrast-enhanced CT, which typically demonstrates a homogeneously enhancing, and less often, a heterogenous, mass in the mesentery, retroperitoneum, or pelvis. Extra-abdominal and abdominal wall desmoids are best imaged with MRI due to its superior soft tissue contrast. During the early cellular stages characterized by greatest growth, desmoid tumors are intermediate to low in T1 signal, predominantly high in T2 signal, and hypervascular on contrast-enhanced images. As they evolve, desmoid tumors become less cellular and more collagenous resulting in a shift to low T2 signal intensity and hypovascularity on postcontrast sequences. The signal characteristics on MRI can be used to monitor medical therapy, especially with targeted therapies, in which responding tumor can undergo changes in signal without concomitant changes in size. FDG-PET also has the potential to monitor responses with these targeted therapies. The decision on which imaging modality to use can also depend on various factors such as renal function, the presence of metallic devices such as pacemakers, the patient's ability to lie within confined spaces for long periods of time, and the concern for radiation exposure.

References

1. McCollough PA, Wolyn R, Rocher LL et al (1997) Acute renal failure after coronary intervention: incidence, risk factors, and relationship to mortality. Am J Med 103:368–375
2. Niwa T, Takemura Y, Inoue T et al (2008) Implant hyperthermia resonant circuit produces heat in response to MRI unit radiofrequency pulses. Br J Radiol 81:69–72. http://bjr.birjournals.org/cgi/reprint/81/961/69.pdf
3. Elsayes KM, Broski SM, Makramalla A (2010) Radiological reasoning: multiple mesenteric masses. Am J Roentgenol 194:S73–S78
4. Dinauer PA, Murphey MD, Flemming DJ, Kransdorf MJ, Fanburg-Smith JC (1998) Imaging of fibromatosis with pathologic correlation (abstr). Radiology 209:312

5. Clark SK, Neale KF, Ladgrebe JC et al (1999) Desmoid tumours complicating familial adenomatous polyposis. Br J Surg 86:1185–1189
6. Chugh R, Maki RG, Thomas DG, Reinke D, Wathen JK, Patel S et al (2006) A SARC phase II multicenter trial of imatinib mesylate (IM) in patients with aggressive fibromatosis. ASCO Meeting Abstracts 24:9515
7. Robbin MR, Murphey MD, Temple HT, Kransdorf MJ, Choi JJ (2001) Imaging of musculoskeletal fibromatosis. Radiographics 21:585–600
8. Kransdorf MJ, Murphey MD (1997) Imaging of soft tissue tumors. Philadelphia, W.B. Saunders
9. Morcos SK, Thomsen HS, Webb JAW (1999) Contrast media safety committee of the European Society of Urogenital Radiology. Contrast-media induced nephrotoxicity: a consensus report. Eur Radiol 9:1602–1613
10. Azizi L, Balu M, Belkacem A et al (2005) MRI features of mesenteric desmoid tumors in familial adenomatous polyposis. Am J Roentgenol 184:1128–1135
11. Castellazzi G, Vanel D, Le Cesne A et al (2009) Can the MRI signal of aggressive fibromatosis be used to predict its behavior? Eur Radiol 69:222–229
12. Elicker BM, Cypel YS, Weinreb JC (2006) IV contrast administration for CT: a survey of practices for the screening and prevention of contrast nephropathy. Am J Roentgenol 186:1651–1658
13. Kawashima A, Goldman SM, Fishman EK et al (1994) CT of intra-abdominal desmoid tumors: is the tumor different in patients with Gardner's disease? Am J Roentgenol 162:339–342
14. Casillas J, Sais GJ, Greve JL, Iparraguirre MC, Morillo G (1991) Imaging of intra- and extra-abdominal desmoid tumors. Radiographics 11:959–968
15. Haldemann Heusler RC, Wight E, Marincek B (1995) Oral superparamagnetic contrast agent (ferumoxsil): tolerance and efficacy in MR imaging of gynecologic diseases. J Magn Reson Imaging 5(4):385–391
16. Kransdorf MJ, Murphey MD (2006) Benign fibrous and fibrohistiocytic tumors. In: Imaging of soft tissue tumor. Philadelphia, Lippincott Williams & Wilkins, pp 189–256
17. Katayama H, Yamaguchi K, Kozuka T, Takashima T, Seez P, Matsuura K (1990) Adverse reactions to ionic and nonionic contrast media: a report from the Japanese committee on safety of contrast media. Radiology 175:621–628
18. Solomon R (2005) The role of osmolality in the incidence of contrast-induced nephropathy: a systematic review of angiographic contrast media in high risk patients. Kidney Intl 68:2256–2263
19. Sundaram M, McGuire MH, Schajowicz F (1987) Soft-tissue masses: histologic basis for decreased signal (short T2) on T2-weighted MR images. Am J Roentgenol 148:1247–1250
20. Benz MR, Tchekmedyian N, Eilber FC, Federman N, Czernin J, Tap WD (2009) Utilization of PET in the management of patients with sarcoma. Curr Opin Oncol 21(4):345–351
21. Einstein DM, Tagliabue JR, Desai RK (1991) Abdominal desmoids: CT findings in 25 patients. Am J Roentgenol 157:275–279
22. Radiation Exposure in x-ray and CT examinations (2010) Radiology Info.org. Oak, Radiology Society of North America
23. Kasper B, Dimitrakopoulou-Strauss A, Strauss LG, Hohenberger P (2010) PET in patients with aggressive fibromatosis/desmoid tumors undergoing therapy with imatinib. Eur J Nucl Mol Imaging 37:1876–1882
24. Broome DR, Girguis MS, Baron PW, Cottrell AC, Kjellin I, Kirk GA (2007) Gadodiamide-associated nephrogenic system fibrosis: why radiologists should be concerned. Am J Roentgenol 188:586–592
25. Basu S, Nair N, Banavali S (2007) Uptake characteristics of FDG in deep fibromatosis and abdominal desmoids: potential clinical role of FDG-PET in the management. Br J Radiol 80(957):750–756
26. Healy JC, Reznek RH, Clark SK et al (1997) MR appearances of desmoid tumors in familial adenomatous polyposis. Am J Roentgenol 169:465–472

27. Little MP, Wakeford R, Tawn EJ et al (2009) Risks associated with low doses and low dose rates of ionizing radiation: why linearity may be (almost) the best we can do. Radiology 251:6–12
28. Altun E, Martin DR, Wertman R et al (2009) Nephrogenic systemic fibrosis: Change in incidence following a switch in gadolinium agents and adoption of a gadolinium policy—report from two U.S. universities. Radiology 253:689–696
29. Parfey PS, Griffiths SM, Barrett BJ et al (1989) Contrast material-induced renal failure in patients with diabetes mellitus, renal insufficiency, or both: a prospective controlled study. N Engl J Med 320:143–149
30. Sheth S, Horton KM, Garland MR et al (2003) Mesenteric neoplasms: CT appearances of primary and secondary tumors and differential diagnosis. Radiographics 23:457–473
31. Murphey MD, Ruble CM, Tyszko SM, Zbojniewicz AM, Potter BK, Miettinen M (2009) Musculoskeletal fibromatoses: radiologic-pathologic correlation. Radiographics 29:2143–2183
32. McCarthy CS, Becker JA (1992) Multiple myeloma and contrast media. Radiology 183:519–521
33. Lautin EM, Freeman NJ, Shoenfeld AH et al (1991) Radiocontrast-associated renal dysfunction: incidence and risk factors. Am J Roentgenol 157:49–58
34. Kreuzberg B, Koudelova J, Ferda J, Treska V, Spidlen V, Mukensnabl P (2007) Diagnostic problems of abdominal desmoid tumors in various locations. Eur J Radiol 62:180–185
35. American College of Radiology (2008) Nephrogenic systemic fibrosis. In: Manual on contrast media, Version 6. Reston, American College of Radiology, pp 53–57
36. Vandevenne JE, De Schepper AM, De Beuckeleer L et al (1997) New concepts in understanding evolution of desmoid tumors: MR imaging of 30 lesions. Eur Radiol 7:1013–1019
37. Marckmann P, Skov L, Rossen K et al (2006) Nephrogenic systemic fibrosis: Suspected causative role of gadodiamide used for contrast-enhanced magnetic resonance imaging. J Am Soc Nephrol 17:2359–2362
38. Rihal CS, Textor SC, Grill DE et al (2002) Incidence and prognostic importance of acute renal failure after percutaneous coronary intervention. Circulation 105:2259–2264
39. Lee JC, Thomas JM, Phillips S et al (2006) Aggressive fibromatosis: MRI features with pathologic correlation. Am J Roentgenol 186:247–254
40. Basu S (2010) PET and PET/CT in gastrointestinal stromal tumours: the unanswered questions and the potential newer applications. Eur J Nucl Med Mol Imaging 37(7):1255–1258. doi:10.1007/s00259-010-1404-6 (18 Mar)
41. Froehlich JM, Daenzer M, von Weymarn C et al (2009) Aperistaltic effect of hyoscine *N*-butylbromide versus glucagon on the small bowel assessed by magnetic resonance imaging. Eur Radiol 19(6):1387–1393
42. Li A, Wong CS, Wong MK, Lee CM, Au Yeung MC (2006) Acute adverse reactions to magnetic resonance contrast media: gadolinium chelates. Br J Radiol 79:368–371
43. Brooks AP, Reznek RH, Nugent K et al (1994) CT appearances of desmoid tumours in familial adenomatous polyposis: further observations. Clin Radiol 49:601–607
44. Brenner DJ, Hall EJ (2007) Computed tomography—an increasing source of radiation exposure. N Engl J Med 357:2277–2284

Chapter 6
Surgical Management of Desmoid Tumors

Paxton V. Dickson and Raphael Pollock

Contents

Abstract Although unable to metastasize, the locally aggressive growth pattern of desmoids can result in significant morbidity for patients burdened with these tumors. Moreover, their diverse anatomic location, propensity for recurrence, and unpredictable biologic behavior present unique challenges for surgeons and other physicians involved in their management. A well-coordinated, multidisciplinary approach involving the input of surgical and nonsurgical specialists is needed to develop an individualized treatment strategy appropriate for each specific patient. When surgery is planned, appropriate imaging and preoperative biopsy is obligatory. The true impact of surgical margin negativity as well as the role of adjuvant therapies (i.e., radiation, antiinflammatory drugs, antiestrogen agents, and cytotoxic chemotherapy) in preventing tumor recurrence remains uncertain. Although radical resection to achieve negative histologic margins is the laudable objective of many oncologic surgical procedures and in some circumstances may be applicable to des-

P. V. Dickson (✉)
Department of Surgical Oncology, The University of Texas; MD Anderson Cancer Center, Houston, Texas 77030, USA
e-mail: PVDickson@mdanderson.org

C. Litchman (ed.), *Desmoid Tumors*,
DOI 10.1007/978-94-007-1685-8_6, © Springer Science+Business Media B.V. 2012

moid surgical management, excessively mutilating resections that result in significant functional impairment do not appear to be warranted in this disease.

This chapter examines the surgical management of desmoid tumors with a focus on general considerations for the surgeon as well as detailed discussions of the management of limb and limb girdle, abdominal wall and truncal, and intra-abdominal tumors.

Keywords Desmoid tumor • Fibromatoses • Surgery • Margin status

6.1 Introduction

Surgical therapy remains the cornerstone of desmoid tumor management. These tumors have a heterogeneous clinical presentation; they occur in all age groups, in a variety of anatomic locations, and in either a sporadic form or in association with familial adenomatous polyposis (FAP). Although histologically benign, desmoids are often locally aggressive with invasion of surrounding tissues which may result in disfigurement, functional impairment, pain, and occasionally mortality [1]. Moreover, the natural history of desmoids is unpredictable in that tumors may demonstrate rapid growth and progression, periods of prolonged stabilization, and occasionally spontaneous regression. Following surgical resection, there is a significant propensity for local recurrence. Several unresolved issues related to the management of desmoid tumors such as the importance of resection margin negativity on local recurrence [2], the role of nonsurgical therapies [3], and the aforementioned clinical heterogeneity present unique challenges for the surgeon. This chapter examines the surgical management of desmoid tumors with a focus on general considerations for the surgeon as well as detailed discussions of the management of limb and limb girdle, abdominal wall and truncal, and intra-abdominal tumors.

6.2 General Considerations for the Surgeon

6.2.1 Preoperative Evaluation

Prior to operating on any soft tissue mass, a preoperative history and physical examination, appropriate imaging, and in most circumstances, a biopsy should be obtained. If desmoid tumor is suspected, it is important to establish the diagnosis preoperatively as this will impact decisions regarding the timing as well as the extent of surgical resection.

An ongoing or recent pregnancy, the use of oral contraceptives, a history of familial adenomatous polyposis, or antecedent trauma to the site of the tumor are features in the patient's history that should raise the possibility of a diagnosis of desmoid in a patient presenting with a soft tissue mass. In general, cross-sectional imaging with CT or MRI should be obtained to establish the extent of tumor growth and its relation to other structures. The differential diagnosis of masses that may present in a similar fashion is broad; depending on the site, it may include a variety of soft tissue sarcomas (i.e., schwannomas, fibrosarcomas, gastrointestinal stromal tumors), intramuscular lipomas, carcinomas, inflammatory masses, or lymphoma. Because physical examination and imaging does not confirm the diagnosis of desmoid, preoperative core needle or incisional biopsy with interpretation by a specialist in soft tissue tumors is advisable. If a tissue diagnosis of desmoid is obtained, the patient should be questioned for a family history of colorectal polyps, and preoperative proctoscopy or flexible sigmoidoscopy should be considered to evaluate for the possibility of Gardner's syndrome.

6.2.2 *Individualized Multidisciplinary Approach*

It is paramount for surgeons involved in the care of patients with desmoid tumors to appreciate that optimal treatment is achieved through a patient-specific, multidisciplinary approach [4]. The varied anatomic locations, unpredictable biologic behaviors, and high rates of local recurrence prohibit adopting a standard surgical approach for desmoid tumors. In general, wide resection to achieve negative surgical margins is desired, but not at the expense of causing severe deformity or loss of function. Consideration of radiotherapy, systemic treatments, or observation is warranted in patients in whom complete surgical extirpation would be associated with major morbidity. Moreover, prior to a radical tumor resection involving the extremities or abdominal wall, consultation with the reconstructive surgery service should be obtained so that the implications of radiation as a possible component of desmoid treatment, as well as the potential need for additional surgery in the event of desmoid recurrence can be incorporated into the overall respective strategy. At the M.D. Anderson Cancer Center (MDACC), the management of desmoid patients is coordinated through deliberations at a biweekly multidisciplinary soft tissue tumor conference with input from dedicated expert surgical specialists, radiotherapists, medical oncologists, pathologists, and radiologists. In light of the rarity of these tumors, as well as the importance of providing an individualized multidisciplinary approach if local recurrence and morbidity are to be minimized, referral of patients to recognized centers of excellence is recommended prior to the initiation of any irrevocable therapeutic decisions.

6.2.3 *Margin Status*

When a decision is made to resect a desmoid tumor, an important consideration for the surgeon is the issue of resection margin status. Obtaining microscopically negative margins (R0 resection) is the preferred objective in oncologic surgery, including resection of desmoid tumors. However, the actual impact of residual microscopic disease on desmoid tumor local recurrence remains less than certain. There are few large series of greater than 100 patients that have addressed the issue of resection margin status, and all are single institution retrospective analyses.

In 1989, Posner et al reported on 131 desmoid patients treated at Memorial Sloan-Kettering Cancer Center (MSKCC) between 1965 and 1984. On multivariate analysis, it was found that tumor resection with positive or close (within millimeters) margins were at significant risk of recurrence [5]. In a study from Massachusetts General Hospital (MGH), Spear et al reported on 105 patients treated for desmoid tumor [6]. Of 51 tumors managed with surgery alone, 5-year local control rates were 50% for patients with gross residual disease, 56% for those with microscopically positive margins, and 77% when negative margins were achieved. On multivariate analysis of factors influencing local control, margin status (negative vs. positive) was statistically significant. Interestingly, in contrast to the MSKCC experience, this analysis found no difference in local recurrence when comparing widely negative surgical margins versus microscopically negative margins (< 1 mm). In an early report from MDACC, of 122 patients who underwent surgery alone for their disease, margin positivity was found to significantly correlate with local relapse; 54% in margin-positive patients versus 27% for margin-negative patients [7]. These larger reports are consistent with several smaller studies indicating that margin positivity results in a higher rate of local recurrence in desmoid tumor [8–10].

Conversely, other studies have found that microscopically positive resection margins did not affect local recurrence. Merchant et al (MSKCC) reported on 103 patients who underwent macroscopically negative resections. On final pathology, 45 patients had a positive microscopic margin, and of these, only ten patients (22%) developed local recurrence. This was not statistically different from the 14 of 58 patients (24%) of patients that had negative resection margins [11]. Similarly, the experience reported from the Instituto Nazionale Tumori in Italy found that in patients with primary desmoids, there was no difference in 5- and 10-year disease-free survival in patients with positive resection margins (79 and 74%) versus those with negative margins (82 and 77%) [12]. Finally, a contemporary report from MDACC examined patients treated from 1995–2005, showing that margin status did not significantly impact local recurrence and that disease-free survival in both margin-positive and margin-negative patients was equivalent to those with margin-negative status from the earlier study from this institution [4].

It is important to realize that each of these studies is a retrospective analysis of heterogeneous groups of patients. Most of these reports included patients with tumors at various anatomic sites, both primary and recurrent disease, and patients with sporadic, as well as FAP-associated desmoids. Furthermore, it is possible that margin positivity had a variable influence on the choice of subsequent adjuvant therapies (i.e., radiation, hormonal, or cytotoxic chemotherapy) in different centers, or even within the same center. Therefore, in considering these data for surgical planning purposes, it is important to appreciate that microscopically positive mar-

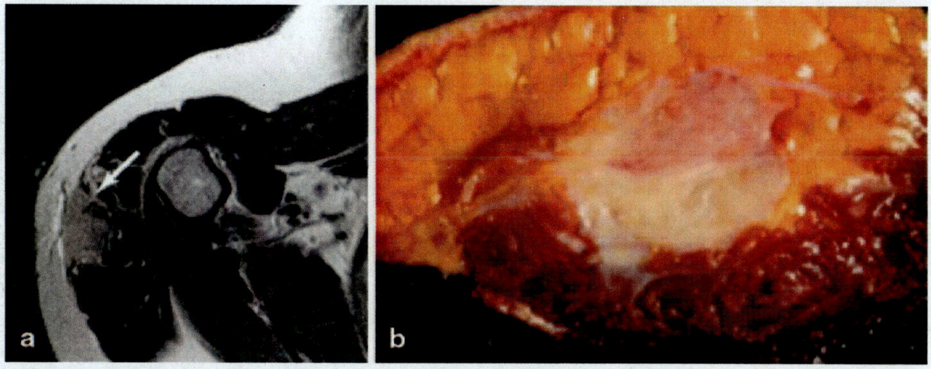

Fig. 6.1 This figure depicts a small desmoid tumor of the shoulder girdle on MRI (**a**) and ex-vivo following resection (**b**)

gins do not necessarily portend recurrence, and that mutilating or highly morbid operations to achieve negative margins are consequently not warranted in this disease.

6.3 Extra-abdominal Desmoids

6.3.1 Limb and Limb Girdle

Most reports identify the limb girdles and proximal extremities as the most common site of desmoid tumors. The locally aggressive nature of these lesions and their relationship to critical neurovascular structures in these anatomic locations present a challenge for the surgeon operating with curative intent, if attempting to adhere to the principle of preserving structure and concomitant function.

In the upper extremity and shoulder girdle, the tumors are often present in the deltoid, scapular region, supraclavicular fossa, posterior cervical triangle, axilla, and upper arm [1] (Fig. 6.1). Vital structures in this area include the brachial plexus as well as the subclavian, axillary, and brachial vessels. Tumors of this region may grow quite large in size and cause significant symptoms such as pain, swelling, and sensory-motor deficits. Reports focusing on the surgical management of shoulder girdle desmoid tumor reveal the difficulty of resection and the resultant morbidity when operating on these infiltrative tumors [13, 14].

In an early series, Enzinger and Shiraki reported on the presentation, surgical therapy, and outcome of 30 patients with desmoid tumors of the shoulder girdle [13]. In their study, all patients presented with a palpable mass: 50% of patients had pain or tenderness at presentation and 17% had impaired range of motion. The location and aggressiveness of tumors described in their series highlight the challenges faced by the surgeon. For patients with tumors centered in the supraclavicular fossa, complete resection often required sacrifice of a portion of the brachial plexus or major vessels. Axillary and chest wall tumors tended to invade local musculature and encase neurovascular bundles; two patients had tumors that penetrated the chest wall and invaded the subpleural space. The extent of surgery was reported as local excision, wide local excision, or amputation. Forty-three percent of patients were cured following their primary operation whereas 57% of patients experienced one or more recurrences. Of the 30 patients treated with surgical resection, four patients had amputations (one for primary lesion and three for recurrent disease). With a minimum of 10 years follow-up, all patients were alive and without evidence of progressive disease. In patients who presented with recurrence, the majority had simple local excision as their initial operation, prompting the authors to recommend radical surgery for these tumors. However, two patients with recurrence refused further surgery and experienced spontaneous tumor regression without any further therapy, demonstrating the unpredictable biology of these tumors.

In a more contemporary series from MSKCC, Gaposchkin et al reported on 15 patients with desmoids and low-grade fibrosarcomas involving the brachial plexus [14]. Their objective was to define the functional and oncologic outcomes in these patients using a nerve-sparing surgical approach, often knowingly leaving gross or microscopic residual disease. At presentation, nine patients were completely intact neurologically; six had neural deficits. Twelve patients underwent gross total resection at initial operation; however, 11 of these had microscopically positive margins on final pathologic analysis. Three patients had subtotal (R2) tumor resection with residual gross macroscopic tumor. Eight of the 15 patients (53%) required reoperation for recurrent disease (including the one patient with histologically negative margins). Some individuals required multiple operations, with a single patient eventually undergoing a forequarter amputation. At follow-up, 11 patients were without evidence of disease, and three had persistent but stable disease (one patient died from other causes). Importantly, in analysis of functional outcomes for these patients, only three (20%) remained neurologically intact following tumor treatment (some received adjuvant radiation), six patients had significant functional impairment of their extremity, and nine (60%) suffered from chronic pain syndromes. These results further exemplify the difficulties in predicting which patients will recur and consequently support conservative surgical approaches.

Published experiences in the management of pelvic and pelvic girdle desmoids consist mostly of anecdotal case reports or small subsets of patients contained within larger series [15–19]. Important structures such as the femoral and obturator neurovascular bundles, the sciatic nerve and gluteal vessels, as well as the pelvic viscera may be encased or compressed by tumor. Furthermore, the rigid confines of the bony pelvis can render surgical resection remarkably challenging (Fig. 6.2). A study from the Mayo Clinic describes the surgical management of desmoids of the female pelvis [19]. Although only seven patients are presented, this report emphasizes the technical issues and potential significant morbidity encountered when operating tumors in this location. Tumors ranged in size from 5–27 cm and were densely adherent to the pelvic sidewall or pelvic floor musculature. Operations generally resulted in significant blood loss (mean 2,088 ml). In addition to surgical excision of the mass, concomitant procedures included intestinal resection, vascular

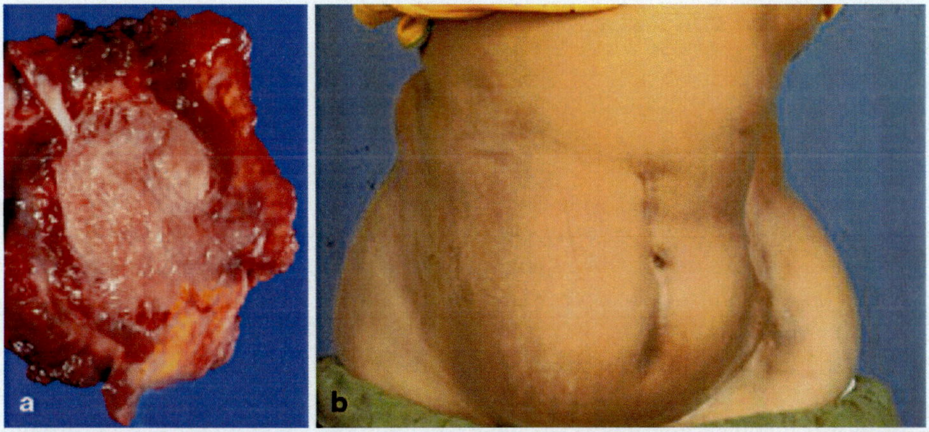

Fig. 6.2 A pelvic girdle desmoid which has eroded into the bony pelvis (**a**). Resection can result in significant deformity (**b**)

resection and reconstruction, resection of portions of the bony pelvis, and nephrectomy and partial ureterectomy. There were three recurrences in this series; as with other studies, recurrence did not correlate with margin status. It is recommended that exenterative surgery for desmoids in this location be contemplated with extreme caution, and that management be directed toward alleviating symptoms while minimizing morbidity rather than achieving R0 resection per se.

In general, desmoid tumors of the distal extremities are less common than more proximal locations, but no less challenging to manage [20–24]. Such tumors may invade or encase entire muscle groups as well as the major neurovascular bundles as they course through the epitrochlear and popliteal regions. Occasionally, these tumors will invade the axial skeleton and can result in significant pain secondary to cortical bone erosion. As with resection of other extremity soft tissue masses, an incision oriented along the long axis of the limb is critical to minimize normal tissue sacrifice with preservation of function. If a tension-free primary closure is not possible, soft tissue reconstruction utilizing skin grafting or myocutaneous flaps may be needed. Accordingly, the plastic and reconstructive surgery service should be consulted in the preoperative setting so that all options can be considered and explained to the patient. Reconstructive strategies should be planned to accommodate the tissue effects of radiation therapy, which may be integral to the management of this desmoid presentation and/or future recurrences.

In summary, limb girdle and extremity desmoids should be managed using function- and structure- preserving operations. Sacrifice of critical neurovascular structures in an effort to achieve negative margin status is not warranted. An overly aggressive surgical approach may lead to unnecessary morbidity while not significantly reducing the risk of recurrence. Amputation is only indicated in select patients who are contending with a painful, nonfunctional extremity for whom no other palliative options are feasible, especially given the occasional spontaneous regression of desmoid tumors [25, 26].

6.3.2 Head and Neck

Desmoids may also occur in the head and neck where compression of craniofacial structures and/or the airway can lead to significant morbidity and potential mortality. Other important structures in this area include cervical vertebrae, the brachial plexus, the phrenic, vagus, and spinal accessory nerves, and the carotid artery and jugular vein. Although typically presenting as a painless mass, desmoids of this region may result in symptoms such as pain and sensory or motor deficits. Management of these tumors often necessitates technically challenging operations requiring the expertise of head and neck surgeons, neurosurgeons, and plastic and reconstructive surgeons [27–29]. Moreover, careful preoperative airway assessment by anesthesiology providers is critical given the possibility of obstruction by tumor. Any historical report of hoarseness or voice change should prompt evaluation of vocal cord function using laryngoscopy or video stroboscopy. As with desmoids at other sites, the impact of margin status on tumor recurrence is questionable, with recurrences noted after either R0 or R1 resections. While margin-free (R0) resection is preferred, this should not be contemplated at the expense of vital neurovascular or aerodigestive structure sacrifice.

6.3.3 Abdominal Wall and Chest Wall Desmoids

The abdominal wall is another common location of desmoid tumors. This location includes tumors arising within the musculoaponeurotic structures that lie between the costal margins and the inguinal ligaments and iliac crest anterolaterally and the lateral borders of the paravertebral muscles posteriorly. Although tumors in this region do not typically invade or encase large neurovascular bundles in a manner reminiscent of limb girdle and extremity desmoids, they can nonetheless grow to quite large dimensions (Fig. 6.3), penetrating the peritoneum and invading underlying viscera. Surgical approaches to desmoid tumors in this anatomic locus frequently require full-thickness resection of the abdominal wall with carefully planned reconstruction [30–32].

Desmoid tumors of the abdominal wall are grossly and microscopically indistinguishable from those occurring in the extremities or limb girdles. The impact of hyperestrogenemic states on desmoid development and growth appears to be particularly applicable to lesions of the abdominal wall, although desmoids occurring in any location may be so affected. Abdominal wall desmoids occur predominantly in younger women of childbearing age either during or shortly after pregnancy [30–33]. Further supporting a possible role of estrogen-related etiology for abdominal wall desmoids, there are reports of spontaneous tumor regression in postmenopausal women with intact desmoids in this region of the body [34, 35]. Another interesting feature of abdominal wall desmoids is their association with antecedent trauma. Several reports document the development of abdominal wall desmoids at the site

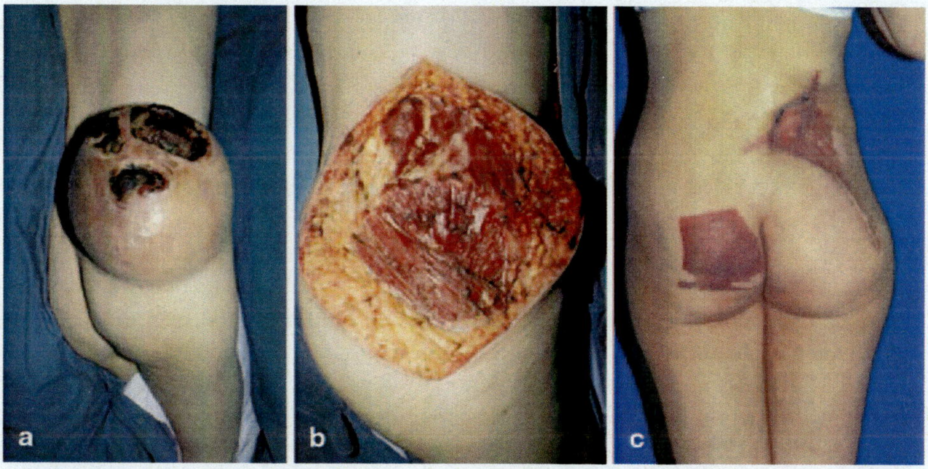

Fig. 6.3 A patient with a large desmoid of the abdominal wall (**a**), following resection (**b**), and reconstruction which utilized a split thickness skin graft for soft tissue coverage (**c**)

of surgical scars [1, 31, 36, 37]. While this is not the situation for most patients with abdominal wall desmoids, it is possible that occult or incidental injury to abdominal wall musculoaponeurotic structures may serve as the inciting event in the development of these tumors in some patients.

As with desmoids in any location, appropriate preoperative biopsy and imaging are critical to confirm the diagnosis and facilitate surgical planning. Abdominal wall desmoids are optimally imaged using cross-sectional MRI or CT to establish relative tumor size and relation to adjacent anatomic structures.

Abdominal wall desmoids are optimally managed by achieving a negative margin surgical resection using intraoperative frozen-section analysis. Attempts at enucleating or "shelling out" these tumors are not advised in that desmoids are notorious for infiltrative microscopic growth along fascial planes. In most circumstances, full-thickness excision of the abdominal wall including the tumor and a 1–2-cm margin of normal surrounding tissue is both desired and attainable. Although thin, the parietal peritoneum serves as a definitive deep margin except in situations where there is underlying visceral involvement. The surgical specimen should be oriented for pathologic evaluation by the surgeon. Because the surrounding soft tissues typically retract toward the tumor following excision, it is helpful to pin or "thumbtack" the skin and muscle of the margins to approximate the true size of the specimen, as it lies in situ. Although the impact of obtaining negative surgical margins of resection on subsequent desmoid recurrence is not unequivocally defined for all anatomic locations, a reasonable objective of negative margins greater than 1 cm for tumors of the abdominal wall can usually be achieved and may account for the lower rates of recurrence observed for such tumors [30].

Following tumor resection, abdominal wall closure is performed either primarily or more commonly with synthetic or biologic mesh in a manner similar to hernia repair. As an early example of such a strategy, in 1932, Bessesen reported the excision of an abdominal wall desmoid located in an appendectomy scar of a 41-year-old female [36]. He then used a piece of tensor fascia lata harvested from the patient's right thigh as an overlay buttress to a primary closure. Abdominal wall desmoids can grow to several centimeters in maximal dimension such that resection results in a significant acquired abdominal wall defect (Fig. 6.3). Consultation with the plastic and reconstructive surgery service is often warranted, and should be obtained in the preoperative setting to optimize surgical planning. Although abdominal wall desmoids may have a lower frequency of recurrence compared to those of the limbs and limb girdles [1, 30, 32], planning of primary tumor resection and abdominal wall reconstruction should take into account the possibility of recurrence so that the initial operation does not preclude the use of reconstructive options that might be needed in the future. Following full-thickness abdominal wall resection for a primary tumor, the most commonly used reconstruction includes a mesh closure to bridge the musculoaponeurotic defect. Because the underlying viscera are exposed, several authors have described circumferentially tacking omentum to cover the resultant defect, creating a "neoperitoneum," prior to placement of synthetic mesh such as polypropylene [30, 32, 37]. This technique is less imperative if a composite dual mesh or bioprosthetic is used, in that it is much less likely that intestine will adhere to such substrates. In situations where tumor resection results in large defects that do not permit skin and soft tissue coverage of a mesh closure, pedicled or free myocutaneous flaps may be required [38].

Desmoids may also develop on the chest wall and nearby structures [39, 40]. Abbas et al reported on the surgical management of 53 patients with desmoids of the chest wall treated at the Mayo Clinic [39]. These tumors were managed with radical excision, often involving full-thickness chest wall resection. In addition to required rib resections, associated procedures included partial resection of the skeletal boundaries of the chest (scapula, clavicle, sternum, and/or vertebrae), pulmonary wedge resections, and even forequarter amputation in conjunction with full-thickness chest wall excision. Complications included pneumonia, hemorrhage, chyle leak, wound infection, and axillary vein thrombosis. As with resection of abdominal wall desmoids, reconstruction is often performed with synthetic or biologic mesh, and myocutaneous flaps may be required for soft tissue coverage. In the Mayo series, the 5-year probability of recurrence was 37.5% and was associated with positive margins, reoperation, and postoperative radiation therapy in that patients receiving radiation were more likely to have undergone incomplete resection. This report emphasizes the potential challenges for the surgeon in managing these tumors, and the authors advocate a radical approach. Nonetheless, the unique biology of desmoids should be kept in mind; as with resection for tumors at other sites, surgical resection that results in significant functional impairment should be avoided if possible.

6.4 Intra-abdominal Desmoid

Intra-abdominal desmoid tumors primarily arise within the mesentery (Fig. 6.4), and include sporadic cases as well as those associated with Gardner's syndrome. As with desmoids in other locations, such tumors may also be seen in patients with hy-

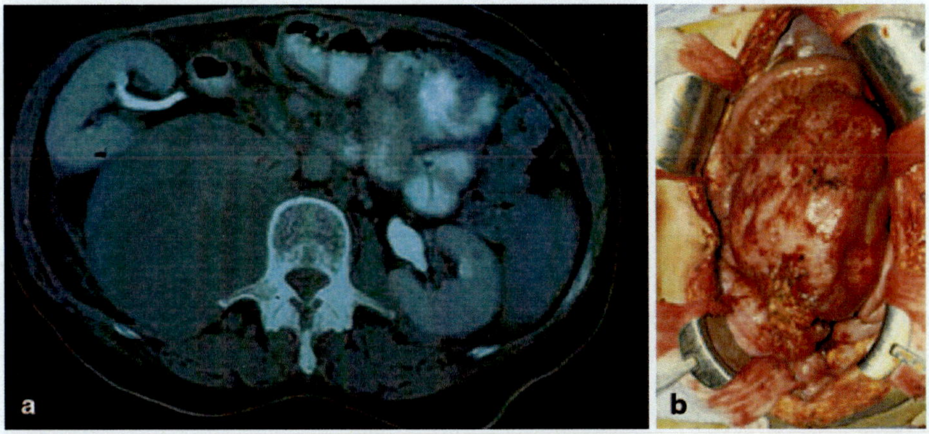

Fig. 6.4 A large intra-abdominal desmoid within the root of the mesentery as seen on CT (**a**) and at operation (**b**)

perestrogenemic states or who have undergone prior abdominal surgery [1]. These lesions most commonly involve the small bowel mesentery; however, they may also originate from the ileocolic and colonic mesentery, omentum, or other peritonealized structures. The majority of such desmoids present as a single lesion, although they can be multifocal, especially in patients with Gardner's syndrome [1, 41, 42]. Moreover, patients with Gardner's syndrome appear to have tumors that possess both a higher propensity for recurrence, as well as a tendency to synchronously or metachronously develop concomitant extra-abdominal or abdominal wall desmoids [41, 42].

Intra-abdominal desmoids may present as a painless mass or can result in significant symptoms due to invasion or compression of visceral structures. Intestinal obstruction, fistula formation, perforation, bleeding, and ischemia are well-documented sequelae of such tumors and can account for significant morbidity and occasional mortality in these patients [1, 43, 44]. Adding to management challenges, meaningful surgery for intra-abdominal desmoids often requires intestinal and/or visceral vascular resections that carry the risk of rendering a patient nutritionally crippled. Two recent series focusing on the management of intra-abdominal desmoids lend support for conservative surgical approaches to these tumors, reserving operation for patients with symptomatic disease and radiographic evidence consistent with resectability [43, 44].

In a review of the MSKCC experience, Smith et al identified 70 patients with intra-abdominal desmoid tumors in which only 24 (34%) were selected for surgical resection. Moreover, only 16 of these patients were able to undergo complete gross resection, whereas eight were demonstrated to be unresectable at the time of surgery. In those patients undergoing resection, surgical morbidity included postoperative intestinal ischemia in two patients (resulting in death in one and dependence on parenteral nutrition in the other), frequent bowel movements requiring close gastroenterology follow-up in three patients as well as one patient with chronic lower extremity edema and foot drop resulting from radical surgery for a pelvic disease component. Although most patients undergoing resection had histologically positive margins (R1), the majority (62%) had not developed recurrence as of the date of most recent follow-up. Interestingly, at 10-year follow-up, there was no difference in survival between patients with resectable and unresectable tumors, again highlighting the enigmatic and unpredictable biology of this disease. Based on these results, the authors concluded that although gross resection is frequently curative if achievable, surgery for intra-abdominal desmoids is potentially associated with significant postoperative morbidity. In patients with asymptomatic or minimally symptomatic disease, a period of "watchful waiting," with or without the addition of medical therapy clearly appears warranted.

Another recent study from the Brigham and Women's Hospital and Dana-Farber Cancer Institute evaluated the outcome of 52 consecutive mesenteric desmoid patients managed with selective use of surgery and/or chemotherapy [43]. All patients underwent CT scan with intravenous and enteral contrast to evaluate the extent of disease and facilitate classification of tumor as either localized or infiltrative. Patients were selected for surgery if resection of all gross disease with preservation of adequate intestinal length was considered feasible based on this preoperative imaging. Patients with tumors deemed to be unresectable were either observed or treated using anthracycline-based chemotherapy. Surgery was offered if subsequent imaging suggested resectability. In the aggregate, 44 patients underwent surgical therapy with a 16% perioperative morbidity rate; however, no patient was rendered parenteral nutrition-dependent and there were no surgical mortalities. Very few of these patients could be resected with histologically negative margins. Nonetheless, at time of most recent follow-up, 50 of 52 patients in this study had either no evidence of desmoids or radiographically stable disease. The encouraging results of these studies emphasize the importance of careful patient selection to balance risk of disease sequelae versus potential benefits (as well as morbidity) of surgical intervention. A general policy of astute patient assessment underlying prudently considered use of surgery versus alternatives clearly appears warranted in these patients.

6.5 Conclusions

Although they are unable to metastasize, the locally aggressive growth pattern of desmoids can result in significant morbidity for patients burdened with these tumors. Moreover, their diverse anatomic location, propensity for recurrence, and unpredictable biologic behavior present unique challenges for surgeons and other physicians involved in their management. A well-coordinated, multidisciplinary approach involving the input of surgical and nonsurgical specialists is needed to develop an individualized treatment strategy appropriate for each specific patient. When surgery is planned, appropriate imaging and preoperative biopsy is obligatory. The true impact of surgical margin negativity as well as the role of adjuvant therapies (i.e., radiation, antiinflammatory drugs, antiestrogen agents, and cytotoxic chemotherapy) in preventing tumor recurrence remains uncertain. Although radical resection to achieve negative histologic margins is the laudable objective of many oncologic surgical procedures and in some circumstances may be applicable to desmoid surgical management, excessively mutilating resections that result in significant functional impairment do not appear to be warranted in this disease.

References

1. Goldblum JR, Weiss SW (2001) Fibromatoses. In: Strauss M (ed) Enzinger and Weiss' soft tissue tumors. Mosby, St. Louis. pp 309–316
2. Melis M, Zager JS, Sondak VK (2008) Multimodality management of desmoid tumors: how important is a negative surgical margin? J Surg Oncol 98(8):594–602
3. de Bree E et al (2009) Desmoid tumors: need for an individualized approach. Expert Rev Anticancer Ther 9(4): 525–535
4. Lev D et al (2007) Optimizing treatment of desmoid tumors. J Clin Oncol 25(13):1785–1791
5. Posner MC et al (1989) The desmoid tumor. Not a benign disease. Arch Surg 124(2):191–196
6. Spear MA et al (1998) Individualizing management of aggressive fibromatoses. Int J Radiat Oncol Biol Phys 40(3):637–645
7. Ballo MT et al (1999) Desmoid tumor: prognostic factors and outcome after surgery, radiation therapy, or combined surgery and radiation therapy. J Clin Oncol 17(1):158–167
8. Dalen BP, Bergh PM, Gunterberg BU (2003) Desmoid tumors: a clinical review of 30 patients with more than 20 years' follow-up. Acta Orthop Scand 74(4):455–459
9. Faulkner LB et al (1995) Pediatric desmoid tumor: retrospective analysis of 63 cases. J Clin Oncol 13(11):2813–2818
10. Goy BW et al (1997) The role of adjuvant radiotherapy in the treatment of resectable desmoid tumors. Int J Radiat Oncol Biol Phys 39(3):659–665
11. Merchant NB et al (1999) Extremity and trunk desmoid tumors: a multifactorial analysis of outcome. Cancer 86(10):2045–2052
12. Gronchi A et al (2003) Quality of surgery and outcome in extra-abdominal aggressive fibromatosis: a series of patients surgically treated at a single institution. J Clin Oncol 21(7):1390–1397
13. Enzinger FM, Shiraki M (1967) Musculo-aponeurotic fibromatosis of the shoulder girdle (extra-abdominal desmoid). Analysis of thirty cases followed up for ten or more years. Cancer 20(7):1131–1140
14. Gaposchkin CG et al (1998) Function-sparing surgery for desmoid tumors and other low-grade fibrosarcomas involving the brachial plexus. Neurosurgery 42(6):1297–1301; discussion 1301–1303
15. Cormio G et al (1997) Fibromatosis of the female pelvis. Ann Chir Gynaecol 86(1):84–86
16. Das Gupta TK, Brasfield RD, O'Hara J (1969) Extra-abdominal desmoids: a clinicopathological study. Ann Surg 170(1):109–121
17. Fishman A, Girtanner RE, Kaplan AL (1996) Aggressive fibromatosis of the female pelvis. A case report and review of the literature. Eur J Gynaecol Oncol 17(3):208–211
18. Kirk JA (1977) Sarcoma-like benign pelvic tumors: three case reports. Am J Obstet Gynecol 128(4):393–396
19. Mariani A et al (2000) Surgical management of desmoid tumors of the female pelvis. J Am Coll Surg 191(2):175–183
20. Agrawal PS, Jagtap SM, Mitra SR (2008) Extra-abdominal desmoid tumour of the leg. Singapore Med J 49(1):e6–7
21. Chew C, Reid R, O'Dwyer PJ (2004) Evaluation of the long term outcome of patients with extremity desmoids. Eur J Surg Oncol 30(4):428–432
22. Duteille F, Dautel G, Sommelet D (1999) Desmoid tumours of the hand. J Hand Surg Br 24(5):628–630

23. Phillips SR, A'Hern R, Thomas JM (2004) Aggressive fibromatosis of the abdominal wall, limbs and limb girdles. Br J Surg 91(12):1624–1629
24. Shido Y et al (2009) Surgical treatment for local control of extremity and trunk desmoid tumors. Arch Orthop Trauma Surg 129(7):929–933
25. Bonvalot S et al (2008) Extra-abdominal primary fibromatosis: aggressive management could be avoided in a subgroup of patients. Eur J Surg Oncol 34(4):462–468
26. Lewis JJ et al (1999) The enigma of desmoid tumors. Ann Surg 229(6):866–72; discussion 872–873
27. Collins BJ, Fischer AC, Tufaro AP (2005) Desmoid tumors of the head and neck: a review. Ann Plast Surg 54(1):103–108
28. Hoos A et al (2000) Desmoid tumors of the head and neck—a clinical study of a rare entity. Head Neck 22(8):814–821
29. Zhu YX et al (2008) Treatment of desmoid tumour in head and neck. Zhonghua Er Bi Yan Hou Tou Jing Wai Ke Za Zhi 43(6):432–434
30. Bertani E et al (2009) Desmoid tumors of the anterior abdominal wall: results from a monocentric surgical experience and review of the literature. Ann Surg Oncol 16(6):1642–1649
31. Brasfield RD, Das Gupta TK (1969) Desmoid tumors of the anterior abdominal wall. Surgery 65(2):241–246
32. Pencavel T et al (2010) The surgical management of soft tissue tumours arising in the abdominal wall. Eur J Surg Oncol 36(5):489–495
33. Johner A et al (2009) Abdominal wall desmoid tumors associated with pregnancy: current concepts. Expert Rev Anticancer Ther 9(11):1675–1682
34. Reitamo JJ, Scheinin TM, Hayry P (1986) The desmoid syndrome. New aspects in the cause, pathogenesis and treatment of the desmoid tumor. Am J Surg 151(2):230–237
35. Shields CJ et al (2001) Desmoid tumours. Eur J Surg Oncol 27(8):701–706.
36. Bessesen DH (1932) Desmoid tumor of the abdominal wall. Am J Surg 16:513–514
37. Sutton RJ, Thomas JM (1999) Desmoid tumours of the anterior abdominal wall. Eur J Surg Oncol 25(4):398–400
38. Kadoch V et al (2010) Latissimus dorsi free flap for reconstruction of extensive full-thickness abdominal wall defect. A case of desmoid tumor. J Visc Surg 147(2):e45–48
39. Abbas AE et al (2004) Chest-wall desmoid tumors: results of surgical intervention. Ann Thorac Surg 78(4):1219–1223; discussion 1219–1223
40. Varghese TK Jr et al (2003) Desmoid tumor of the chest wall with pleural involvement. Ann Thorac Surg 76(3):937–939
41. Anthony T et al (1996) Desmoid tumors. J Am Coll Surg 182(4):369–377
42. Jones IT et al (1986) Desmoid tumors in familial polyposis coli. Ann Surg 204(1):94–97
43. Bertagnolli MM et al (2008) Multimodality treatment of mesenteric desmoid tumours. Eur J Cancer 44(16):2404–2410
44. Smith AJ et al (2000) Surgical management of intra-abdominal desmoid tumours. Br J Surg 87(5):608–613

Chapter 7
Systemic Therapy in the Treatment of Desmoid Tumors

Andrea Marrari and Suzanne George

Contents

Abstract Desmoid tumors respond to systemic medical therapies, from antiinflammatory drugs to standard chemotherapy agents. Liposomal doxorubicin, doxorubicin-based regimens, methotrexate in combination with vincristine, and vinorelbine have all demonstrated notable responses in this disease. Recently, molecular-targeted agents have shown antitumor activity, giving patients with desmoid tumor and their care providers multiple therapeutic options.

However, the selection of the most appropriate treatment according to disease behavior, location, and patients' characteristics remains a field of debate. Given the rarity of the disease, randomized studies in the management of desmoid tumor have never been carried out.

In this chapter we describe the systemic regimens that have demonstrated activity in desmoid tumors, along with their response rate and expected toxicity.

S. George (✉)
Department of Medical Oncology, Center for Sarcoma and Bone Oncology, Dana-Farber Cancer Institute, Boston, MA, USA
e-mail: suzanne_george@dfci.harvard.edu

C. Litchman (ed.), *Desmoid Tumors*,
DOI 10.1007/978-94-007-1685-8_7, © Springer Science+Business Media B.V. 2012

We also present an approach to the selection of a given regimen, according to the specific presentation of the disease.

Keywords Desmoid tumor • Chemotherapy • Molecular-targeted agents • Hormones • Antiinflammatory drugs

7.1 Introduction

Desmoid tumor (DT; also known as desmoid fibromatosis, desmoid-like fibromatosis, or fibromatosis) is a local disease which does not metastasize [1]. Because of this, surgery has historically been regarded as the mainstay of treatment [2, 3]. Unfortunately, despite surgery, DT may recur. Reported local recurrence rates vary between 20 and 60% at five years from surgery [4–6].

In addition, some DT are not amenable to local therapy due to the location of the tumor and potential morbidity associated with a surgical approach. Although consideration of observation alone may be appropriate in some DT, in other clinical situations the tumor may be actively growing, and/or symptomatic, or threatening vital structures, thereby requiring therapy when surgery is not feasible. This, together with an increased understanding of the wide range of biologic variability of DT, has spurred further interest into exploring nonsurgical treatments for DT.

There are a number of systemic therapies which have been studied in DT. These include antiinflammatory agents, conventional chemotherapeutic agents, hormones, and molecular-targeted agents. Since DT is a rare disease, no direct comparison between drugs has ever been made, and the majority of the literature in this realm is based on small retrospective series. However, even with this limited dataset, some clear trends are evident in the literature and there are several agents which demonstrate benefit in this disease. In addition, there is notable interest in newer, targeted therapies, which may allow for additional systemic treatment options for DT.

The aim of this chapter is to summarize the current available data on systemic therapies in the management of DT.

7.2 Traditional Chemotherapy

Desmoid tumor is a slow-growing disease comprised of benign appearing tumor cells, without metastatic potential. For this reason, its sensitivity to chemotherapy has long been questioned.

However, based on a number of recent reports in the literature, the chemosensitivity of DT now has been reliably established. Anthracyclines as well as methotrexate in combination with vinca alkaloids have demonstrated significant activity in this disease.

7.2.1 Anthracyclines: Liposomal Doxorubicin and Doxorubicin-based Regimens

Doxorubicin is one of the most commonly used agents in the field of sarcoma and one of the most active drugs in DT [6–8]. Single-agent doxorubicin is fairly well tolerated. Mouth sores, asthenia, alopecia, and myelosuppression are commonly seen. Cardiac toxicity is a known concern related to anthracyclines, however the risk can be minimized by close monitoring of cumulative dose. Liposomal doxorubicin has a more favorable toxicity profile, with notably less myelosuppression, low risk of alopecia, but a more unique risk of hand foot syndrome.

The effectiveness of doxorubicin has been evaluated in several studies. Seiter et al described the use of doxorubicin in a patient affected by intrabdominal DT [9]. The patient demonstrated a reduction of more than 50% of her disease. When the maximum dose of doxorubicin was achieved, treatment was stopped. Interestingly, the patient did well for 4 years after cessation of therapy, suggesting that responses to doxorubicin can be long lasting.

Similar results have been demonstrated with liposomal doxorubicin in larger cohorts (Fig. 7.1). In a recent retrospective study of 52 patients with mesenteric DT, 10 patients were treated with liposomal doxorubicin. All patients have unresectable, progressing disease at the time of initiation of liposomal doxorubicin. In this series, 9 of 10 patients treated (90%) developed disease stabilization or regression, which lasted beyond cessation of systemic therapy [8]. Constantinidou administered liposomal doxorubicin to 12 patients affected by DT [10]. After a mean number of six cycles, 4 patients experienced a dimensional reduction of their disease while the drug prevented the further growth of DT in additional seven patients, thereby demonstrating a disease control in 11 of 12 patients treated. Moreover, all the patients experienced clinical improvements in mobility and relief of pain. Although the follow-up is relatively short, some of the responses were long lasting, and tumor control was demonstrated beyond cessation of therapy. Toxicity consisted in mild-to-moderate palmar-plantar erythema, mucositis, and fatigue. Dose reduction was necessary in six cases, but apparently it did not compromise the activity of the drug.

A small series of liposomal doxorubicin in DT in children has also been published [11]. In this series, four pediatric patients received liposomal doxorubicin for DT. Although this was a very small series, all 4 patients treated demonstrated disease control, again demonstrating activity of liposomal doxorubicin in this disease.

Since doxorubicin is a relatively well-tolerated drug, combination chemotherapy in DT has been attempted. Doxorubicin and dacarbazine have been frequently used together [12–17]. In the most recent study by Gega et al [12], seven patients with FAP (familial adenomatous polyposis)—associated mesenteric DT were treated with doxorubicin plus dacarbazine. All patients received either four or five cycles of therapy. All patients experienced disease control, similar to other series, which lasted beyond cessation of therapy. At a median follow-up of 74 months, all patients remained without disease progression. In this series, three of the seven patients experienced severe drug-related toxicities. Therefore, doxorubicin-based

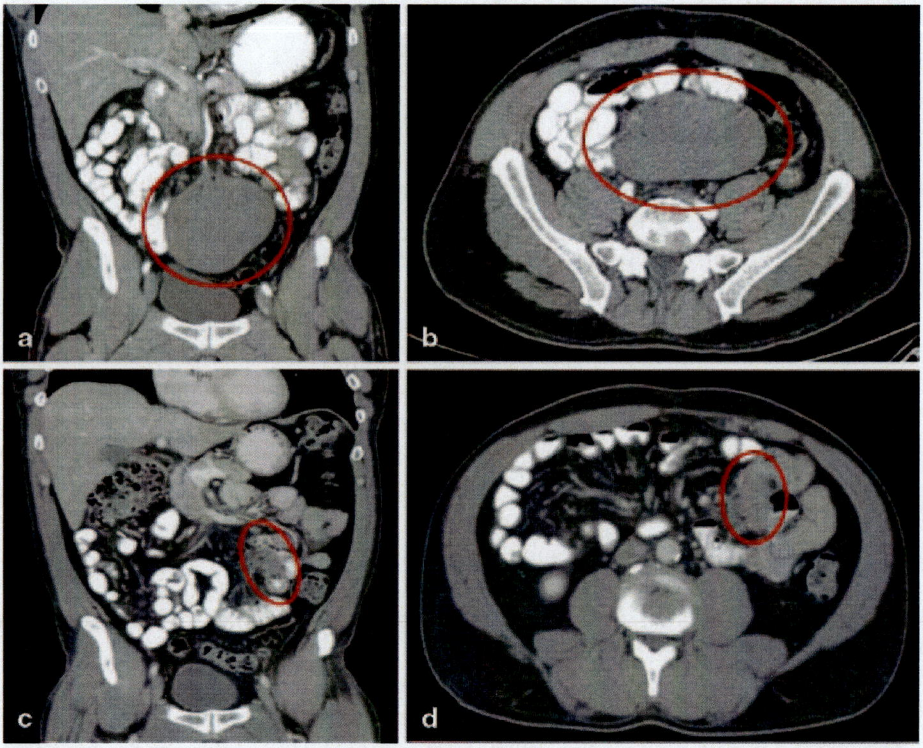

Fig. 7.1 Response to liposomal doxorubicin. CT scan before (images **a** and **b**) and after (images **c** and **d**) six cycles of liposomal doxorubicin administered as 40 mg/mq every four weeks in a 52-year-old patient with an intra-abdominal DT

therapy is highly effective in disease control in DT. Combination therapy with doxorubicin plus dacarbazine has increased toxicity when compared to single-agent liposomal doxorubicin. There have been no direct comparisons of these regimens.

Esorubicin, another doxorubicin analog, has been evaluated in a group of soft tissue and bone sarcoma [18]. Interestingly, the only responder patient was a patient with DT, achieving long-lasting partial response.

7.2.2 Methotrexate and Vinblastine/Vinorelbine

Weiss and colleagues first described the activity of methotrexate and vinblastine in DT in 1989 [19]. Methotrexate is a drug commonly used to treat neoplastic and non-neoplastic conditions while vinblastine is chemotherapeutic agent used in a variety of malignancies. Eight adult patients, suffering from DT not amenable to conservative surgical treatment, received weekly low-dose methotrexate and vinblastine.

Treatment was administered as long as responses were noted, with some patients receiving chemotherapy for up to 12 months. All patients benefited from chemotherapy with two complete responses, five partial responses, and one stable disease. Some of the responses were long lasting and continued beyond cessation of therapy.

When used at low dose, even for a long period of time, methotrexate and vinblastine are generally well tolerated. Nausea, myelosuppression, and transient hepatic toxicity were recorded. Peripheral neuropathy may be permanent. In the attempt to decrease the neurotoxicity associated with vinblastine, vinorelbine, a closely related compound characterized by a better toxicity profile, has been successfully employed, without reducing the activity of the combination [20].

These encouraging results have prompted further studies on the combination of methotrexate and vinblastine, both in the adult and in the pediatric setting. Azzarelli treated 30 patients with locally advanced primary or recurrent DT with methotrexate and vinblastine, every 7–10 days for 12 months [21]. All patients experienced clinical benefit from chemotherapy. Toxicity was reported to be mild and manageable.

A significant challenge with this regimen is patient compliance to such a long treatment plan. Nineteen patients (63%) stopped treatment within the first six months of therapy. Interestingly all the patients who received less than 20 cycles of therapy experienced a progression of their disease within a year. Conversely, only one patient who had more than 40 cycles progressed in the same timeframe, suggesting a possible correlation between the number of cycles of chemotherapy and disease control. No patients with intra-abdominal DT were enrolled in this study. However, the results of a retrospective analysis on the efficacy of this combination on 29 patients with mesenteric DT have been presented by the same group, suggesting comparable results for abdominal and nonabdominal locations [22].

Given the tolerability of the combination and the low incidence of acute and chronic toxicity, methotrexate and vinblastine has been utilized also in the pediatric population. In 1998, Skapek described 10 pediatric patients with unresectable DT [23]. Treatment duration varied between two months and almost three years. All patients responded to chemotherapy. Similar results were reported by other groups. Reich and coworkers reported on one patient who experienced the complete response of disease during methotrexate and vinblastine but subsequently developed disease recurrence 15 months after the end of treatment [24]. Methotrexate and vinblastine were restarted at the time of recurrence, and a new complete response was achieved after four weeks of treatment.

The largest pediatric experience with methotrexate and vinblastine is a multiinstitutional clinical study within the Pediatric Oncology Group enrolling 28 patients with recurrent DT or with DT not amenable of conservative surgery [25]. In this prospective phase II trial, 8 patients (31%) achieved an objective response, and an additional 10 patients experienced stable disease as best response. Eighteen patients developed disease progression after a median of 9.4 months and 8 patients remained with disease control after a median of 43 months. This implies that this combination

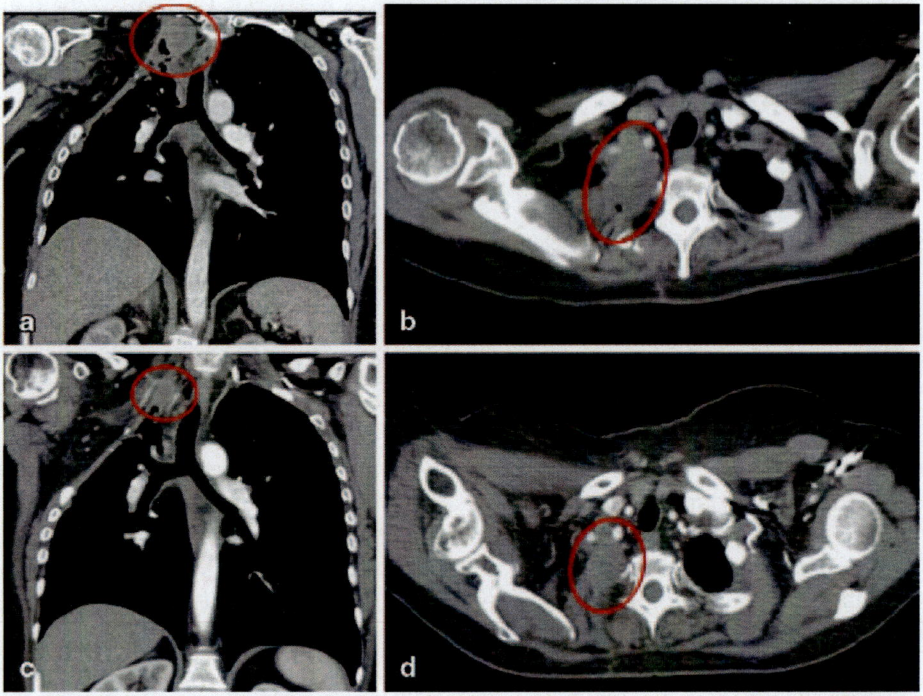

Fig. 7.2 Response to vinorelbine monotherapy. CT scan before (images **a** and **b**) and after five cycles (images **c** and **d**) of vinorelbine administered as 30 mg/mq every two weeks in a 56-year-old patient with a recurrent DT of the right apical chest wall

is effective initially in the majority of patients, and that a subset of patients may go on to experience long-term disease control.

Methotrexate and vinorelbine have also been reported to demonstrate activity as single agents in DT, although the number of patients treated is quite small [4, 5] (Fig. 7.2).

7.3 Other Therapies

Molecular-targeted agents, antiinflammatory drugs, hormonal agents, and interferons have all shown various degrees of activity in DT. However, the mechanisms through which these compounds conduct their antitumor activity are not completely understood. This accounts for the unpredictable tumor response seen in the clinical setting. The identification of predictive markers of response to these agents is one of the major challenges to be addressed in next few years. The utilization of these markers will result in minimization of unnecessary toxicity, optimization of resources, and individualization of tumor treatment based upon tumor-specific characteristics.

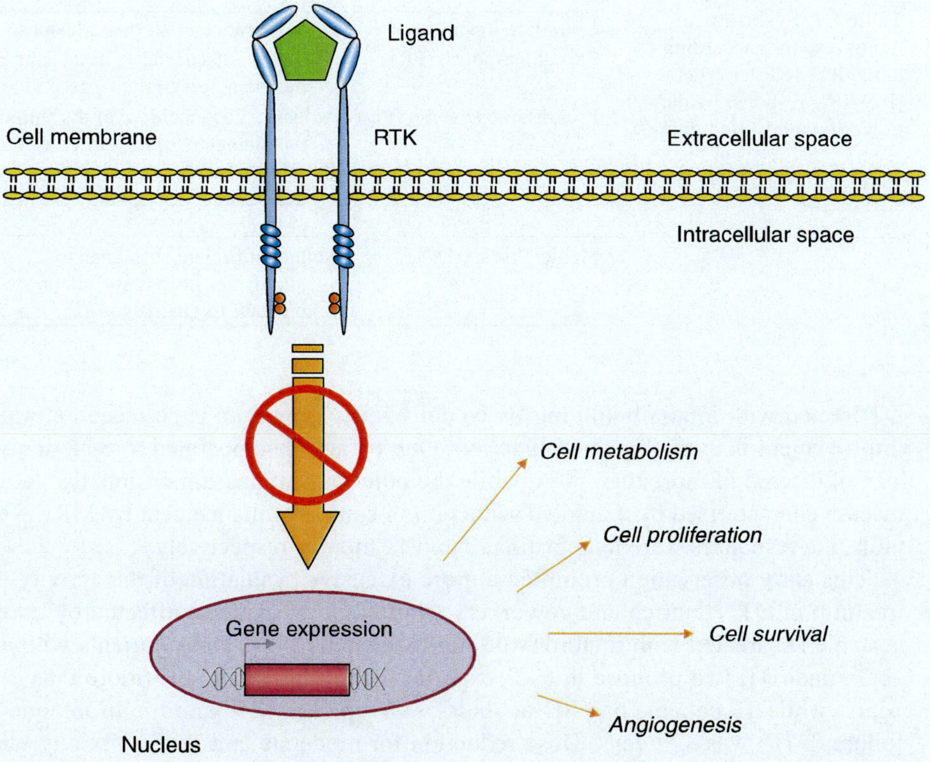

Fig. 7.3 In nonneoplastic cells, the activity of receptor tyrosine kinases (in *blue*) is tightly regulated. Following binding with their ligand (in *green*), they control cell proliferation, metabolism, motility, and survival. In tumor cells, the activity of kinases is often deregulated. This results in tumor growth. Kinase inhibitors exert their antitumor activity by blocking the receptor, thus preventing the generation of proliferative signals

7.3.1 Molecular-Targeted Agents

A tremendous advancement in understanding tumor cell biology has been made over the last decade. Kinases proved to be key regulators of cell growth, differentiation, and motility, processes that are deregulated in tumor cells. These discoveries have prompted the development of a new class of drugs, called receptor kinase inhibitors, which possess the ability to interfere with these molecules in cancer cells [26] (Fig. 7.3).

Imatinib was the first tyrosine kinase inhibitor approved in 2001 for patients with chronic myelogenous leukemia and subsequently for gastrointestinal stromal tumor [27, 28]. It inhibits a relative small number of kinases, such as KIT, PDGFR, ABL, and ARG.

The efficacy of imatinib in CML is related to its ability to inhibit signals from BCR-ABL while in GIST from c-KIT. The first report on the activity of imatinib in DT dates back to 2002. Mace and colleagues described 2 patients with unresectable

Table 7.1 Evaluation of tumor response according to the RECIST 1.1 criteria. (RECIST: response evaluation criteria in solid tumors)

Complete Response (CR)	Disappearance of all target lesions
Partial Response (PR)	At least a 30% decrease in the sum of the diameters of the target lesions
Progressive Disease (PD)	At least a 20% increase in the sum of the diameters of the target lesions The appearance of one or more new lesions denotes disease progression
Stable Disease (SD)	Neither sufficient shrinkage to qualify for PR nor sufficient increase to qualify for PD

DT treated with imatinib 400 mg twice daily [29]. They both experienced a rapid improvement in symptoms and function. One patient demonstrated a reduction in size of disease of more than 50%, while the other patient had dimensionally stable disease characterized by a marked reduction in contrast enhancement by MRI. Notably, the responses were long lasting, 9 and 11 months respectively.

This early observation prompted a more extensive evaluation of the activity of imatinib in DT. Heinrich and coworkers reported on 19 patients affected by unresectable DT treated with imatinib 400 mg twice daily [30]. Three patients with an abdominal DT, two of those in FAP, experienced a long-lasting PR (more than 1.5 years) while 13 patients had SD as their best response. Median time to treatment failure (TTF) was 325 days. Dose reduction for moderate and severe toxicity was common. Hematologic, gastrointestinal, and dermatologic toxicities were the most common, not dissimilar from those observed in CML or GIST patients on the same drug dosage.

Experiences utilizing imatinib in DT from the French Sarcoma Group [31] and the Sarcoma Alliance for Research through Collaboration (SARC) [32] have also been reported. In the former study, 40 patients with progressing DT received imatinib 400 mg daily for a median duration of treatment of 12 months (range 1–35). Dose escalation to 400 mg twice daily was allowed if the patient experienced disease progression at 400 mg daily. The primary end point of the study was the non-progressive disease rate at three months, which included RECIST defined CR, PR, and SD. According to the statistical design of the study, imatinib would have been considered effective if at least 7 out of 35 evaluable patients did not progress. After three months of therapy, 1 CR, 3 PR, 28 SD, and 3 PR were observed. The median PFS was 25 months (Table 7.1).

In the SARC study, 51 patients received a daily dose of imatinib according to their body surface area, ranging from 100 to 300 mg twice daily. The primary end point of the study was the clinical benefit rate at 16 weeks, defined as CR and PR within 16 weeks or SD lasting more than 16 weeks. After four months of therapy, the clinical benefit rate was 84%, due to 43 patients achieving SD. Unlike the study of the French Sarcoma Group, a documented progression of disease was not required for study enrollment. This is an intrinsic weakness of this study given the natural history of the disease, which is frequently characterized by long-lasting spontaneous stabilization of disease. The 3-year PFS was 58% while median PFS was not reached. Interestingly, three patients (5.9%) developed a PR after 19, 22, and 26 months of treatment.

The mechanism of action of imatinib in DT is still unclear. Imatinib is a receptor tyrosine kinase inhibitor which targets KIT and PDGFR. Contrasting results have been obtained in studies attempting to demonstrate the expression of these target kinases and to elucidate their actual involvement in the pathogenesis of the disease [29–37].

Sunitinib is a receptor tyrosine kinase inhibitor that possesses a broader spectrum of target kinases than imatinib. In addition to KIT and PDGFR, sunitinib inhibits VEGFRs and RET. Sunitinib treatment is often associated with hypertension, thyroid dysfunction, and mucocutaneous toxicity [38]. Skubitz et al recently reported a case of DT which demonstrated disease control with sunitinib following resistance to imatinib [39]. In this report, a 22-year-old woman with a multifocal, multiply recurrent DT of the left thigh treated with sunitinib experienced a dramatic radiological response, which paralleled improvements of symptoms and motility. Interestingly when imatinib was substituted for sunitinib due to tolerance, the disease progressed. Sunitinib was then reintroduced, reestablishing tumor response. No biological insights on the potential mechanism of action have been reported.

Preliminary findings on the use of sorafenib in DT appear promising. Sorafenib, which gained FDA approval for metastatic renal cell cancer and hepatocellular carcinoma, is a broad spectrum kinase inhibitor, targeting KIT, PDGF, VEGFR, RET, and RAF [40–42]. Unlike imatinib and sunitinib, it targets the MAP-kinase pathway, which is often deregulated in cancer [43]. At the 2010 American Society of Clinical Oncology Meeting, Gounder and colleagues presented their retrospective experience on 14 unresectable DT patients treated with sorafenib [44]. Patients received sorafenib 400 mg daily. All patients benefited from the drug. According to RECIST 1.1, 9 patients achieved PR and 5 SD. Desmoids located in the extremities appeared to have benefited the most from therapy than abdominal ones. Median follow-up in this report was short, 14 months, but these early data are intriguing.

7.3.2 Antiinflammatory Agents

The utility of antiinflammatory drugs in the treatment of DT was a serendipitous finding. A patient with an unresectable DT of the chest received radiation therapy, achieving a dimensional reduction in size of his disease. Unfortunately, radiation-induced pericarditis ensued and indomethacin was administered. Surprisingly, indomethacin induced the complete disappearance of the DT [45]. Although this response could have been attributed to a delayed response to radiation therapy, this unexpected response prompted further evaluation of the activity of antiinflammatory drugs in DT [46].

Several antiinflammatory agents have been studied in DT. Nishida et al administered meloxicam to 22 patients affected by sporadic DT [47]. Among 20 evaluable patients, 19 benefited from the drug. Interestingly, the immunohistochemical analysis performed on their surgical specimens revealed that COX-2 was expressed in all the samples, suggesting that it may play a role in DT development [47, 48]. Another antiinflammatory drug whose activity has been explored in DT is sulindac. Sulindac, a long-acting analog of indomethacin, has been administered to patients affected by intra-abdominal DT in the context of FAP, confirming the activity of these compounds in this population of patients [49].

Antiinflammatory drugs are generally well tolerated, though prolonged administration can precipitate gastrointestinal, cardiovascular, or renal toxicity. Therefore, close medical monitoring is needed.

7.3.3 Hormonal Therapy

The clinical observation that DT occurs predominantly in young female of childbearing age and frequently during or after pregnancy led to the hypothesis that estrogens might have a role in the pathogenesis of the disease.

Different compounds which interfere with estrogens have been tested. The most widely tested agent is tamoxifen. The first description of its activity dates back to1983 and since then many case reports or small retrospective and prospective series have been published [50–52, 46, 49]. The dose of tamoxifen varied widely among the different studies, from 20 mg to 160 mg daily. The drug is usually started at a low dose, in order to evaluate its tolerability, and then escalates if disease progression occurs. Tamoxifen is relatively well tolerated at standard doses, while at higher doses, toxicity may be a limiting factor, with hot flashes, asthenia, and joint pain.

Tamoxifen and antiinflammatory drugs have been used in combination [46, 49, 53, 54]. There has been no direct comparison between antiinflammatory drug, antiestrogen, and antiinflammatory + antiestrogen lacks. Current concensus is that combination therapy is not superior to single-agent therapy.

7.3.4 Interferon

The largest reported experience of IFN in DT comes from Leitchner and coworkers who administered interferon α (IFN-α) 3.5×10^6 IU, three times weekly [55]. Given the in vitro evidence of an antiproliferative effect of IFN-α and tretinoin, 7 patients also received 30 mg tretinoin daily. Nine patients received the treatment prophylactically to prevent local recurrence while 4 patients received the treatment to control progressive disease. After a median follow-up of 27 months, 2 PD occurred in the former group after 7 and 9 months of treatment. Both patients received IFN-α alone.

In the latter group no PD was noted after more than 30 months of combination treatment with IFN-α and tretinoin.

7.3.5 *Colchicine*

The activity of colchicine in DT is likely due to its ability to interfere with collagen production. Malagon described one patient affected by DT of the right buttock who received 3 mg colchicine daily and achieved pain relief and PR after three weeks of therapy [56]. Surgery was then performed and adjuvant colchicine was started at 1 mg/day. Two years postsurgery the patient was free from local recurrence. Other reports on the activity of colchicine in DT are scarce. Skapek reported on three patients who had previously received colchicine [23]. Two of them experienced progressive disease while the third patient interrupted colchicine because of gastrointestinal toxicity.

7.4 Conclusions

The options of surgery or observation alone have historically represented the mainstay of treatment of DT. In some clinical situations, such as when the tumor is growing and/or symptomatic or when surgery is not possible due to the anatomic location of the tumor, systemic therapy can play an important role in disease control.

Although large clinical trials are not available in DT, several small series confirm the activity of systemic therapy in this disease. Low doses of traditionally less toxic regimens, such as liposomal doxorubicin and the combination of methotrexate and vinblastine, have shown clear activity to date, with disease control achievable in most patients treated. Importantly, this disease control is often durable beyond the cessation of therapy, even in patients with documented progression at the time of systemic therapy initiation. COX-2 inhibitors and hormonal therapy also have shown evidence of disease control. In addition, more recent studies suggest activity of kinase inhibitors in DT. Clearly more study is needed to establish the relevant target, and also to identify which patients are most likely to benefit from this approach. Although many of the systemic therapies studied to date have relatively favorable toxicity profiles, DT have a wide variety of clinical behaviors and may remain quiescent for years without any therapy. Therefore, assessment of tumor location, growth rate, and local options, typically by an experienced multidisciplinary team, remains critical to identifying patients most likely to benefit from systemic therapy. In the future, improved understanding of the biology and the biologic diversity of DT will likely lead to additional systemic therapy options, and, most importantly, will lead to the identification of patients most likely to benefit from systemic therapies.

References

1. Lazar AJ, Hajibashi S, Lev D (2009) Desmoid tumor: from surgical extirpation to molecular dissection. Curr Opin Oncol 21:352
2. Casali PG, Blay JY, Aglietta M et al (2010) Soft tissue sarcomas: ESMO clinical practice guidelines for diagnosis, treatment and follow-up. Ann Oncol 21:v198
3. Demetri GD, Antonia S, Benjamin RS et al (2010) The NCCN soft tissue sarcoma clinical practice guidelines in oncology. JNCCN 8:630
4. Gronchi A, Casali PG, Mariani L et al (2003) Quality of surgery and outcome in extra-abdominal aggressive fibromatosis: a series of patients surgically treated at a single institution. J Clin Oncol 21(7):1390–1397
5. Merchant NB, Lewis JJ, Woodruff JM et al (1999) Extremity and trunk desmoid tumors: a multifactorial analysis of outcome. Cancer 86(10):2045–2052
6. Lev D, Kotilingam D, Wei C et al (2007) Optimizing treatment of desmoid tumors. J Clin Oncol 25:1785
7. De Camargo VP, Keohan ML, D'Adamo DR et al (2010) Clinical outcomes of systemic therapy for patients with deep fibromatosis (desmoid tumor). Cancer 116:2258
8. Bertagnolli MM, Morgan JA, Fletcher CD et al (2008) Multimodality treatment of mesenteric desmoid tumours. Eur J Cancer 44:2404
9. Seiter K, Kemeny N (1993) Successful treatment of a desmoid tumor with doxorubicin. Cancer 71:2242
10. Constantinidou A, Jones RL, Scurr M et al (2009) Pegylated liposomal doxorubicin, an effective, well-tolerated treatment for refractory aggressive fibromatosis. Eur J Cancer 45:2930
11. Wehl G, Rossler J, Otten JE et al (2004) Response of progressive fibromatosis to therapy with liposomal doxorubicin. Onkologie 27:552
12. Gega M, Yanagi H, Yoshikawa R et al (2006) Successful chemotherapeutic modality of doxorubicin plus dacarbazine for the treatment of desmoid tumors in association with familial adenomatous polyposis. J Clin Oncol 24:102
13. Patel SR, Evans HL, Benjamin RS (1993) Combination chemotherapy in adult desmoid tumors. Cancer 72:3244
14. Goepfert H, Cangir A, Ayala AG, Eftekhari F (1982) Chemotherapy of locally aggressive head and neck tumors in the pediatric age group. Desmoid fibromatosis and nasopharyngeal angiofibroma. Am J Surg 144:437
15. Schnitzler M, Cohen Z, Blackstein M et al (1997) Chemotherapy for desmoid tumors in association with familial adenomatous polyposis. Dis Colon Rectum 40:798
16. Okuno SH, Edmonson JH (2003) Combination chemotherapy for desmoid tumors. Cancer 97:1134
17. Lynch HT, Fitzgibbons R, Chong S et al (1994) Use of doxorubicin and dacarbazine for the management of unresectable intra-abdominal desmoid tumors in Gardner's syndrome. Dis Colon Rectum 37:260
18. Giaccone G, Donadio C, Calcinati A (1989) Phase II study of esorubicin in the treatment of patients with advanced sarcoma. Oncology 46:285
19. Weiss AJ, Lackman RD (1989) Low-dose chemotherapy of desmoid tumors. Cancer 64:1192
20. Weiss AJ, Horowitz S, Lackman RD (1999) Therapy of desmoid tumors and fibromatosis using vinorelbine. Am J Clin Oncol 22:193
21. Azzarelli A, Gronchi A, Bertulli R et al (2001) Low-dose chemotherapy with methotrexate and vinblastine for patients with advanced aggressive fibromatosis. Cancer 92:1259
22. Dileo P, Sala P, Piovesan C et al (2008) Efficacy of methotrexate + vinblastine in intra-abdominal desmoid (mesenteric aggressive fibromatosis): retrospective analysis of 29 patients from a single institution (abstract). J Clin Oncol 26:569s
23. Skapek S, Hawk BJ, Hoffer FA et al (1998) Combination chemotherapy using vinblastine and methotrexate for the treatment of progressive desmoid tumor in children. J Clin Oncol 16:3021

24. Reich S, Overberg-Schmidt US, Buhrer C et al (1999) Low-dose chemotherapy with vinblastine and methotrexate in childhood desmoid tumors. J Clin Oncol 17:1086
25. Skapek SX, Ferguson WS, Granowetter L et al (2007) Vinblastine and methotrexate for desmoid fibromatosis in children: results of a Pediatric Oncology Group Phase II Trial. J Clin Oncol 25:501
26. Krause DS, Van Etten RA (2005) Tyrosine kinases as targets for cancer therapy. N Engl J Med 353:172
27. Cohen MH, Williams G, Johnson JR et al (2002) Approval summary for imatinib mesylate capsules in the treatment of chronic myelogenous leukemia. Clin Cancer Res 8:935
28. Dagher R, Cohen M, Williams G et al (2002) Approval summary: imatinib mesylate in the treatment of metastatic and/or unresectable malignant gastrointestinal stromal tumors. Clin Cancer Res 8:3034
29. Mace J, Sybil Biermann J, Sondak V et al (2002) Response of extraabdominal desmoid tumors to therapy with imatinib mesylate. Cancer 95:2373
30. Heinrich MC, McArthur GA, Demetri GD et al (2006) Clinical and molecular studies of the effect of imatinib on advanced aggressive fibromatosis (desmoid tumor). J Clin Oncol 24:1195
31. Penel N, Le Cesne A, Bui BN et al (2010) Imatinib for progressive and recurrent aggressive fibromatosis (desmoid tumors): an FNCLCC/French Sarcoma Group phase II trial with a long-term follow-up. Ann Oncol 22(2):452–457
32. Chugh R, Wathen JK, Patel SR et al (2010) Efficacy of imatinib in aggressive fibromatosis: results of a phase II multicenter Sarcoma Alliance for Research through Collaboration (SARC) Trial. Clin Cancer Res 16:4884
33. Kurtz JE, Asmane I, Voegeli AC et al (2010) A V530I mutation in c-KIT exon 10 is associated to imatinib response in extraabdominal aggressive fibromatosis. Sarcoma 10.1155/2010/458156
34. Seinfeld J, Kleinschmidt-Demasters BK, Tayal S et al (2006) Desmoid-type fibromatoses involving the brachial plexus: treatment options and assessment of c-KIT mutational status. J Neurosurg 104:749
35. Dufresne A, Bertucci F, Penel N et al (2010) Identification of biological factors predictive of response to imatinib mesylate in aggressive fibromatosis. Br J Cancer 103:482
36. Gonçalves A, Monges G, Yang Y et al (2006) Response of a KIT-positive extra-abdominal fibromatosis to imatinib mesylate and KIT genetic analysis. J Natl Cancer Inst 98:562
37. Tamborini E, Negri T, Miselli F et al (2006) Re: response of a KIT-positive extra-abdominal fibromatosis to imatinib mesylate and KIT genetic analysis. J Natl Cancer Inst 98:1583
38. Chow LQ, Eckhardt SG (2007) Sunitinib: from rational design to clinical efficacy. J Clin Oncol 25:884
39. Skubitz KM, Manivel JC, Clohisy DR et al (2009) Response of imatinib-resistant extra-abdominal aggressive fibromatosis to sunitinib: case report and review of the literature on response to tyrosine kinase inhibitors. Cancer Chemother Pharmacol 64:635
40. Rini BI (2006) Sorafenib. Expert Opin Pharmacother 7:453
41. Llovet JM, Ricci S, Mazzaferro V et al (2008) Sorafenib in advanced hepatocellular carcinoma. N Engl J Med 359:378
42. Escudier B, Eisen T, Stadler WM et al (2007) Sorafenib in advanced clear-cell renal-cell carcinoma. N Engl J Med 356:125
43. Dhillon AS, Hagan S, Rath O et al (2007) MAP kinase signalling pathways in cancer. Oncogene 26:3279
44. Gounder MM, Antonescu C, Hameed MR et al (2010) Activity of sorafenib against desmoid tumor/deep fibromatosis (DT/DF). J Clin Oncol 28:15s (suppl; abstr 10013)
45. Waddell WR, Gerner RE (1980) Indomethacin and ascorbate inhibit desmoid tumors. J Surg Oncol 15:85
46. Klein WA, Miller HH, Anderson M, DeCosse JJ (1987) The use of indomethacin, sulindac, and tamoxifen for the treatment of desmoid tumors associated with familial polyposis. Cancer 60:2863

47. Nishida Y, Tsukushi S, Shido Y et al (2010) Successful treatment with meloxicam, a cyclo-oxygenase-2 inhibitor, of patients with extra-abdominal desmoid tumors: a pilot study. J Clin Oncol 28:107
48. Signoroni S, Frattini M, Negri T et al (2007) Cyclooxygenase-2 and platelet-derived growth factor receptors as potential targets in treating aggressive fibromatosis. Clin Cancer Res 13:5034
49. Tsukada K, Church JM, Jagelman DG et al (1992) Noncytotoxic drug therapy for intra-abdominal desmoid tumor in patients with familial adenomatous polyposis. Dis Colon Rectum 35:29
50. Kinzbrunner B, Ritter S, Domingo J, Rosenthal CJ (1983) Remission of rapidly growing desmoid tumors after tamoxifen therapy. Cancer 52:2201
51. Sportiello DJ, Hoogerland DL (1991) A recurrent pelvic desmoid tumor successfully treated with tamoxifen. Cancer 67:1443
52. Wilcken N, Tattersall MH (1991) Endocrine therapy for desmoid tumors. Cancer 68:1384
53. Hansmann A, Adolph C, Vogel T et al (2004) High-dose tamoxifen and sulindac as first-line treatment for desmoid tumors. Cancer 100:612
54. Lackner H, Urban C, Kerbl R et al (1997) Noncytotoxic drug therapy in children with unresectable desmoid tumors. Cancer 80:334
55. Leithner A, Schnack B, Katterschafka T et al (2000) Treatment of extra-abdominal desmoid tumors with interferon-alpha with or without tretinoin. J Surg Oncol 73:21
56. Dominguez-Malagon HR, Alfeiran-Ruiz A, Chavarria-Xicotencatl P et al (1992) Clinical and cellular effects of colchicine in fibromatosis. Cancer 69:2478

Chapter 8
Radiation Therapy for Desmoid Tumors

Hani O. Al-Halabi, Yen-Lin Chen, John T. Mullen, Sam S. Yoon, Francis J. Hornicek and Thomas F. DeLaney

Contents

Abstract Radiation therapy uses high-energy ionizing radiation beams to treat malignant cancers as well as a variety of benign tumors and medical conditions. James Ewing was the first to report the successful use of radiotherapy in the management of unresectable desmoid tumors in 1928 [1]. Since then several studies have shown excellent control rates with radiation, which indicate a role for radiotherapy in the multidisciplinary management of these nonmalignant tumors [2–6]. Currently, radiation can be used as the primary treatment for desmoids, as an adjunct to surgery, and as the treatment of recurrent disease.

H. O. Al-Halabi (✉)
Department of Radiation Oncology, McGill University, Montreal, Canada
e-mail: hani.elhalabi@mail.mcgill.ca

C. Litchman (ed.), *Desmoid Tumors*,
DOI 10.1007/978-94-007-1685-8_8,

Surgery has generally been the standard initial modality for treating patients with desmoid tumors, although experience is accumulating with a more conservative approach of initial observation, deferring surgery or other treatment until there is evidence of progression [7, 8]. Optimizing local control is the key element for the curative treatment of these benign tumors, given their inability to metastasize and the expectation of long-term survival for most patients. This underlies the rationale for combining surgical resection and radiotherapy with the goal of improving local control and to limit the morbidity associated with recurrence in some patients. Despite the large number of published series examining the effect of adding radiation to surgery, there is a lack of consensus on the indications for such an approach. Furthermore, due to the low incidence of desmoids, there are no randomized controlled trials comparing the effect of different treatment modalities in the management of desmoid tumors. In the absence of such high-level evidence, the application of radiation in the management of desmoids is based upon effectiveness seen in retrospective and phase II studies. In most of these studies, radiation has been used largely in patients who have recurred after initial surgery and as primary treatment in those patients who are medically inoperable or those in whom resection presents unacceptable morbidity [9–12]. However, because there are other treatment modalities available for the management of desmoids, the use of radiotherapy must be considered carefully in light of the potential long-term side effects of radiotherapy including the risk of secondary malignancy, particularly in younger patients. Table 8.1 outlines the principles of irradiating nonmalignant diseases, which applies to the use of radiation in this disease [13]. Ultimately, treatment decisions are individualized to each patient depending on a range of patient and tumor characteristics [8, 14]. In Fig. 8.1, we outline a treatment algorithm that we have found useful in managing patients with desmoid tumors.

In this chapter, we discuss separately the role of radiation in the treatment of primary and recurrent desmoid tumors. We will also review the basics of radiation treatment planning and the different radiation techniques that can be applied.

Keywords Primary radiation therapy for unresected desmoid • Radiation therapy for recurrent desmoid • Adjuvant (postoperative) radiation therapy • Neoadjuvant (preoperative) radiation therapy • Radiotherapy dose • Radiotherapy for pediatric desmoid • Radiotherapy treatment planning • Brachytherapy • Intraoperative radiotherapy • Radiation therapy toxicity • Follow-up guidelines after radiation therapy • Margin status

8.1 Introduction

Radiation therapy has been in use for the treatment of cancer for more than 100 years since the discovery of x-rays by Wilhelm Röntgen in 1895 [15]. Radiation therapy primarily works by causing damage to cellular DNA. In clinical practice worldwide, photon beam radiation is the major form of radiation used in external beam radiotherapy. These beams consist of high-energy penetrating x-rays.

Table 8.1 Principles of radiation therapy for non-malignant diseases

1	Estimate the natural history of disease without therapy
2	Consider potential consequences of not treating the patient
3	Review data about alternative therapies and their therapeutic results
4	Conduct a risk-benefit analysis in comparison to other possible measures
5	Prove that the indication is justified if conventional therapies have failed, if risks and consequences of other therapies are greater, and if nontreatment would have more dramatic consequences than irradiation for the patient
6	Consider the individual potential long-term radiogenic risks
7	Inform each patient about all relevant details of radiotherapy: volume treated, dose (dose per fraction and total dose), treatment duration, treatment efficacy, side effects, and relevant radiogenic effects
8	Obtain written consent for radiotherapy treatments from the patient following thorough patient education
9	Ensure long-term follow-up to document treatment results and manage potential toxicity
10	In case of doubt, request a competent second opinion and present for tumor board opinion

Charged particles have also been used. Traditionally these charged particles have been primarily electrons, but in recent years in some specialized centers, protons and heavier ions such as carbon ions can also be employed for external beam radiotherapy. Photon beam radiation can directly or indirectly ionize atoms that form the DNA chain. Ionization refers to the ejection of electrons from atomic orbit by the interaction of the radiation with the atom, resulting in chemically reactive ions or free radicals. Indirect ionization occurs as a result of the ionization of water which forms free radicals, notably hydroxyl radicals that damage the DNA. Damage to both DNA strands with resultant double strand breaks in the DNA that constitute a chromosome is considered to be the dominant lethal event from radiation. Cell death occurs when it attempts to divide (i.e., reproductive cell death), thus abrogating cellular growth and proliferation. Normal cells are equipped with machinery that repairs sublethal DNA damage in response to radiation, thereby allowing continued cellular growth and division. This process is less efficient in transformed cells compared to most healthy differentiated cells, resulting in higher radiation sensitivity in tumor cells. Some tumor and benign cells, such as lymphomas and lymphocytes, may undergo apoptosis or programmed cell death in response to radiation therapy. Following the administration of radiation, tumor cells may be rapidly killed (as occurs with apoptosis), may remain alive but be unable to replicate, or may die following one or several rounds of attempted replication, depending upon the radiation dose and the type of cell [16]. These effects can occur over a long period of time ranging from weeks to months, which explains the latency and variability in tumor responses to radiation seen in clinical practice.

As for any tumor treated with radiation, the dose of radiotherapy used for the treatment of desmoids should be high enough to permanently eradicate all tumor cells while ideally sparing as much surrounding normal tissue as possible. In practice, the potential for normal tissue injury by radiation limits the total dose that can be delivered safely to the tumor. As a result, the recommended doses are intended to maximize the therapeutic ratio of radiation to give a high probability of tumor control with an acceptable probability of normal tissue damage. Because desmoid tumors can arise at a variety of anatomic sites with differing adjacent normal tissues which have variable radiation sensitivities, the doses employed for radiotherapy must be tailored to the individual patient. Minimizing long-term sequelae of radiotherapy is important when using radiation to treat benign tumors such as desmoids [16, 17].

External beam photon radiotherapy was historically generated using x-ray tubes and cobalt units which contained a radioactive Co^{60} source. Over the past few decades, megavoltage linear accelerators have replaced the older cobalt units in most radiotherapy clinics around the developed world. Linear accelerators are able to generate photon beams of variable energy which penetrate more efficiently without a physical radiation source. Recent advances including three-dimensional conformal treatment planning and intensity-modulated radiotherapy have allowed the delivery of high radiation doses to the target, while minimizing the dose delivered to normal structures [18–20]. This has served to improve the therapeutic ratio of radiotherapy for many cancers and benign conditions.

8.2 Management of Primary Desmoid Tumors

As a general rule, treatment of desmoid tumors is indicated in patients with progressive and symptomatic disease. Observation is a valid treatment option when the consequences of treatment (surgery or radiation) are expected to be more damaging than tumor progression [10, 3, 26, 27]. Complete surgical resection remains the mainstay of managing desmoids when medically and technically feasible. Radiotherapy is an effective alternative to surgery and can be used in the adjuvant setting under certain conditions as discussed below [4, 12]. Ideally the management of desmoid tumors should be based on a multidisciplinary approach where cases are reviewed by a multidisciplinary tumor board in order to formulate the best possible treatment plan for individual patients.

8.3 Adjuvant Radiotherapy

Despite adequate surgical resection, local failure occurs in at least 20% of patients [5]. In a review that included 780 patients from 22 series published prior to 1999, Nuyttens et al. [5] reported a local failure rate of 39% in patients treated with resection alone. Given the possible morbidity associated with recurrent disease, adjuvant radiotherapy has been administered to some patients to improve local control over surgery alone. To avoid overtreatment of patients who would not have had disease recurrence even when treated with surgery alone, the goal of many studies has been identifying risk factors that predict for local failure. Several clinical factors have been implicated, such as patient age, tumor size, disease site, extent of surgical resection and margin status, number of prior surgeries, and the association with familial adenomatous polyposis (FAP) [14]. Unfortunately, there is no unanimous agreement on the validity of these factors amongst different series and the indications for adjuvant radiation therapy are subject to interpretation of the available data.

In the absence of randomized data, it is difficult to accurately estimate the potential benefits of adjuvant treatment. As shown in Table 8.2, several studies demonstrate better control of local disease with the addition of surgery and radiotherapy. Investigators from the University of Washington reported the local control results for 54 patients who underwent surgery, of whom 35 received adjuvant radiation. The 5-year local control rate was 53% with surgery alone and 81% in patients who received combined treatment, thus advocating for a role for adjuvant radiation therapy in some patients [4]. Similarly, the results of 189 patients treated at the MD Anderson Cancer Center were reported by Ballo et al. [7] to show a 10-year actuarial relapse rate of 25% for combined treatment compared to 33% in patients treated with surgery alone. Local control outcomes were also superior for the combined modality treatment arm in the review by Nuyttens et al. [5] (75% vs. 61%).

Conversely, a number of series did not show a clear advantage to adjuvant radiation. Investigators from Milan published the outcomes of 203 patients with desmoid tumors who underwent gross total resection. Forty of these patients received adjuvant radiation therapy; there was no statistically significant benefit to the addition of radiation in terms of local control [28]. Merchant et al. [25] from Memorial Sloan-Kettering Cancer Center reported a contemporary series of 105 patients with extra-abdominal desmoid tumors treated primarily with surgical management over 15 years. There was no benefit seen in the 31 patients who received adjuvant radiation as compared to surgery alone (both local control 77%). More recently, Gluck et al. [10] reported the experience of the University of Michigan in the treatment of 95 patients treated for desmoids using surgery, radiation, or both. While the 3-year local control rate was higher in the surgery alone arm at 84.6% as compared to 69% in 28 patients treated with adjuvant radiation, this difference did not reach statistical significance. In addition, reported toxicity is higher in patients who received combined compared to single modality treatment [7]. It is likely that there is significant selection bias for which patients are chosen for radiation therapy. Nevertheless, these studies support management with definitive surgical intervention and make consideration of adjuvant radiation therapy at the time of initial treatment a less than clear decision.

8.3.1 Margin Status

The significance of margin status as an important risk factor for local recurrence following surgery remains controversial. Many studies report lower rates of relapse in patients following radical resections with negative margins compared to patients

Table 8.2 Local control rates for surgery, radiation, and combined treatment from selected series

Investigators (Reference)	Total patients	Overall local control	Surgery: patients	Surgery: local control	S+RT[a]: patients	S+RT[a]: local control	Radiation: patients	Radiation: local control	Median follow-up (years)
Milan [28]	203	73%	163	72%	40	78%	–	–	11.25
Seoul [57]	24	88.5%	–	–	–	–	–	–	5.75
Heidelberg [58]	28	73%	–	–	26	–	2	–	3.8
U Florida [11]	65	83%	–	–	65	83%	–	–	6
Denmark [38]	72	73%	44	69%	28	78%	–	–	8
U Wash [4]	54	72%	19	53%	35	81%	–	–	3.25
MSKCC[b] [25]‖ (intraabd)	24	73%	24	73%	–	–	–	–	5.17
MSKCC[b] [25] (extraabd)	105	75%[b]	74	77%[b]	31	77%[b]	–	–	4.08
MGH [27]	107	74%	51	69%	41	72%	15	93%	5
MDACC[c] [2]	75	78%	–	–	52	82%	23	69%	7.5
MDACC[c] [7] (with Surgery)	189	70%	122	66%	46	80%	21	76%	9.5
Germany [12]	345	–	–	–	262	79.6%	83	81.4%	3.58
RCN[d] [9]	106	73%	38	84%[d]	68	95%[d]	–	–	6
MDACC[c] [3]	115	74%[e]	–	–	74	80%[e]	41	68%[e]	10.1
U Michigan[f] [10]	95	–	54	84.6%[f]	28	69%[f]	14	92.3%[f]	3.16

Results for 5 years unless otherwise indicated

[a] S+RT: surgery and radiation

[b] Memorial Sloan-Kettering Cancer Center; data presented are local recurrence-free survival, all patients reported at 5 years

[c] MD Anderson Cancer Center

[d] Rare Cancer Network, data presented are progression-free survival

[e] Long-term data reported at 10 years

[f] University of Michigan, data reported at 3 years

with microscopic or macroscopic disease after surgery. In a recent abstract, Singh et al. [29] reported an update of data from the University of California on 137 patients treated with surgery, showing a significant increase in local failure in the presence of positive margins (31%) compared to negative margins (11%). The compiled results of Nuyttens et al. [5] showed that despite improved local control rates with combined modality therapy, patients with positive margins had higher recurrence rates. The local control was 72% versus 41% with surgery alone and 94% versus 75% with surgery plus radiation for patients with negative or positive margins, respectively. The updated experience from Massachusetts General Hospital (MGH) reported by Spear et al. [27] had similar findings regarding margin status in 107 patients with desmoid tumors and revealed an improvement in local control rates with the addition of radiation to surgery. At 5 years, local control rates for the surgery alone and surgery plus radiation groups were 50% and 59% for gross residual disease, 56% and 78% for microscopically positive margins, and 77% and 100% for true negative margins. The importance of surgical margin was also emphasized in the MD Anderson series reported by Ballo et al. [7] where margin status was the single most significant factor to predict recurrence in multivariate analysis for patients treated with surgery. However, other reports, such as the one from Milan and Memorial Sloan-Kettering failed to show an increased risk of recurrence in association with positive margin [24, 28, 25].

It is important to recognize that the difference in results reported may be the result of several factors including the retrospective nature of the series, the low statistical power associated with the small sample size in most series, as well as potential differences in margin assessment and positive margin definitions between the different series. The adverse effects of positive margins may also have been offset by the fact that a large number of patients with positive margins historically received adjuvant radiation.

Collectively, these reports reaffirm a potential role for adjuvant radiation in cases where complete surgical resection is not feasible. As such, radical disfiguring surgery with potential functional loss should be avoided and replaced with more conservative surgery followed by adjuvant radiotherapy. These data are generally interpreted as not supportive of the use of radiation in the adjuvant setting after gross total resections with negative pathologic margins (R0 resections). For microscopic residual disease (R1 resections), conservative approach with deferral of adjuvant radiation is generally advised for patients' margins as long as local progression, if it occurred, would not risk significant morbidity. It should be noted that even in those series that did show a higher rate of recurrence in patients with positive margins in the absence of radiation, recurrence is not inevitable in these patients and is no greater than 50% in many series [26, 5, 27, 30]. Management with observation alone allows at least half of these patients to be spared the potential risks of radiation therapy such as secondary malignancies, which is of concern, particularly in younger patients who make up the majority of patients with desmoid tumors. Adjuvant radiotherapy following subtotal resection of desmoids is more reasonable and is indicated at our center and many others [7, 4, 12, 5]. For patients in whom subtotal resection is anticipated, it may be preferable to avoid surgery and proceed with observation or medical therapy, reserving definitive radiotherapy without an attempt at subtotal excision for disease progression [10, 12].

8.3.2 Primary Versus Recurrent Disease

Many authors have reported more locally aggressive behavior in tumors previously surgically resected as compared with primary tumors. Zlotecki et al. [11] reported the outcomes of 65 patients with desmoid and showed worse 5-year local-regional control rates for recurrent tumors (75%) than for primary tumors (96%) regardless of the type of therapy they received. Similar results were obtained in the updated experience from Massachusetts General Hospital reported by Spear et al. [27]. More recently, Gluck et al. [10] reported recurrence in 9 out of 23 (39.1%) patients who had undergone prior definitive surgery as opposed to recurrence in only 10 out of 72 (13.9%) patients with primary tumors ($p=0.01$). The increased risk of recurrence associated with recurrent disease may be compounded in the presence of positive margins. The poor prognosis associated with having both risk factors was suggested by Nuyttens et al. [5] and Goy et al. [24], and radiotherapy is recommended in this situation. However, regardless of margins achieved, postoperative radiation therapy is generally recommended in older adult patients with recurrent disease if the patient has not received it previously because of the high risk of recurrence and lessened concern of the long-term sequelae of radiotherapy.

8.3.3 Other Factors

Tumor location has been associated with an increased risk of local recurrences in some series, but the results are inconsistent. Some studies suggest intra-abdominal tumors have the highest recurrence rate, followed by extremity, and then trunk/abdominal wall tumors while others suggest desmoids in the extremities have a higher rate of recurrence [7, 31, 32]. Moreover, tumors originating in the head and neck region were shown to carry a higher risk of local failure [10]. The most plausible explanation for these observations is the proximity of tumors in these areas to critical structures which limits the feasibility of obtaining adequate surgical resection with negative margins. Otherwise, it is possible that tumors within these sites have biological differences that account for more locally aggressive behavior [33]. Adjuvant radiation is indicated in the treatment of desmoids originating in these sites if the risk of morbidity associated with a recurrence is high or difficult to manage surgically. Intra-abdominal and mesenteric tumors occur more frequently in FAP/Gardner's syndrome patients. These patients are frequently not ideal radiation therapy candidates because of the often generous area that would need to be treated and the potential for significant renal, hepatic, and bowel toxicities from radiotherapy as a result of tumor proximity to these organs [34, 35]. Younger age, female sex, and tumor size are other factors implicated with a higher risk of treatment failure but their significance is less pronounced [7, 9, 28, 14, 4]. Consideration should be given to their value in relation to the more pertinent risk factors, namely margin status and disease presentation.

In summary, it is possible to select a subset of patients with a higher risk of local failure following surgical resection that may benefit from adjuvant radiation. These include patients with positive margins, recurrent tumors previously treated with surgery, and tumors in unfavorable locations such as the extremities and/or the head and neck. Despite these guidelines, treatment is ultimately based on individualized assessment and decision process with considerations of potential morbidities with surgery and radiation as well as with future therapy if the tumor should recur.

8.3.4 Neoadjuvant Radiation

The use of neoadjuvant (preoperative) radiation is a novel approach in the management of desmoid tumors. The goal of preoperative radiation is improving resectability by shrinking the tumor and potentially reducing rates of local recurrence in extra-abdominal desmoids. The experience with this approach is limited to a few series. In the largest report from the Princess Margaret Hospital, 58 patients received preoperative radiation and had a local control rate of 81% after a median follow-up of 69 months. This was associated with a low risk of wound healing complications at 3.4% [36]. In two other small series from the same institution, a total of 43 patients with potentially resectable desmoid tumors received neoadjuvant doxorubicin with concurrent radiation followed by resection 4 to 8 weeks later. In the latter study, 16 of 30 patients received 1 year of postoperative therapy with high-dose tamoxifen and an NSAID. With a median follow-up of 71 and 45 months in the two studies, respectively, there were only five local recurrences (11%) [37]. While these results are promising, confirmation with larger, ideally prospective, randomized trials is needed before this approach can be considered standard.

8.4 Primary Radiotherapy

Primary radiation therapy is an appropriate treatment option for symptomatic patients with unresectable tumors, patients who are not medically fit to undergo surgery, and in those who decline surgery. Over the last decade, the use of primary radiation has been favored in the treatment of tumors to avoid functional loss where anticipated surgical morbidity is excessive [3, 4, 9, 12]. The latter is particularly true for tumors that would require amputation for adequate surgical management.

The majority of reports on the efficacy of primary radiotherapy in controlling desmoid tumors are encouraging with control rates ranging between 68 and 93% amongst different studies as shown in Table 8.2. The Patterns of Care Study conducted by the German Cooperative Group on Radiotherapy for Benign Diseases reported the largest experience on the use of radiotherapy in the treatment of desmoid tumors [12]. A total of 204 patients with primary or recurrent unresectable tumors were treated with primary radiation; after a median follow-up of 43 months, a local control rate of 81.4% was observed. The control rates for radiation alone have been equivalent or even better than results for postoperative radiation in all series that compared the two modalities [7, 10, 3–5, 27]. This suggests that for tumors that are not amenable to complete resection and thus require the administration of adjuvant radiation for optimal control, surgery could be omitted to avoid the added toxicity associated with combined modality treatment.

Successfully treated tumors regress slowly following radiation. Physicians and patients should be aware of the potential for slight lesion enlargement during radiation therapy. Complete regression occurs in up to 17% of cases and is not commonly seen earlier than 1–2 years and may require as many as 5–8 years. The lesion may regress partially and then stabilize at a smaller size over a long period of time [14, 12].

It can be concluded from these data that desmoids are radiosensitive tumors. Although radiation is an option for nonsurgical definitive therapy of desmoids, its use must be balanced against the potential for late radiation effects such as secondary malignancies, particularly in younger patients. Figure 8.1 outlines a treatment algorithm that we have found useful in managing patients with desmoid tumors using radiotherapy.

8.5 Radiotherapy for the Management of Recurrent Disease

Recurrences typically occur within the first 2 years following primary therapy and are rarely seen beyond 5 years [3, 7, 38]. Radical surgical resection with the goal of obtaining negative resection margins is one treatment option for the successful surgical salvage of recurrences. This, however, can be associated with significant surgical morbidity and should be avoided if radiation can be offered. Radiotherapy is indicated for nonresectable recurrences and in the postoperative setting if microscopically positive margins or gross residual disease remains [9, 39, 10]. The expected 5-year local control rates for recurrent lesions treated with surgery and adjuvant radiation ranges between 75 and 81% while local failure can be as high as 100% when radiation is omitted [9, 12]. Fontanesi et al. [39] reported the outcomes of 11 patients treated with postoperative radiation following resection with positive margins or gross residual disease and showed a 76% local control rate with a median follow-up of more than 6 years.

In the setting of a recurrence, radiation should be considered for patients who were not previously treated with radiotherapy. It remains unclear in this setting whether there is any difference in outcome between definitive radiation therapy to doses of 56–58 Gy versus the alternative strategy of surgery and adjuvant or neoadjuvant radiotherapy to doses of ~50 Gy. Shown in Fig. 8.2 is a patient who was

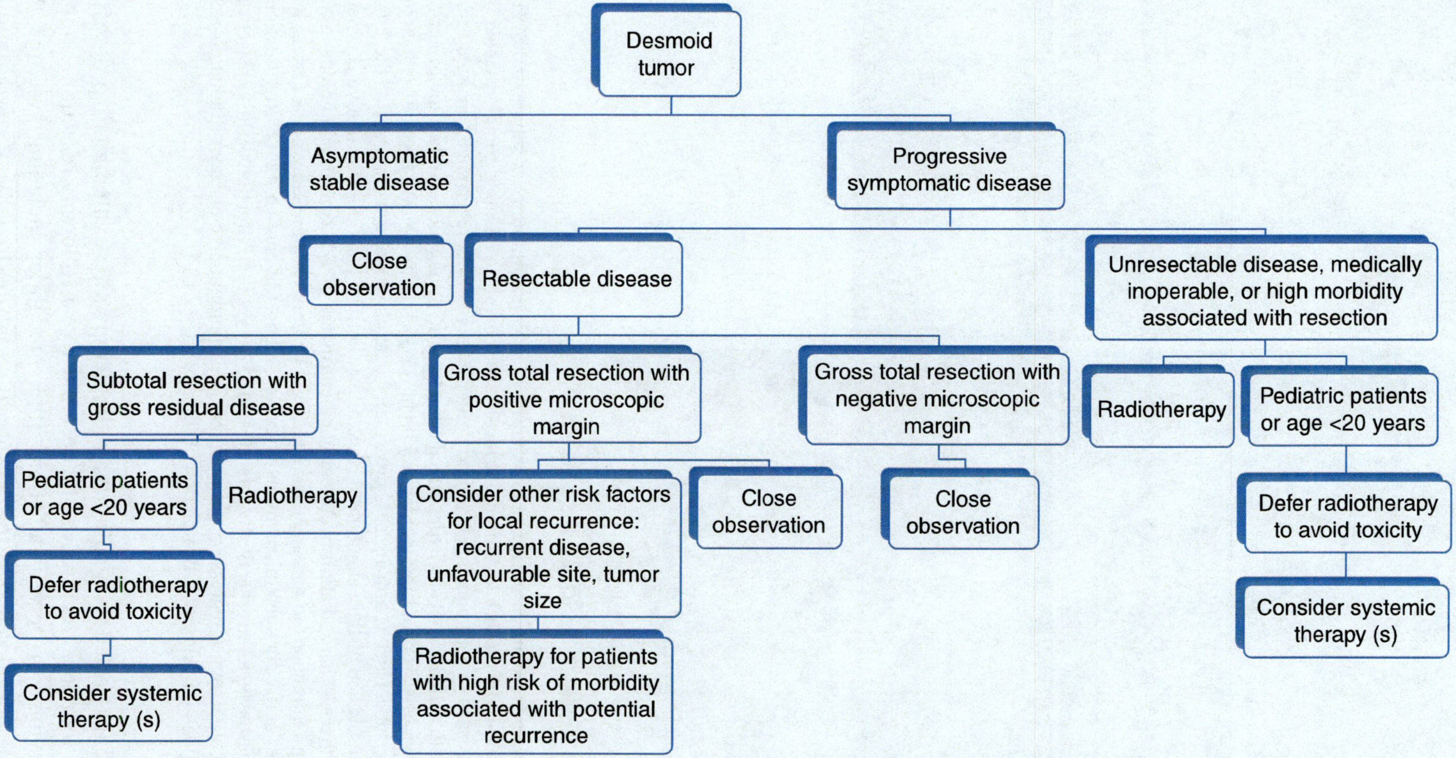

Fig. 8.1 Suggested treatment algorithm for the use of radiation therapy for the management of desmoid tumors

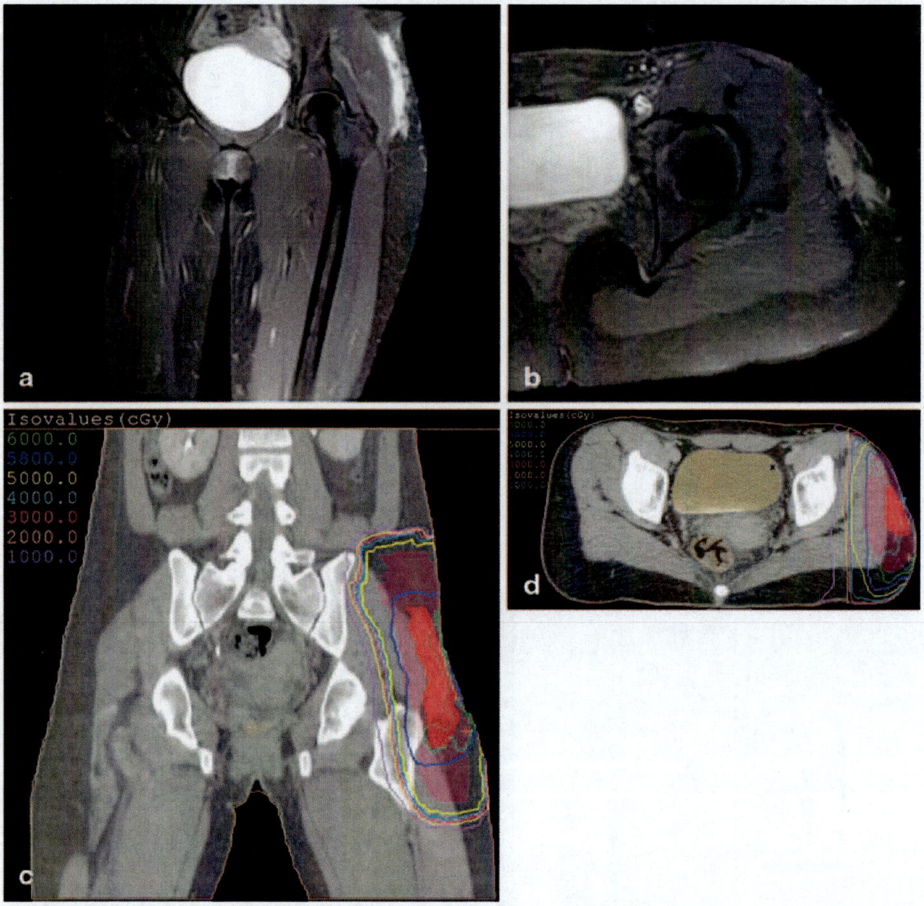

Fig. 8.2 Shown are the coronal (**a**) and axial (**b**) T1, post-gadolinium, fat-suppressed MRI images of a 24-year-old woman who suffered a local recurrence of a desmoid tumor resected one year earlier. Because of her young age, the initial management of her recurrence consisted of systemic therapy with sulindac, but she experienced symptomatic progression. At the time of her radiation therapy, her MRI showed the lobulated 3.0-cm AP × 1.2-cm TV × 9.8-cm SI enhancing mass within the subcutaneous soft tissues, proximally extending along the margin of the left gluteus medius muscle and distally along the surface of the iliotibial band. Representative coronal (**c**) and axial (**d**) slices of her radiation treatment plan, consisting of 3-D conformal photons to a dose of 50.4 Gy in 28 fractions to the larger clinical target volume encompassing gross disease and adjacent tissues at risk for subclinical involvement and a boost of another 7.2 Gy in 4 fractions to the gross disease which thus received a total dose of 57.6 Gy in 32 fractions. She experienced complete pain relief, tumor regression, and remains free of progressive disease or radiation-associated complications 1.5 years after completion of therapy

successfully treated with definitive radiotherapy after symptomatic progression on sulindac for a local recurrence of a desmoid 1 year following resection. For patients who previously received radiation, other modalities including systemic therapy should be considered first for salvage to avoid the toxicity of reirradiation. Otherwise, more focal treatment including brachytherapy can be considered to avoid exceeding normal tissue radiation tolerance.

8.6 Radiotherapy Dose

A compilation of available data in desmoid tumors suggest an optimal radiation dose between 50 and 60 Gy [7, 24, 3, 5, 33, 40, 41]. Several studies failed to elicit a significant dose–response relation with respect to improvement in local control for adjuvant and primary radiation [9, 10]. Doses between 50 and 54 Gy can be used to eradicate microscopic residual disease, whereas doses >54 Gy are recommended for gross residual disease. Doses exceeding 60 Gy are associated with increased radiation morbidity without any added benefit for local control [7]. Radiation morbidity is more pronounced in cases involving periosteal stripping, bone curettage, or where lymphatic drainage has been compromised. Radiotherapy is typically delivered in daily fractions (5 days per week) over a period of 5–7 weeks in 1.8–2 Gy per fraction. Only one study reported by the Rare Cancer Network has shown a statistically significant benefit in local control with the use of daily fractions >2 Gy [9].

Treatment failures following radiation are typically seen within the field of radiation and are more common than marginal recurrences [7, 24, 5]. As discussed above, there is no evidence to suggest that higher radiation doses would result in a different pattern of failure.

8.7 Radiotherapy for Pediatric Desmoid Tumors

Elucidating the appropriate management of pediatric desmoid tumors is limited by the small number of published data in the literature. Studies suggested that these tumors are less biologically responsive to radiation compared to their adult counterparts. Merchant et al. [42] reviewed the St. Jude Children's Hospital experience in the treatment of pediatric desmoids and reported failure in 12 out of 13 patients who received adjuvant radiation (median dose of 50 Gy) following subtotal resection. Dissimilar to the experience in adults, these results demonstrate the inability of adjuvant radiation to compensate for incomplete resection in children. In contrast, results from the University of California in San Francisco showed better outcomes for pediatric patients treated with adjuvant radiation following gross total resection with microscopically positive margins compared to surgery alone [43]. The same study reported complete tumor regression in 9 out of 13 treated with radiation alone either in the primary or salvage setting.

It is difficult to establish any conclusions from these small studies, and complete surgical resection remains the gold standard for treatment of these difficult to control tumors in children. Low doses of the chemotherapeutic agents methotrexate and vinblastine produce impressive responses, particularly in children, and probably are the next step for management of pediatric patients [44]. If recurrence or progression occurs after systemic therapy(s) and radiotherapy is considered for the treatment of recurrent or inoperable disease, pediatric patients should be considered for proton beam radiation whenever possible. Proton therapy has an important role in the treatment of pediatric cancers given its unique physical characteristics that minimize the dose of radiation delivered to normal structures beyond the target. The "integral" or total-body dose of radiation with protons is often ~60% lower than with photons and appears to be associated with a lower risk of long-term complications and potential for secondary malignancy in children. These concerns are more important in children than in adults as they are more susceptible to late radiation toxicity because of their developing tissues and expected longer period of survival time following radiotherapy [45].

8.8 Treatment Planning

Management with external beam radiotherapy involves a workflow of steps required to plan and deliver treatment. Prior to initiating the process of treatment planning, patients undergo diagnostic imaging of the tumor site in order to clearly demarcate the extent of disease and possible invasion of local structures. For patients undergoing surgery, obtaining pre- and postoperative imaging is recommended in order to observe the initial disease extension and possible residual disease which must be included in the treatment volume. Desmoid tumors form soft tissue masses that are known to infiltrate muscles, deep tissue, and extend along muscle planes. Magnetic resonance imaging (MRI) is the gold standard for imaging extra-abdominal desmoid tumors, especially lesions in the head and neck, trunk, and extremities. It allows visualization of soft tissue extension and local invasion with better resolution than computed tomography (CT scans). Bone invasion is sometimes better visualized using a CT scan. Intra-abdominal lesions are best imaged with CT scans [17].

Radiotherapy treatment planning has been revolutionized by the ability to delineate tumors and adjacent normal structures in three dimensions using specialized CT scanners and planning software. Upon the decision to pursue radiotherapy in the treatment of desmoid tumors, patients undergo a specialized CT scan that allows the virtual simulation of the radiation treatment plan. Patients are immobilized prior to or at the time of simulation in order to elicit a treatment position that can be daily reproduced throughout treatment. The radiation oncologist is able to accurately delineate the tumor volume targeted for treatment on the CT slices. Very commonly the planning software allows fusion of the planning CT slices with corresponding images from the patient's diagnostic MRI to improve the ability to delineate tumor extension.

8.8.1 Treatment Volumes

In general, three volumes are generated during radiotherapy planning specific to the treatment of desmoids. The gross tumor volume (GTV) is a volume that encompasses the gross palpable or visible extent of the disease as outlined on physical exam and radiographic imaging. The clinical target volume (CTV) is a volume that encompass the GTV in addition to regions of suspected microscopic disease. Given the infiltrative nature of desmoids, the CTV for the treatment of desmoids is generated by adding a security margin around the GTV, which can range from 2–5 cm in any direction not bounded by a facial barrier or tissue plane that would block spread of tumor (such as the pleura or peritoneum) [12]. The CTV should not extend beyond these and other anatomic barriers (bone and air). The M.D. Anderson group [7] reported that there was no evidence that radiation margins exceeding 5 cm beyond the tumor or surgical field improved local-regional control. Finally, another safety margin is added onto the CTV to generate the planning target volume (PTV) which ensures that the GTV and CTV receive the prescribed dose in light of uncertainties related to organ, patient motion, and daily setup variability. The margin for PTV may vary depending on the immobilization, on-treatment imaging, and other quality assurance techniques used [46].

Following the delineation of radiotherapy treatment volumes, radiation beams are designed to cover the target volume while minimizing the volume of normal tissue radiated. The exact number and geometry of radiation beams varies depending on the site and volume of PTV targeted. The advent of three-dimensional conformal radiotherapy (3DCRT) has revolutionized treatment planning in radiotherapy. In 3DCRT, the profile of each radiation beam is shaped to fit the profile of the target from using a multileaf collimator (MLC). This conforms the treatment volume to the shape of the tumor, reducing the relative toxicity of radiation to the surrounding normal tissues and allowing a higher dose of radiation to be delivered to the tumor compared to conventional techniques [18, 46]. Additional sparing of normal structures can be achieved using intensity-modulated radiotherapy (IMRT) which involves high-precision delivery of radiation with variable intensity and improves the ability to conform the treatment volume to concave tumor shapes. One way to conceptualize IMRT is to think of it as the obverse of the CT, which is a map of radiation absorption obtained by rotating a constant, symmetric source of radiation around the patient and measuring the transmitted radiation with detectors and back projecting the absorbing structure. For IMRT, the radiation oncologist defines the desired "map" of high-dose radiation absorption in the tumor and constraints on the adjacent normal tissues; this is achieved by asymmetric radiation delivery from selected angles or in circumferential tomographic fields of variable intensity produced by moving blocking fingers (or "leaves") of 0.5 to 1 cm in size in and out of the radiation fields [20, 46].

Various types of quality assurance procedures are conducted prior to and throughout the radiotherapy treatments to ensure appropriate target coverage. These include review of the designated target volumes by radiation oncology and, in some cases, surgical colleagues prior to or during the first week of radiotherapy and imaging of the radiotherapy fields generated by the three-dimensional treatment planning system in the patient prior to and generally at least weekly during radiotherapy to ensure the accuracy of treatment. Image guided radiotherapy (IGRT) is growing in popularity and involves the use of various imaging modalities prior to the daily delivery of radiation treatments to ensure that patients are treated accurately and in accordance to the original treatment plan [47].

8.9 Other Radiotherapy Techniques

8.9.1 Brachytherapy

As opposed to external beam radiotherapy, brachytherapy involves the delivery of radiation from radioactive sources placed within or adjacent to the treatment target. This typically allows the delivery of high radiation doses locally and minimizes the volume of normal tissue receiving radiation due to the rapid dose fall off associated with distance from the radiation source [48]. Brachytherapy can be applied as monotherapy for resected desmoids provided adequate margins around the tumor bed are covered or may be added to external beam radiation to boost the dose to the tumor [49]. Consideration should be made for the use of brachytherapy in recurrent disease especially in patients who previously received external beam radiation. Patients with desmoid tumors involving the bony structures of the hand or feet were shown to be poor candidates for brachytherapy due to high-toxicity profile [39].

Interstitial brachytherapy implants are the most commonly used form of brachytherapy applied in the treatment of desmoid tumors. These are generally implants of sterile afterloading catheters inserted into the tumor bed and adjacent tissues at time of surgery. The geometry of the implant is optimized to ensure adequate coverage of the target [48]. Radiotherapy treatment usually starts 5 days following surgery to avoid wound healing complications. The dose of radiotherapy used in brachytherapy depends on the indication for treatment. Patients receiving brachytherapy as radiation monotherapy after surgery are typically treated with a high-dose-rate dose of 30–36 Gy delivered twice daily over a period of 5 days or 45 Gy over 4–5 days by conventional dose rate brachytherapy [39, 50].

8.9.2 Intraoperative Radiotherapy

Intraoperative radiotherapy (IORT) is the delivery of radiation at time of surgery. This technique is intended to facilitate tumor dose escalation without increasing normal tissue toxicity by direct tumor/tumor bed visualization and exclusion of dose limiting normal structures either by operative mobilization or direct shielding. Electron beam radiation is typically used, which is less penetrating than photons and provides adequate coverage of the residual disease/tumor bed surface. IORT is delivered in the operating room following resection and is usually in combination with pre or postoperative external beam radiation. Roeder et al. [51] recently reported the experience of using IORT for desmoids at the University of Heidelberg, using a median intraoperative dose of 12 Gy generally in conjunction with 45 Gy of external beam radiotherapy and showed a 3-year local control rate of 91% within regions treated with IORT. Generally, IORT is recommended in the adjuvant treatment of intra-abdominal desmoids for positive margins and following incomplete resection.

8.10 Toxicity

Treatment with radiotherapy can be associated with acute and long-term sequelae that are dependent on a number of factors including age, treatment site, radiation dose, and the volume treated, combination with surgery, previous radiation, and inherent host biological factors that determine radiation sensitivity [7, 28, 3, 12]. Acute side effects are conventionally defined as those occurring within 90 days of initiating radiotherapy treatments, while toxicities occurring after 90 days are considered late side effects. In general, acute toxicity tends to be reversible and resolves after a period of recovery following the completion of radiation, whereas late toxicities are often chronic and much less treatable or reversible [16, 14, 46].

Overall, late radiation toxicity is relatively uncommon, and its incidence is higher amongst patients treated by surgery and radiation. In the series reported by Ballo et al. [7] from the MD Anderson Cancer Center, 13 of 75 patients developed “significant” complications. Radiation dose correlated with the incidence of complications. Doses of 56 Gy or less produced a 5% 15-year complication rate, compared to a 30% incidence with higher doses ($p<0.05$).

The exact profile of toxicity caused by radiation depends largely on the site being treated since the effects of radiation are local. Potential complications include soft tissue necrosis, skin hyperpigmentation, bone fractures and osteonecrosis, radiation enteritis, peripheral neuropathy, soft tissue fibrosis, lymphedema, wound infection and cellulitis, limb shortening and limitation of motion, bone hypoplasia, and chronic pain. Fatigue, usually mild and transient, is encountered by patients during treatment and is the most common systemic effect seen in response to radiation [14]. The severity of radiation toxicity can be assessed based on a number of radiation toxicity scoring criteria including the Radiation Therapy Oncology Group (RTOG) [52], European Organization for Research and Treatment of Cancer (EORTC) [52, 53], and the National Cancer Institute Common Terminology Criteria for Adverse Events (CTCAE) toxicity schemas [54].

The risk of secondary malignancy is dependent on the age and sex of the patient. Younger patients have a higher life-time risk of developing a secondary malignancy compared to older patients. Jansen et al. [55] reported the life-time relative risk for tumor induction for various age groups treated with radiation for benign disease. The relative risk for male patients treated under the age of ten reached 25%/sievert compared to 13%/sievert for patients in the 21–30 age group and 7%/sievert for patients in the 31–40 age group. The risk is slightly higher for women across all age groups. Radiation should be avoided as much as possible in patients below 20 years of age.

8.11 Posttreatment Surveillance

There is no standard protocol for follow-up of patients with desmoid tumors. The NCCN (National Comprehensive Cancer Network) follow-up guidelines call for follow-up examinations every 3–6 months for 2–3 years and then annually [56]. Surveillance MRI scan is typically the imaging study of choice for extra-abdominal tumors with CT scans used for intra-abdominal desmoids. In addition to early detection of potential recurrences, follow-up is important for understanding and managing treatment-related toxicities.

8.12 Conclusions

Treatment recommendations with regard to the role of radiation therapy in the management of desmoid tumors are based on the available data in the literature, which are retrospective as there have been few data published from prospective clinical trials evaluating the role of radiation therapy in the disease. Surgery has been the mainstay of local tumor management; the current trend in management is to consider initial observation for asymptomatic, nonprogressive tumor, reserving surgery for those patients who become symptomatic or progress while under observation. Radiation is generally not given for patients resected with a positive margin, as only half of the patients will develop recurrent disease. Radiation is generally used for patients who recur following surgery or for patients with symptomatic or progressive primary tumors in which surgical resection is felt to be excessively morbid. For recurrent tumors, radiation therapy can be used either preoperatively or postoperatively. Radiation is given by shrinking field techniques, treating elective volumes to 50 Gy, and boosting gross disease to total doses in the range of 56–58 Gy with conventional fractionation. Local control rates with radiation alone for unresected disease are ~ 75%. Because of the potential late effects of radiation therapy in the pediatric patient that include growth abnormalities and a radiation-associated malignancy, surgery or systemic therapies are the preferred treatments in children.

References

1. Ewing J (1928) Neoplastic disease. WB Saunders, Philadelphia
2. Ballo MT, Zagars GK, Pollack A (1998) Radiation therapy in the management of desmoid tumors. Int J Radiat Oncol Biol Phys 42(5):1007–1014. doi:S0360-3016(98)00285-5 [pii]
3. Guadagnolo BA, Zagars GK, Ballo MT (2008) Long-term outcomes for desmoid tumors treated with radiation therapy. Int J Radiat Oncol Biol Phys 71(2):441–447. doi:S0360-3016(07)04425-2 [pii] 10.1016/j.ijrobp.2007.10.013
4. Jelinek JA, Stelzer KJ, Conrad E, Bruckner J, Kliot M, Koh W, Laramore GE (2001) The efficacy of radiotherapy as postoperative treatment for desmoid tumors. Int J Radiat Oncol Biol Phys 50(1):121–125. doi:S0360301600015704 [pii]

5. Nuyttens JJ, Rust PF, Thomas CR, Jr, Turrisi AT, 3rd (2000) Surgery versus radiation therapy for patients with aggressive fibromatosis or desmoid tumors: a comparative review of 22 articles. Cancer 88(7):1517–1523. doi:10.1002/(SICI)1097-0142(20000401)88:7-1517::AID-CNCR3-3.0.CO;2-9 [pii]
6. Acker JC, Bossen EH, Halperin EC (1993) The management of desmoid tumors. Int J Radiat Oncol Biol Phys 26(5):851–858
7. Ballo MT, Zagars GK, Pollack A, Pisters PW, Pollack RA (1999) Desmoid tumor: prognostic factors and outcome after surgery, radiation therapy, or combined surgery and radiation therapy. J Clin Oncol 17(1):158–167
8. de Bree E, Keus R, Melissas J, Tsiftsis D, van Coevorden F (2009) Desmoid tumors: need for an individualized approach. Expert Rev Anticancer Ther 9(4):525–535. doi:10.1586/era.09.9
9. Baumert BG, Spahr MO, Von Hochstetter A, Beauvois S, Landmann C, Fridrich K, Villa S, Kirschner MJ, Storme G, Thum P, Streuli HK, Lombriser N, Maurer R, Ries G, Bleher EA, Willi A, Allemann J, Buehler U, Blessing H, Luetolf UM, Davis JB, Seifert B, Infanger M (2007) The impact of radiotherapy in the treatment of desmoid tumours. An international survey of 110 patients. A study of the Rare Cancer Network. Radiat Oncol 2:(12). doi:1748-717X-2-12 [pii] 10.1186/1748-717X-2-12
10. Gluck I, Griffith KA, Biermann JS, Feng FY, Lucas DR, Ben-Josef E (2010) Role of radiotherapy in the management of desmoid tumors. Int J Radiat Oncol Biol Phys. doi:S0360-3016(10)00416-5 [pii] 10.1016/j.ijrobp.2010.02.053
11. Zlotecki RA, Scarborough MT, Morris CG, Berrey BH, Lind DS, Enneking WF, Marcus RB Jr (2002) External beam radiotherapy for primary and adjuvant management of aggressive fibromatosis. Int J Radiat Oncol Biol Phys 54(1):177–181. doi:S0360301602029267 [pii]
12. Micke O, Seegenschmiedt MH (2005) Radiation therapy for aggressive fibromatosis (desmoid tumors): results of a national Patterns of Care Study. Int J Radiat Oncol Biol Phys 61(3):882–891. doi:S0360-3016(04)02101-7 [pii] 10.1016/j.ijrobp.2004.07.705
13. Micke O, Seegenschmiedt MH (2002) Consensus guidelines for radiation therapy of benign diseases: a multicenter approach in Germany. Int J Radiat Oncol Biol Phys 52(2):496–513. doi:S0360301601018144 [pii]
14. Hosalkar HS, Fox EJ, Delaney T, Torbert JT, Ogilvie CM, Lackman RD (2006) Desmoid tumors and current status of management. Orthop Clin North Am 37(1):53–63. doi:S0030-5898(05)00077-5 [pii] 10.1016/j.ocl.2005.08.004
15. Rontgen WK (1896) A new form of radiation. Science 3(72):726–729. doi:3/72/726 [pii] 10.1126/science.3.72.726
16. Hall EJ, Giaccia AJ (2005) Radiobiology for the radiologist, 6th edn. Lippincott Williams & Wilkins, Philadelphia
17. Serber W, Bracy, LW, Zhang, M, Hoppe, RT (2004) Radiation treatment of benign disease. In: Perez C, Brady LW, Halperin EG, Schmidt-Ullrich R (eds) Principles and practice of radiation oncology, 4th edn. Lippincott Williams and Wilkins, Philadelphia
18. Bhide SA, Nutting CM (2010) Recent advances in radiotherapy. BMC Med 8:25. doi:1741-7015-8-25 [pii] 10.1186/1741-7015-8-25
19. Connell PP, Hellman S (2009) Advances in radiotherapy and implications for the next century: a historical perspective. Cancer Res 69(2):383–392. doi:69/2/383 [pii] 10.1158/0008-5472.CAN-07-6871
20. Fenwick JD, Riley SW, Scott AJ (2008) Advances in intensity-modulated radiotherapy delivery. Cancer Treat Res 139:193–214
21. Jenkins NH, Freedman LS, McKibbin B (1986) Spontaneous regression of a desmoid tumour. J Bone Joint Surg Br 68(5):780–781
22. Lazar AJ, Hajibashi S, Lev D (2009) Desmoid tumor: from surgical extirpation to molecular dissection. Curr Opin Oncol 21(4):352–359. doi:10.1097/CCO.0b013e32832c9502
23. Lazar AJ, Tuvin D, Hajibashi S, Habeeb S, Bolshakov S, Mayordomo-Aranda E, Warneke CL, Lopez-Terrada D, Pollock RE, Lev D (2008) Specific mutations in the beta-catenin gene (CTNNB1) correlate with local recurrence in sporadic desmoid tumors. Am J Pathol 173(5):1518–1527. doi:ajpath.2008.080475 [pii] 10.2353/ajpath.2008.080475

24. Goy BW, Lee SP, Eilber F, Dorey F, Eckardt J, Fu YS, Juillard GJ, Selch MT (1997) The role of adjuvant radiotherapy in the treatment of resectable desmoid tumors. Int J Radiat Oncol Biol Phys 39(3):659–665. doi:S0360-3016(97)00334-9 [pii]
25. Merchant NB, Lewis JJ, Woodruff JM, Leung DH, Brennan MF (1999) Extremity and trunk desmoid tumors: a multifactorial analysis of outcome. Cancer 86(10):2045–2052. doi:10.1002/(SICI)1097-0142(19991115)86:10-2045::AID-CNCR23-3.0.CO;2-F [pii]
26. Lev D, Kotilingam D, Wei C, Ballo MT, Zagars GK, Pisters PW, Lazar AA, Patel SR, Benjamin RS, Pollock RE (2007) Optimizing treatment of desmoid tumors. J Clin Oncol 25(13):1785–1791. doi:25/13/1785 [pii] 10.1200/JCO.2006.10.5015
27. Spear MA, Jennings LC, Mankin HJ, Spiro IJ, Springfield DS, Gebhardt MC, Rosenberg AE, Efird JT, Suit HD (1998) Individualizing management of aggressive fibromatoses. Int J Radiat Oncol Biol Phys 40(3):637–645. doi:S0360301697008456 [pii]
28. Gronchi A, Casali PG, Mariani L, Lo Vullo S, Colecchia M, Lozza L, Bertulli R, Fiore M, Olmi P, Santinami M, Rosai J (2003) Quality of surgery and outcome in extra-abdominal aggressive fibromatosis: a series of patients surgically treated at a single institution. J Clin Oncol 21(7):1390–1397
29. Singh G, Syed SP, Tome M et al. (2008) Prognostic value of margin status in the treatment of desmoid tumor [abstract]. Int J Radiat Oncol Biol Phys 72(Suppl 1):107–108
30. Melis M, Zager JS, Sondak VK (2008) Multimodality management of desmoid tumors: how important is a negative surgical margin? J Surg Oncol 98(8):594–602. doi:10.1002/jso.21033
31. Kamath SS, Parsons JT, Marcus RB, Zlotecki RA, Scarborough MT (1996) Radiotherapy for local control of aggressive fibromatosis. Int J Radiat Oncol Biol Phys 36(2):325–328. doi:S0360301696003215 [pii]
32. McCollough WM, Parsons JT, Van Der Griend R, Enneking WF, Heare T (1991) Radiation therapy for aggressive fibromatosis. The experience at the University of Florida. J Bone Joint Surg Am 73(5):717–725
33. Stoeckle E, Coindre JM, Longy M, Binh MB, Kantor G, Kind M, de Lara CT, Avril A, Bonichon F, Bui BN (2009) A critical analysis of treatment strategies in desmoid tumours: a review of a series of 106 cases. Eur J Surg Oncol 35(2):129–134. doi:S0748-7983(08)01713-7 [pii] 10.1016/j.ejso.2008.06.1495
34. Latchford AR, Sturt NJ, Neale K, Rogers PA, Phillips RK (2006) A 10-year review of surgery for desmoid disease associated with familial adenomatous polyposis. Br J Surg 93(10):1258–1264. doi:10.1002/bjs.5425
35. Seow-Choen F (2008) The management of desmoids in patients with familial adenomatous polyposis (FAP). Acta Chir Iugosl 55(3):83–87
36. O'Dea FJ, Wunder J, Bell RS, Griffin AM, Catton C, O'Sullivan B (2003) Preoperative radiotherapy is effective in the treatment of fibromatosis. Clin Orthop Relat Res 415:19–24. doi:10.1097/01.blo.0000093892.12372.d4
37. Baliski CR, Temple WJ, Arthur K, Schachar NS (2002) Desmoid tumors: a novel approach for local control. J Surg Oncol 80(2):96–99. doi:10.1002/jso.10104
38. Sorensen A, Keller J, Nielsen OS, Jensen OM (2002) Treatment of aggressive fibromatosis: a retrospective study of 72 patients followed for 1-27 years. Acta Orthop Scand 73(2):213–219. doi:10.1080/000164702753671830
39. Fontanesi J, Mott MP, Kraut MJ, Lucas DP, Miller PR (2004) The role of postoperative irradiation in the treatment of locally recurrent incompletely resected extra-abdominal desmoid tumors. Sarcoma 8(2–3):83–86. doi:10.1080/13577140410001710512
40. Suit H, Spiro I (2001) Radiation in the multidisciplinary management of desmoid tumors. Front Radiat Ther Oncol 35:107–119
41. Suit HD (1990) Radiation dose and response of desmoid tumors. Int J Radiat Oncol Biol Phys 19(1):225–227
42. Merchant TE, Nguyen D, Walter AW, Pappo AS, Kun LE, Rao BN (2000) Long-term results with radiation therapy for pediatric desmoid tumors. Int J Radiat Oncol Biol Phys 47(5):1267–1271. doi:S0360-3016(00)005666 [pii]

43. Jabbari S, Andolino D, Weinberg V, Missett BT, Law J, Wara WM, O'Donnell RJ, Matthay KK, DuBois SG, Goldsby R, Haas-Kogan DA (2009) Successful treatment of high risk and recurrent pediatric desmoids using radiation as a component of multimodality therapy. Int J Radiat Oncol Biol Phys 75(1):177–182. doi:S0360-3016(08)03865-0 [pii] 10.1016/j.ijrobp.2008.10.072
44. Skapek SX, Ferguson WS, Granowetter L, Devidas M, Perez-Atayde AR, Dehner LP, Hoffer FA, Speights R, Gebhardt MC, Dahl GV, Grier HE (2007) Vinblastine and methotrexate for desmoid fibromatosis in children: results of a Pediatric Oncology Group Phase II Trial. J Clin Oncol 25(5):501–506. doi:25/5/501 [pii] 10.1200/JCO.2006.08.2966
45. Miralbell R, Lomax A, Cella L, Schneider U (2002) Potential reduction of the incidence of radiation-induced second cancers by using proton beams in the treatment of pediatric tumors. Int J Radiat Oncol Biol Phys 54(3):824–829. doi:S0360301602029826 [pii]
46. Perez C, Brady, LW, Halperin, EG, Schmidt-Ullrich, R (2004) Principles and practice of radiation oncology, 4th edn. Lippincott, Williams and Wilkins, Philadelphia
47. Dawson LA, Jaffray DA (2007) Advances in image-guided radiation therapy. J Clin Oncol 25(8):938–946. doi:25/8/938 [pii] 10.1200/JCO.2006.09.9515
48. Devlin PM (2006) Brachytherapy: applications and techniques, 1st edn. Lippincott Williams & Wilkins, Philadelphia
49. Assad WA, Nori D, Hilaris BS, Shiu MH, Hajdu SI (1986) Role of brachytherapy in the management of desmoid tumors. Int J Radiat Oncol Biol Phys 12(6):901–906
50. Alektiar KM, Leung D, Zelefsky MJ, Healey JH, Brennan MF (2002) Adjuvant brachytherapy for primary high-grade soft tissue sarcoma of the extremity. Ann Surg Oncol 9(1):48–56
51. Roeder F, Timke C, Oertel S, Hensley FW, Bischof M, Muenter MW, Weitz J, Buchler MW, Lehner B, Debus J, Krempien R (2010) Intraoperative electron radiotherapy for the management of aggressive fibromatosis. Int J Radiat Oncol Biol Phys 76(4):1154–1160. doi:S0360-3016(09)00608-7 [pii] 10.1016/j.ijrobp.2009.03.067
52. Radiation Therapy Oncology Group (RTOG) acute radiation morbidity scoring criteria. http://208.251.169.72/members/toxicity/acute.html. Accessed 3 July 2011
53. Radiation Therapy Oncology Group (RTOG), European Organization for Research and Treatment of Cancer (EORTC) late radiation morbidity scoring schema. http://208.251.169.72/members/toxicity/late.html. Accessed 3 July 2011
54. NCI National Cancer Institute Common Terminology Criteria for Adverse Events (CTCAE) toxicity schemas. http://www.eortc.be/services/doc/ctc/default.html. Accessed 3 July 2011
55. Jansen JT, Broerse JJ, Zoetelief J, Klein C, Seegenschmiedt HM (2005) Estimation of the carcinogenic risk of radiotherapy of benign diseases from shoulder to heel. Radiother Oncol 76(3):270–277. doi:S0167-8140(05)00275-6 [pii] 10.1016/j.radonc.2005.06.034
56. National Comprehensive Cancer Network (NCCN) treatment guidelines. www.nccn.org
57. Park HC, Pyo HR, Shin KH, Suh CO (2003) Radiation treatment for aggressive fibromatosis: findings from observed patterns of local failure. Oncology 64(4):346–352. doi:10.1159/000070292 OCL2003064004346 [pii]
58. Schulz-Ertner D, Zierhut D, Mende U, Harms W, Branitzki P, Wannenmacher M (2002) The role of radiation therapy in the management of desmoid tumors. Strahlenther Onkol 178(2):78–83

Chapter 9
Interventional Radiology

David S. Pryluck and Joseph P. Erinjeri

Contents

Abstract Given the unique challenges encountered in the diagnosis and treatment of desmoid tumors and the high rate of tumor recurrence, clinicians have sought alternative therapies which maximize efficacy and minimize patient morbidity. Interventional radiology and interventional oncology offer several minimally invasive, percutaneous image-guided procedures that are well suited to the challenges that desmoid tumors present. Fine needle aspiration and core needle biopsy are routinely used as an alternative to open surgical biopsy to obtain cytological and histological specimens for definitive tissue diagnosis of desmoid tumors. Chemical ablation, radiofrequency ablation, and cryoablation have been used to treat patients with desmoid tumors which have recurred after surgery, radiation, and/or chemotherapy, and as a palliative option for patients with unresectable lesions. In this chapter, the mechanism of action and rationale for use, as well as technical and clinical considerations of each technique will be discussed.

D. S. Pryluck (✉)
Department of Interventional Radiology, Hospital of the University of Pennsylvania, Philadelphia, PA, USA
e-mail: david.pryluck@uphs.upenn.edu

C. Litchman (ed.), *Desmoid Tumors*,
DOI 10.1007/978-94-007-1685-8_9, © Springer Science+Business Media B.V. 2012

Keywords Cryoablation • Thermal ablation • Radiofrequency ablation • Chemical ablation • Biopsy • Desmoid tumor • Aggressive fibromatosis • Interventional radiology

9.1 Introduction

Interventional radiology and interventional oncology play an increasingly important role alongside traditional surgical oncology, medical oncology, and radiation oncology in the multidisciplinary approach to the diagnosis and treatment of desmoid tumors and other soft tissue malignancies [1]. The purpose of this chapter is to discuss the role of interventional radiology and interventional oncology as it relates specifically to this challenging neoplasm.

As with other soft tissue tumors, a definitive tissue diagnosis of desmoid tumor is required prior to the initiation of therapy. Tissue can be obtained by open or excisional biopsy, both of which are invasive and associated with multiple potential surgical morbidities, including wound breakdown, hemorrhage, and infection [2, 3]. Interventional radiology, however, offers two minimally invasive, image-guided alternatives to surgical biopsy: fine needle aspiration and core needle biopsy. These two procedures will be described and compared, with specific emphasis on each technique's applicability to the diagnosis of desmoid tumors.

Desmoid tumors are typically treated with a combination of surgical resection, systemic chemotherapy, and radiation therapy. However, multiple minimally invasive, percutaneous image-guided therapies are becoming increasingly utilized to meet the unique challenges of the desmoid tumor, including chemical ablation, radiofrequency ablation, and cryoablation. These modalities, which are routinely used in the treatment of other neoplasms including hepatocellular and renal cell carcinoma, are now being applied to the treatment of desmoid tumors. The mechanism of action and rationale for use, as well as the clinical and technical considerations of each technique will be discussed.

9.2 Diagnosis of Desmoid Tumors by Percutaneous Needle Biopsy

Percutaneous needle biopsy (PNB) is the insertion of a needle into an abnormal lesion or organ for the purpose of obtaining cells or tissue for diagnosis [4]. Needle placement is typically under real-time ultrasound or computed tomographic (CT) guidance using a freehand technique. PNB is less invasive than open or excisional biopsy [5], is associated with decreased morbidity [5], and has become the primary method by which pathological diagnosis is obtained before the initiation of therapy [6].

PNB comprises two basic procedures: fine needle aspiration [7] and core needle biopsy [8]. Fine needle aspiration (FNA) involves the use of a thin, hollow needle (22 G or smaller) that is inserted into a lesion to sample cells for cytological analysis. Core needle biopsy (CNB) is a coaxial technique by which a cutting device is inserted through a hollow needle (20 G or larger) which has been placed into a lesion, and a 1-mm cylinder of tissue (a core) is obtained for histological analysis. Although these procedures can be performed in a surgeon's office for palpable lesions [9], FNA and CNB performed using ultrasound or CT guidance ensures precise tissue sampling with direct visualization of the needle tip as it enters a lesion (Fig. 9.1). Image guidance also minimizes the risk of injury to vital structures adjacent to or in the plane of a lesion, including blood vessels, nerves, and nontarget organs, which cannot be seen during "blind" office biopsies.

9.2.1 Fine Needle Aspiration

The FNA cytological findings of fibromatosis have been reviewed in a few small case series and single case reports [10–14]. In the largest series of 17 patients with histologically proven desmoid tumors, Owens et al. described a range of observed cytological features, including the presence of low-to-moderate cellularity of bland spindled cells with bipolar nuclei, dense and metachromatic stromal fragments, and tumor cells embedded within or in close proximity to stroma, and the absence of prominent vascularity, nuclear hyperchromasia, and severe atypia [13]. These cytological features overlap other myofibroblastic proliferations, including nodular fasciitis, scar tissue, myofibroma, low-grade fibromyxoid sarcoma, and low-grade fibrosarcoma. Differentiation among these entities for a specific diagnosis of desmoid tumor can be difficult based on cytology alone. In fact, only one of the 17 patients included in this study received a specific diagnosis of desmoid tumor solely based on FNA cytology. An additional four patients were diagnosed with desmoid tumor based on FNA cytology with immunohistochemical analysis conducted on cell block material or core needle biopsy samples obtained at the time of FNA; two of these patients had a prior history of fibromatosis.

Two larger retrospective studies of patients with soft tissue masses including desmoid tumors evaluated the diagnostic accuracy of preoperative fine needle aspiration. Dey et al. examined 82 histopathologically proven cases of FNA cytology of soft tissue tumors, which included five cases of fibromatosis, only one of which was correctly diagnosed based on FNA [15]. Three of the remaining lesions were diagnosed as benign spindle cell tumors, and one lesion as spindle cell tumor, possibly low-grade malignancy. Jakowski et al. correlated FNA cytology of 141 distal extremity lesions with either tissue biopsy confirmation or clinical follow-up, seven of which were diagnosed as fibromatosis based on FNA cytology [16]. A biopsy tissue diagnosis was available for only one of those lesions, which supported a diagnosis of fibromatosis. The remaining six lesions were reported as being concordant based upon clinical follow-up.

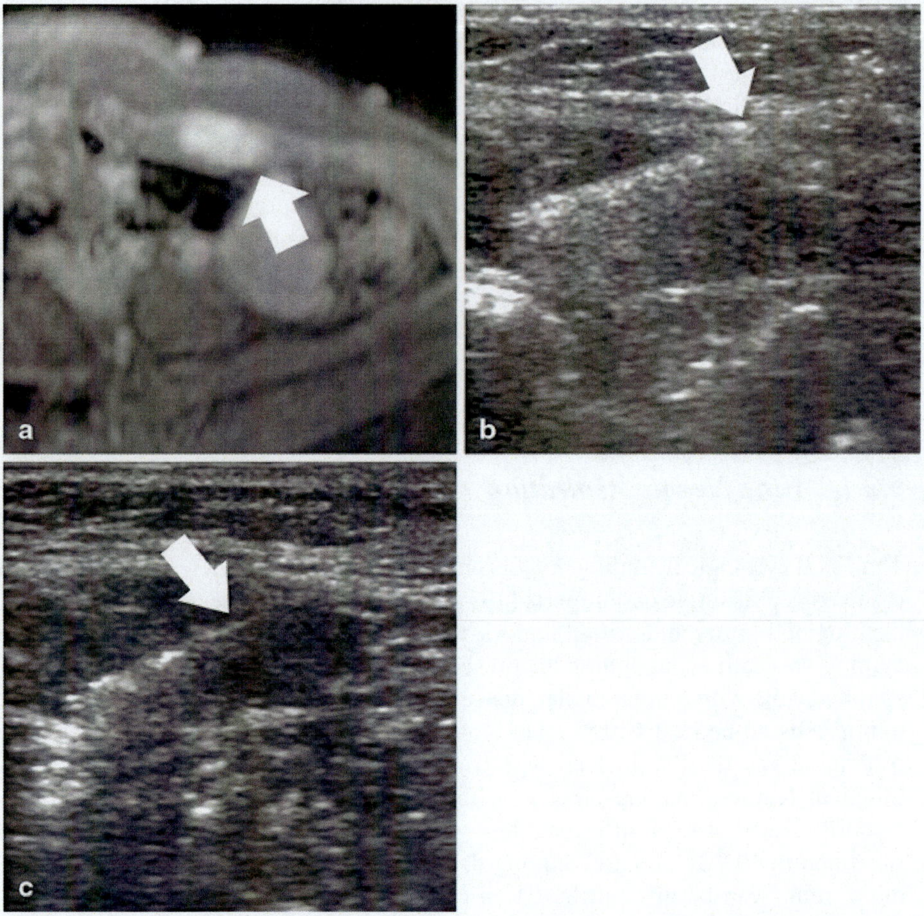

Fig. 9.1 Percutaneous needle biopsy of a left rectus abdominis desmoid tumor in a 37-year-old female who presented with a palpable lump. **a** Axial postcontrast 3D T1-weighted gradient echo demonstrates a 2.6 × 1.7 cm-enhancing lesion embedded within the left rectus abdominis muscle (*arrow*), which corresponds to the palpable abnormality. **b** Fine Needle Aspiration: a 22-G Turner biopsy needle has been advanced into the rectus nodule using real-time ultrasound guidance via an anterior approach (*arrow*). The sampled cytological material demonstrated poor cellularity. **c** Core Needle Biopsy: an 18-G biopsy device has been advanced into the rectus nodule with real-time ultrasound guidance via an anterior approach (*arrow*). Two 23-mm core biopsy specimens were obtained

9.2.2 Core Needle Biopsy

Two retrospective studies evaluated the use of core needle biopsy in the preoperative diagnosis of soft tissue masses which included desmoid tumors. Serpell et al. assessed the accuracy of core needle biopsy in the diagnosis of soft tissue tumors in 45 patients with established or suspected soft tissue sarcomas [17]. In six patients, surgical excision yielded desmoid tumors. Four of these patients had undergone preoperative core needle biopsy, and in all four cases, desmoid tumor was correctly diagnosed by CNB preoperatively. For the cohort of 45 patients, the authors reported that CNB had 94% sensitivity and 100% specificity, and enabled planning of definitive one-stage surgeries in most cases.

Ray-Coquard evaluated 103 soft tissue masses diagnosed preoperatively by CNB, including six desmoid tumors [18]. All six soft tissue masses diagnosed as desmoids by CNB were either totally or partially concordant with postoperative pathology. Positive and negative predictive values, sensitivity and specificity of CNB for malignant criteria, and diagnosis of sarcoma were 100% for the six desmoid tumors in this study.

A single retrospective study compared the accuracy of preoperative FNA and CNB diagnoses of desmoid tumors. Dalén et al. reviewed 95 cases of surgically resected desmoids, 69 of which were evaluated preoperatively by FNA cytology, and 26 by CNB [19]. A correct diagnosis was made in only 35 of the 69 cases sampled by FNA, while 24 of the 26 cases sampled by CNB were correctly diagnosed as desmoid tumor. In the remaining two cases sampled by CNB, desmoid tumor was offered as the most likely diagnosis. Incorrect FNA-based preoperative diagnoses included benign fibroblastic lesion not otherwise specified (NOS), nodular fasciitis, desmoid or nodular fasciitis, spindle cell malignancy, schwannoma, and nondiagnostic. The authors also discussed 15 cases in which an incorrect preoperative diagnosis of desmoid tumor was made by FNA, two of which were later found to be sarcomas on surgical excision.

9.3 Image-Guided Therapy for Desmoid Tumors

9.3.1 Chemical Ablation

9.3.1.1 Mechanism and Rationale

Image-guided percutaneous chemical ablation refers to the direct intratumoral injection of cytotoxic compounds using either ultrasound or CT scan for needle localization [20]. Under conscious sedation, an infusion needle is inserted percutaneously using a freehand technique into the center of the tumor. Typically, a 20–22 G infusion needle is used, although the use of an 18 G needle has also been reported [21]. A liquid cytotoxin, typically ethanol or acetic acid, is gradually infused into the tumor (Fig. 9.2). The volume and concentration of cytotoxin will vary with protocol and tumor mass. Multiple treatment sessions are often required, with interval imaging follow-up by CT or magnetic resonance imaging (MRI).

The cytotoxic effect of ethanol has been attributed to a combination of cytoplasmic dehydration, cell protein denaturation, and small vessel thrombosis, all contributing to coagulative necrosis on histopathological studies [22–24]. The cytotoxic mechanism of acetic acid has been attributed to its effective protein desiccation,

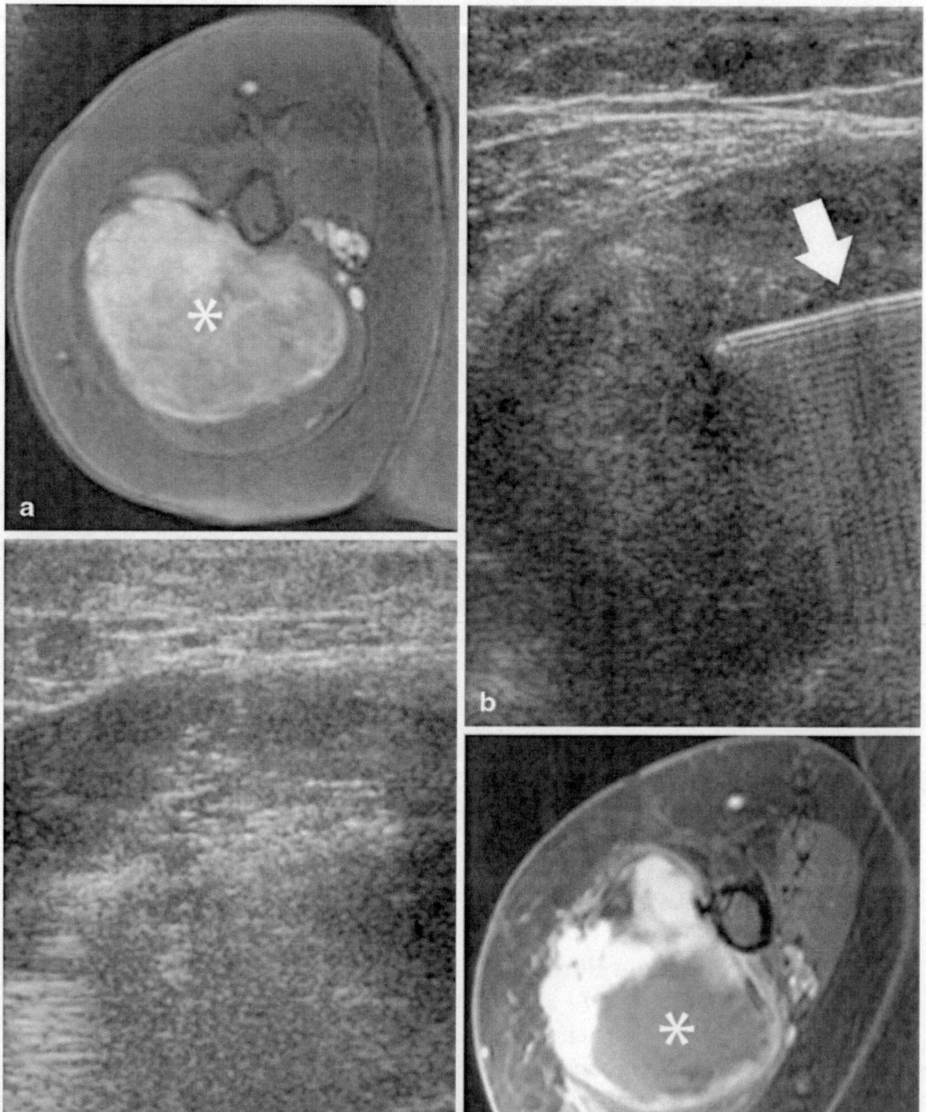

Fig. 9.2 Ultrasound-guided percutaneous chemical ablation with acetic acid of a right upper extremity desmoid tumor in a 44-year-old female. **a** Axial postcontrast T1-weighted gradient echo with fat suppression demonstrates a heterogeneously enhancing desmoid tumor interposed between the distal deltoid muscle and anterolateral aspect of the triceps muscle (*). The triceps muscle is markedly compressed and displaced posteromedially. **b** Under ultrasound guidance, a 20-G infusion needle has been advanced into the hypoechoic desmoid tumor subjacent to the right deltoid muscle using a posterolateral approach (*arrow*). **c** A total of 8 ml of 50% acetic acid has been slowly infused into the mass using aliquots of 0.1–0.2 ml, rendering the tumor center echogenic. **d** Axial postcontrast T1-weighted spin echo with fat suppression following seven treatment sessions of chemical ablation with acetic acid over a 10-month time period demonstrates a large confluent region of tumor nonenhancement (*)

lipid dissolution, and collagen extraction, also resulting in coagulative necrosis [25, 26]. Acetic acid has been shown to promote disruption of collagen by dissociation of intermolecular aldimine bonds, attributed to its low pH [27, 25]. This property enables acetic acid to penetrate collagen-containing portions of tumor, including fibrous septa capsules, during ablation procedures [28].

Early uses of ethanol as a therapeutic agent included the intraarterial injection of renal arteries for renal cell carcinoma embolization [29], coronary vein infusion for sclerotherapy of bleeding esophageal varices [30, 31], bronchial artery embolization for massive hemoptysis [32], and celiac ganglion neurolysis for intractable abdominal pain [33]. Chemical ablation of masses was first described for the treatment of parathyroid hyperplasia as an alternative to surgery, during which ultrasound-guided intraparenchymal injection of absolute ethanol was performed in patients with refractory secondary hyperparathyroidism [34]. In that study, Solbiati et al. demonstrated significant volume reduction and changes in ultrasonographic echo pattern of the injected parathyroid glands, accompanied by improvements in clinical and laboratory indicators of hyperparathyroidism.

Much of the existing medical literature describing percutaneous ethanol injection (PEI) and percutaneous acetic acid injection (PAI) relates to the treatment of hepatocellular carcinoma, with multiple long-term studies demonstrating its efficacy. Livraghi et al. reported mean 5-year survival rates of patients with cirrhosis and single hepatocellular carcinomas with diameters less than or equal to 5.0 cm treated with PEI to be essentially comparable to that of surgical resection [35]. Ohnishi et al. demonstrated 1-, 3-, and 5-year cancer-free survival rates of patients with hepatocellular carcinomas smaller than 3.0 cm after PAI to be comparable to those after hepatic resection [26]. In that study of 91 patients, concentrations of acetic acid ranging from 15 to 50% were utilized, with fewer treatment sessions necessary to ablate lesions of similar sizes when higher concentrations of acetic acid were used [26]. In a prospective, randomized controlled trial, Ohnishi et al. demonstrated chemical ablation using 50% acetic acid to be superior to absolute ethanol in the treatment of hepatocellular carcinomas smaller than 3.0 cm, both in terms of local recurrence and 2-year survival rates [28]. These findings were attributed to a stronger necrotizing effect of acetic acid compared to ethanol, and its ability to penetrate tumoral fibrous septa and capsules. In that study, 50% acetic acid was administered in small volumes (1.8 ± 0.9 ml) during multiple treatment sessions (2.5 ± 0.9), with total volume injected for all sessions combined of 4.3 ± 2.3 ml. Liang et al. subsequently reported single high-dose PAI (4.0–10.5 ml per session of 50% acetic acid) to be both safe and effective in the treatment of small hepatocellular carcinomas [36].

9.3.1.2 Technical and Clinical Considerations

The existing medical literature describing the use of percutaneous chemical ablation in the treatment of desmoid tumors is limited to a single case series of two patients [21]. In the first case, a 26-year-old female with a recurrent 7.0-cm right superior mediastinal desmoid tumor previously treated with wide surgical resection with positive margins, postoperative external beam radiation, and multiple courses of chemotherapy presented with constant right shoulder and upper thoracic pain. CT-guided percutaneous ablation using absolute ethanol was initially attempted, during which there was resistance to insertion of the 22 G infusion needle and no more than 5 ml of ethanol could be injected. Chemical ablation with acetic acid was performed one week later using an 18 G infusion needle, during which a total of 15 ml of 50% acetic acid was injected over 15 min. The concentration and volume of acetic acid were extrapolated based on similar volumes of 50% acetic acid previously used in the percutaneous ablation of small hepatocellular carcinomas. A third session of chemical ablation was performed four weeks later, using 20 ml of 50% acetic acid. Favorable results were reported at four months clinical follow-up, with complete resolution of the patient's right shoulder pain and tumor regression to an ill-defined 2.0-cm area of soft tissue density. The patient remained asymptomatic at 36 months clinical follow-up.

In the second case, a 70-year-old female with a 7.0-cm mesenteric desmoid tumor previously treated with chemotherapy and aborted surgical resection presented with persistent abdominal pain. This patient was also treated with CT-guided percutaneous chemical ablation with acetic acid, three treatment sessions each staged four weeks apart. In the first treatment session, a total of 15 ml of 50% acetic acid was injected over 15 min using a 20 G infusion needle. Favorable results were also reported, with significant improvement in the patient's abdominal pain and diminution of tumor size to 4.5 cm at two months clinical follow-up. Contrast-enhanced CT at that time demonstrated areas of hypoattenuation and nonenhancement centrally within the mass, consistent with tumor necrosis. Stable disease was reported at 24 months clinical follow-up. No complications or adverse side effects were reported in either case.

Acetic acid offers several theoretical advantages compared to ethanol for the ablation of desmoid tumors. Desmoids are largely composed of a collagenous matrix containing sparsely populated fibroblasts and myofibroblasts [37]. Desmoid histology therefore may contribute to its susceptibility to acetic acid, as the cytotoxic effect is mediated through collagen destruction, protein denaturation, and basement membrane dissolution [38]. Also, because of its superior diffusion characteristics through tumor tissue, a smaller volume of acetic acid compared to ethanol is required to achieve the same cytotoxicity with fewer treatment sessions [28, 21]. Ohnishi et al. estimated the necrotizing capability of 50% acetic acid to be more than three times that of absolute ethanol [28]. This suggests that a similar degree of necrosis can be achieved with a smaller dose of acetic acid than absolute ethanol.

A potential disadvantage of PAI and PEI is the potential risk of nontarget tissue injury secondary to cytotoxin diffusion away from the site of delivery into adjacent soft tissues. This risk is particularly relevant in the discussion of desmoid tumor chemical ablation due to its lack of tumor capsulation, locally infiltrative nature, and tendency to encase vital neurovascular structures [21]. The smaller dose of acetic acid required to achieve necrosis improves its safety profile when compared to absolute ethanol. Careful patient selection, as well as the use of controlled, small volume injections under image guidance is necessary to mitigate the risk of nontarget ablation.

9.3.2 *Radiofrequency Ablation*

9.3.2.1 Mechanism and Rationale

Radiofrequency ablation (RFA) involves the use of high-frequency alternating current from a needle electrode into surrounding tissue, which results in frictional heating and tissue necrosis [39, 40]. RFA is based on the principle that the passage of radiofrequency waves through viable tissue causes an elevation in tissue temperature [41, 42]. This concept is also the basis for the development of the Bovie knife (Liebel Florsheim, Cincinnati, OH), used to cauterize bleeding tissue during surgery [43, 42]. Various RFA needle electrodes have been developed, which essentially combine an insulated needle shaft with a noninsulated electrode tip, thereby allowing targeted delivery of radiofrequency pulses.

Although RFA has been performed via laparscopy or laparotomy under general anesthesia, percutaneous RFA using ultrasound or CT guidance has been shown to be an effective minimally invasive alternative [44]. Imaged-guided percutaneous RFA has been reported for the treatment of hepatocellular carcinoma and hepatic metastases [42, 45–47], solid renal masses [48, 49], pulmonary neoplasms [50], and osseous lesions including bony metastases [51], osteoid osteoma [52], eosinophilic granuloma [53], chondroblastoma [54], and chordoma [55]. Imaging follow-up is typically with MRI or CT. Potential complications of RFA include bleeding, infection, tumor seeding from needle electrode placement and manipulation, pneumothorax, thermal injury to nontarget tissues, and grounding pad burns [56].

9.3.2.2 Technical and Clinical Considerations

Discussion in the medical literature of percutaneous radiofrequency ablation for the treatment of desmoid tumors is limited to a single case report and one case series. Tsz-Kan et al. initially described the use of this technique in a 47-year-old female with a history of prior resection of a lower back desmoid tumor, which recurred four months after surgery [57]. The patient was treated with radiofrequency ablation as an alternative to additional surgery or external beam radiation therapy. Under CT-guidance, eight ablations were performed via four puncture sites using a 15-G-active expandable needle electrode, with radiofrequency powers incrementally increasing from 10 to 60 W. MR imaging one day after treatment demonstrated markedly decreased postcontrast enhancement, consistent with tumor necrosis. Although there were no immediate complications at the time of RFA, an abscess developed at the site of tumor necrosis during the first week postablation, which required catheter drainage and antibiotics. Serial follow-up MR imaging demonstrated progressive diminution in tumor size; no evidence of residual tumor was seen at 28 months follow-up.

Ilaslan et al. described the use of radiofrequency ablation to treat five desmoid tumors in four patients: a 59-year-old female with recurrent desmoid tumors of the right calf and thigh following resection, reresection, and external beam radiation; a 5-year-old male subsequently diagnosed with Gardner's syndrome with a recurrent left paraspinal desmoid following excisional biopsy; a 14-year-old female with an enlarging left hip desmoid; and a 32-year-old male with a thoracic paraspinal desmoid [58]. For the latter two patients, RFA was the initial therapy selected. In the case of 14-year-old female with the left hip desmoid, the mass was embedded within the tensor fascia lata muscle, and extended into the gluteus medius and lateral abdominal wall musculature. RFA was selected rather than surgery due to the lesion's location and size, and potential functional morbidity from surgical resection. Three lesions were less than 3.0 cm and required one ablation each; the two remaining lesions were larger than 3.0 cm, and required up to four ablations each with intermittent electrode repositioning. Approximately 1–2 cm of normal adjacent tissue was included in the ablation zone. Immediate complications included superficial cellulitis in one patient, and focal soft tissue necrosis in another patient, which required surgical debridement and skin grafting. Clinical follow-up for all four patients and MR imaging follow-up for two patients demonstrated no evidence of desmoid tumor recurrence following RFA.

As with chemical ablation, careful patient selection is required for successful radiofrequency ablation. RFA should be avoided in lesions located less than 1 cm from a vital neural or visceral structure, due to the risk of thermal injury. Due to similarities in tissue density between desmoid tumors and skeletal muscle, CT guidance may obscure lesion margins when tumors are located within or adjacent to muscle. Superficial lesions are of particular concern, due to the risk of skin burns. Preoperative MRI may be helpful in this situation, as the increased soft tissue resolution may more clearly delineate tumor margins from adjacent soft tissues, and provide anatomical landmarks for CT-guided probe placement and ablation.

The greatest challenge of RFA is the inability to definitively identify ablation margins. During radiofrequency ablation, a temperature gradient is generated within the tissues surrounding an RFA probe, with an exponential decrease in tissue temperature with increasing distance from the probe [59]. The target tumor and adjacent tissues experience variations in temperature depending upon the distance from the RFA probe. Tissue density as well as proximity to adjacent vascular structures can also result in variations in tumor heating, which can greatly impact the size and shape of the ablation zone. Certain tissues demonstrate a slight decrease in attenuation on postablation noncontrast CT, but the changes are so slight that they are not a reliable indicator of complete thermal destruction of the tumor. Contrast-enhanced CT postablation can show abrogation of contrast enhancement within the tumor, which is a more reliable indicator of the ablation margin.

9.3.3 Cryoablation

9.3.3.1 Mechanism and Rationale

Cryoablation is the destruction of living tissue by freezing, performed percutaneously or surgically [60]. Percutaneous cryoablation involves the insertion of multiple modified hollow needles known as cryoprobes into a target lesion, typically under direct visualization using CT, MR, or ultrasound [61]. Alternating cycles of rapid cooling and warming of the cryoprobe tips are then performed. Rapid cooling removes heat from the adjacent tissue by conduction, and induces the formation of extracellular and intracellular ice crystals within the affected tissue [62]. These ice crystals in aggregate form an iceball, which can be directly visualized and monitored using CT, MR, or ultrasound (Fig. 9.3). Rapid warming of the cryoprobe tips induces a thawing effect in the involved tissues. Cryoablation-induced cytotoxicity is mediated through this cyclical rapid freezing and thawing, which results in a confluent coagulative necrosis with eventual fibrosis and scarring [63].

Much of the existing medical literature regarding the use of cryoablation relates to the treatment of hepatic [64], renal [63, 65], pulmonary [66], and prostate [67, 68] malignancies, as well as breast masses [69, 70] and painful osseous metastases [71]. Advantages of cryoablation compared to other heat-based thermal ablation techniques include the ability to directly visualize iceball formation and monitor the ablation zone margins in real-time, as well as the anesthetizing affect of soft tissue cooling, which results in a less painful procedure for the patient. One potential disadvantage is the intense inflammatory response which can be evoked by cryoablation [72]. In its most extreme form, this inflammatory response can precipitate cryoshock, a cytokine-mediated systemic inflammatory response syndrome characterized by hypotension, respiratory distress, multiorgan failure, and disseminated intravascular coagulation (DIC) [73–75]. Although rare, cryoshock has primarily been associated with the ablation of large volume hepatic and renal tumors [73, 76, 77].

9.3.3.2 Technical and Clinical Considerations

The existing medical literature describing the use of cryoablation for the treatment of desmoid tumors is limited to a single retrospective case series of five patients with extra-abdominal desmoids: a 9-year-old female with a painful 3.0-cm lower back desmoid that recurred following prior surgical resection and chemotherapy; a 32-year-old female with a painful 4.9-cm right scapular desmoid previously treated with chemotherapy; a 41-year-old female with a painful 6.1-cm left scapular desmoid previously treated with chemotherapy; a 21-year-old male with a history of Familial Adenomatous Polyposis (FAP) and a painful 9.1-cm chest wall desmoid that invaded several thoracic neural foramina and encased several spinal nerve roots and recurred following prior surgical resection; and an 18-year-old male with a history of FAP and a painful 10.0-cm desmoid tumor that involved the left posterior neck, supraclavicular, and axillary regions including the brachial plexus and subclavian vessels, and had failed prior surgical resection, chemotherapy, and radiation therapy [78]. The former three patients were referred for local tumor control, and complete tumor coverage with the cryoablation zones was achieved. The latter two patients were referred for palliation of pain symptoms caused by inoperable lesions which had encased major neural structures. Incomplete tumor coverage with the cryoablation zones occurred in these two cases, in order to protect the involved

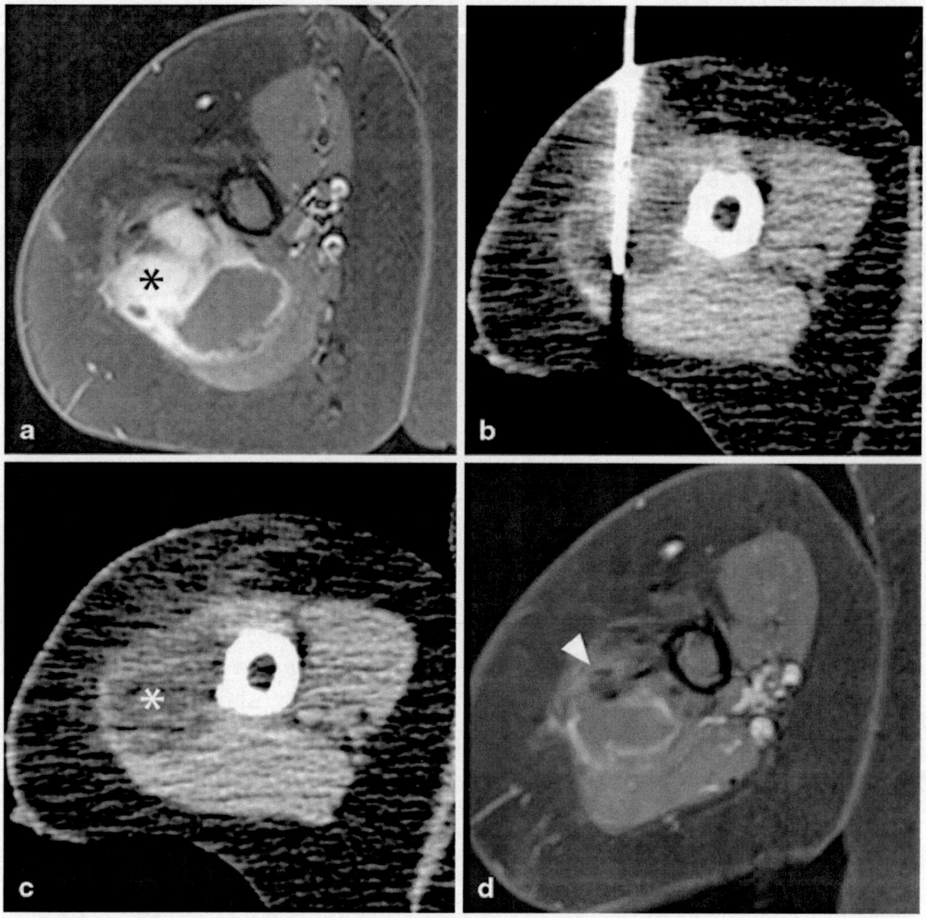

Fig. 9.3 Percutaneous cryoablation of a right upper extremity desmoid tumor in a 44-year-old female status post prior percutaneous chemical ablation. **a** Axial postcontrast T1-weighted spin echo with fat suppression demonstrates a right upper extremity desmoid tumor with lateral enhancing (*) and medial nonenhancing components, interposed between the deltoid and triceps muscles. **b** Under CT guidance, two cryoprobes have been advanced into the mass using a posterolateral approach. A 10-min freeze was performed, followed by an 8-min active thaw, followed by a second 5-min freeze. A single cryoprobe with real-time visualization of the hypodense ice ball formation is demonstrated in this image. **c** The cryoprobes have been removed, and the hypodense intratumoral ice ball remains (*). **d** Axial postcontrast T1-weighted spin echo with fat suppression following three cryoablation treatment sessions over a 12-month time interval demonstrates decrease in tumor size and enhancement (*arrowhead*)

nerves from thermal injury. No immediate complications were reported with any of the cryoablation procedures.

Favorable long-term results were reported in the three patients in whom complete tumor coverage with the ablation zones was achieved, including diminution in tumor size and pain relief; complete tumor regression was observed in two patients [78]. For the remaining two patients with FAP and neural encasement by tumor, partial pain relief was initially observed two weeks following cryoablation. At long-term follow-up however, although one lesion had decreased in size from 9.1 to 4.9 cm at 58 months, the other lesion which initially measured 10.0 cm had enlarged at 36 months with marked growth of the untreated portions in the left supraclavicular and axillary regions. Also, local pain symptoms returned to pretreatment, moderate levels for both patients. Additional cryoablation treatment sessions were not pursued in either case.

Although this was a small retrospective case series, several inferences regarding the use of percutaneous cryoablation for the treatment of desmoid tumors can be made. Cryoablation appears to be a viable alternative to surgery for local control of lesions which do not involve major neurovascular structures. For patients who have desmoid tumors that do involve major nerves or blood vessels, both surgery and cryoablation share the same limitations in terms of ability to remove or destroy sufficient tumor volume without neural or vascular injury, and achievement of long-term pain relief. In the two reported cases of patients with FAP and neural encasement by tumor, failure to achieve long-term pain relief was likely due to the incomplete treatment of those portions of tumor which involved neural structures.

9.4 Discussion

Several factors can impact both the potential success of an image-guided ablation procedure and concomitant risk of nontarget tissue injury in desmoid tumor patients. These factors include size, location, and lesion proximity to adjacent nerves, blood vessels, or visceral organs. Patients with small superficial desmoid tumors are ideal candidates for percutaneous ablation. For example, a desmoid tumor of the anterior abdominal wall rectus sheath could easily be accessed using either CT or ultrasound guidance without significant risk of damage to adjacent nontarget tissues. Larger lesions in a similar location or located superficially within the extremities away from neurovascular structures would also likely be ideal candidates for ablation, although the number of treatment sessions required is proportional to tumor volume. Lesions that are extremely superficial with respect to the skin surface can be challenging, due to the risk of cutaneous thermal injury. Several techniques can be employed during ablation to mitigate this risk, including thickening of the skin with saline injections, and warming or cooling the skin overlying the ablation site. Lesions which have eroded through the skin surface will require primary closure and should be treated surgically.

Desmoids tend to enlarge and grow laterally along fascial planes, often insinuating around nerves, blood vessels, muscles, and tendons. Desmoids intimately associated with vital neural or vascular structures such as the sciatic nerve in the lower extremity or brachial plexus in the axilla are not necessarily precluded from being ablation candidates, but selection of the appropriate ablation technique becomes more relevant of a consideration. For example, chemical ablation is considered to be far less cytotoxic than radiofrequency ablation or cryoablation. Although the lower cytoxicity of chemical ablation may be considered disadvantageous for the treatment of a large bulky extremity lesion, this factor makes chemical ablation more favorable for the treatment of a smaller desmoid tumor which abuts the sciatic nerve, brachial plexus, or other vital neural or vascular structure. With controlled injection of small aliquots of ablatant, the risk of injury to adjacent nontarget tissues can be reduced. In addition, the use of intraoperative nerve monitoring during the ablation of perineural lesions may prove useful in minimizing neural injury [72].

Larger lesions may potentially benefit from combination ablation therapies, either used in series or parallel. Of the thermal ablation techniques, radiofrequency ablation conveys a larger kill zone than cryoablation, and can be used to ablate larger tumor volumes in less time and with fewer treatment sessions. However, it can be difficult or impossible to identify the exact temperature achieved at the visualized margin during radiofrequency ablation. The ability to more accurately visualize ablation zone margins during cryoablation enables finer control over the ablation zone and flexibility in ablating portions of tumor which may come in close proximity to neurovascular structures. Potential synergies may exist in using a combination of thermal ablation techniques for difficult to treat lesions, such as a large lower extremity desmoid tumor which encroaches upon the sciatic nerve. The bulk of such a lesion could be treated with radiofrequency ablation, while cryoablation could be used to treat the perineural component, thereby mitigating the risk of nontarget vital tissue injury while capitalizing on the larger kill zone of radiofrequency ablation.

Once a lesion has encased a vital structure, complete surgical resection with negative margins is often impossible to achieve. Even with negative surgical margins, desmoid tumors have a propensity to recur [79]. For recurrent desmoid tumors which are technically resectable, a surgeon may opt to watch and wait, and consider repeat surgery only when symptoms occur or to preempt the consequence of rapid tumor growth given the relative high morbidity of surgical therapy. However, owing to the relatively low morbidity of image-guided ablation, there may also be a role for early percutaneous ablation as a therapeutic option in patients who have failed primary surgical resection and/or radiation. In this scenario, the goal of ablation is local tumor control and growth retardation, and to delay or even obviate the need for a subsequent higher morbidity surgical intervention or chemotherapy. This would represent a paradigm shift away from ablation being used predominantly as a final salvage therapy after sometimes years of surgery, radiation, and chemotherapy. This shift in treatment strategy may enable patients with recurrent desmoid tumors to avoid the potential morbidity associated with multiple surgeries or chemotherapy regimens. It has also been observed that over a period of 10–15 years, some desmoid tumors may spontaneously regress [80]. Percutaneous ablation may therefore provide a low morbidity therapeutic option that can be repeated over years to decrease tumor volume and arrest growth, until which time the desmoid "burns out" and regresses on its own.

9.5 Conclusion

Interventional radiology and interventional oncology offer several percutaneous image-guided techniques that may provide low morbidity options for the diagnosis and treatment of desmoid tumors. Core needle biopsy is an effective, accurate, and minimally invasive alternative to open surgical biopsy. Fine needle aspiration cytology can be nonspecific for the diagnosis of desmoid tumors, overlaps with other myofibroblastic lesions resulting in false positive and false negative evaluations, and may potentially fail to diagnose more aggressive malignancies, such as soft tissue sarcoma. Although the existing medical literature is limited, chemical ablation, radiofrequency ablation, and cryoablation offer additional opportunities for local tumor control, either as an adjunct to surgery, chemotherapy, and radiation, or as an alternative therapeutic option. Although prospective trials are difficult due to the rarity of this neoplasm, additional research is needed to further define the role of these techniques in the management of desmoid tumors.

References

1. Kwan SW, Kerlan RK Jr, Sunshine JH (2010) Utilization of interventional oncology treatments in the United States. J Vasc Interv Radiol 21:1054–1060
2. Mankin HJ, Lange TA, Spanier SS (1982) The hazards of biopsy in patients with malignant primary bone and soft-tissue tumors. J Bone Joint Surg Am 64:1121–1127
3. Rougraff BT, Aboulafia A, Biermann JS, Healey J (2009) Biopsy of soft tissue masses: evidence-based medicine for the musculoskeletal tumor society. Clin Orthop Relat Res 467:2783–2791
4. Gupta S, Wallace MJ, Cardella JF, Kundu S, Miller DL, Rose SC (2010) Quality improvement guidelines for percutaneous needle biopsy. J Vasc Interv Radiol 21:969–975
5. Mitsuyoshi G, Naito N, Kawai A, Kunisada T, Yoshida A, Yanai H, Dendo S, Yoshino T, Kanazawa S, Ozaki T (2006) Accurate diagnosis of musculoskeletal lesions by core needle biopsy. J Surg Oncol 94:21–27
6. Brown DB, Gonsalves CF (2008) Percutaneous biopsy before interventional oncologic therapy: current status. J Vasc Interv Radiol 19:973–979
7. Domanski HA (2007) Fine-needle aspiration cytology of soft tissue lesions: diagnostic challenges. Diagn Cytopathol 35:768–773
8. Yao L, Nelson SD, Seeger LL, Eckardt JJ, Eilber FR (1999) Primary musculoskeletal neoplasms: effectiveness of core-needle biopsy. Radiology 212:682–686
9. Adams SC, Potter BK, Pitcher DJ, Temple HT (2010) Office-based core needle biopsy of bone and soft tissue malignancies: an accurate alternative to open biopsy with infrequent complications. Clin Orthop Relat Res 468:2774–2780
10. Zaharopoulos P, Wong JY (1992) Fine-needle aspiration cytology in fibromatoses. Diagn Cytopathol 8:73–78
11. Raab SS, Silverman JF, McLeod DL, Benning TL, Geisinger KR (1993) Fine needle aspiration biopsy of fibromatoses. Acta Cytol 37:323–328
12. Powers CN, Berardo MD, Frable WJ (1994) Fine-needle aspiration biopsy: pitfalls in the diagnosis of spindle-cell lesions. Diagn Cytopathol 10:232–240; discussion 241
13. Owens CL, Sharma R, Ali SZ (2007) Deep fibromatosis (desmoid tumor): cytopathologic characteristics, clinicoradiologic features, and immunohistochemical findings on fine-needle aspiration. Cancer 111:166–172

14. Saleh H, Kapadia R (2008) Aspiration biopsy cytology of extraabdominal desmoid tumor concurrently occurring in a patient with tumoral calcinosis. Diagn Cytopathol 36:624–627
15. Dey P, Mallik MK, Gupta SK, Vasishta RK (2004) Role of fine needle aspiration cytology in the diagnosis of soft tissue tumours and tumour-like lesions. Cytopathology 15:32–37
16. Jakowski JD, Mayerson J, Wakely PE Jr (2010) Fine-needle aspiration biopsy of the distal extremities: a study of 141 cases. Am J Clin Pathol 133:224–231
17. Serpell JW, Pitcher ME (1998) Pre-operative core biopsy of soft-tissue tumours facilitates their surgical management. Aust N Z J Surg 68:345–349
18. Ray-Coquard I, Ranchere-Vince D, Thiesse P, Ghesquieres H, Biron P, Sunyach MP, Rivoire M, Lancry L, Meeus P, Sebban C, Blay JY (2003) Evaluation of core needle biopsy as a substitute to open biopsy in the diagnosis of soft-tissue masses. Eur J Cancer 39:2021–2025
19. Dalen BP, Geijer M, Kvist H, Bergh PM, Gunterberg BU (2006) Clinical and imaging observations of desmoid tumors left without treatment. Acta Orthop 77:932–937
20. Goldberg SN, Grassi CJ, Cardella JF, Charboneau JW, Dodd GD, 3rd, Dupuy DE, Gervais D, Gillams AR, Kane RA, Lee FT, Jr., Livraghi T, McGahan J, Phillips DA, Rhim H, Silverman SG (2005) Image-guided tumor ablation: standardization of terminology and reporting criteria. Radiology 235:728–739
21. Clark TW (2003) Percutaneous chemical ablation of desmoid tumors. J Vasc Interv Radiol 14:629–634
22. Livraghi T, Festi D, Monti F, Salmi A, Vettori C (1986) US-guided percutaneous alcohol injection of small hepatic and abdominal tumors. Radiology 161:309–312
23. Shiina S, Tagawa K, Unuma T, Takanashi R, Yoshiura K, Komatsu Y, Hata Y, Niwa Y, Shiratori Y, Terano A et al. (1991) Percutaneous ethanol injection therapy for hepatocellular carcinoma. A histopathologic study. Cancer 68:1524–1530
24. Bartolozzi C, Lencioni R (1996) Ethanol injection for the treatment of hepatic tumours. Eur Radiol 6:682–696
25. Miller E, Rhodes RK (1982) Preparation and characterization of the different types of collagen. In: Cunningham LW, Frederiksen DW (eds) Methods in enzymology, vol 82, structural and contractile proteins, extracellular matrix. Academic Press, New York
26. Ohnishi K, Nomura F, Ito S, Fujiwara K (1996) Prognosis of small hepatocellular carcinoma (less than 3 cm) after percutaneous acetic acid injection: study of 91 cases. Hepatology 23:994–1002
27. Timpl R, Wiedemann H, Delden VV, Furthmayr H, Kuhn K (1981) A network model for the organization of type IV collagen molecules in basement membranes. Eur J Biochem 120:203–211
28. Ohnishi K, Yoshioka H, Ito S, Fujiwara K (1998) Prospective randomized controlled trial comparing percutaneous acetic acid injection and percutaneous ethanol injection for small hepatocellular carcinoma. Hepatology 27:67–72
29. Ellman BA, Parkhill BJ, Curry TS, Marcus PB, Peters PC (1981) Ablation of renal tumors with absolute ethanol: a new technique. Radiology 141:619–626
30. Yune HY, Klatte EC, Richmond BD, Rabe FE (1982) Absolute ethanol in thrombotherapy of bleeding esophageal varices. Am J Roentgenol 138:1137–1141
31. Yune HY, O'Connor KW, Klatte EC, Olson EW, Becker GJ, Strickler SA (1985) Ethanol thrombotherapy of esophageal varices: further experience. Am J Roentgenol 144:1049–1053
32. Naar CA, Soong J, Clore F, Hawkins IF Jr (1983) Control of massive hemoptysis by bronchial artery embolization with absolute alcohol. Am J Roentgenol 140:271–272
33. Haaga JR, Kori SH, Eastwood DW, Borkowski GP (1984) Improved technique for CT-guided celiac ganglia block. Am J Roentgenol 142:1201–1204
34. Solbiati L, Giangrande A, De Pra L, Bellotti E, Cantu P, Ravetto C (1985) Percutaneous ethanol injection of parathyroid tumors under US guidance: treatment for secondary hyperparathyroidism. Radiology 155:607–610
35. Livraghi T, Torzilli G (1991) Percutaneous alcoholization of the small hepatocarcinoma. Ann Ital Chir 62:19–23
36. Liang HL, Yang CF, Pan HB, Lai KH, Cheng JS, Lo GH, Chen CK, Lai PH (2000) Small hepatocellular carcinoma: safety and efficacy of single high-dose percutaneous acetic acid injection for treatment. Radiology 214:769–774

37. Goellner JR, Soule EH (1980) Desmoid tumors. An ultrastructural study of eight cases. Hum Pathol 11:43–50
38. Clark TW, Soulen MC (2002) Chemical ablation of hepatocellular carcinoma. J Vasc Interv Radiol 13:S245–S252
39. Dupuy DE, Goldberg SN (2001) Image-guided radiofrequency tumor ablation: challenges and opportunities—part II. J Vasc Interv Radiol 12:1135–1148
40. Goldberg SN, Dupuy DE (2001) Image-guided radiofrequency tumor ablation: challenges and opportunities—part I. J Vasc Interv Radiol 12:1021–1032
41. d'Arsonval MA (1891) Action physiologique des courants alternaties. Societe de Biologie 43:283–289
42. McGahan JP, Dodd GD 3rd (2001) Radiofrequency ablation of the liver: current status. Am J Roentgenol 176:3–16
43. Cushing H (1928) Electro-surgery as an aid to the removal of intracranial tumors. Surg Gynecol Obstet 47:751–784
44. Wong J, Lee KF, Lee PS, Ho SS, Yu SC, Ng WW, Cheung YS, Tsang YY, Ling E, Lai PB (2009) Radiofrequency ablation for 110 malignant liver tumours: preliminary results on percutaneous and surgical approaches. Asian J Surg 32:13–20
45. Wood TF, Rose DM, Chung M, Allegra DP, Foshag LJ, Bilchik AJ (2000) Radiofrequency ablation of 231 unresectable hepatic tumors: indications, limitations, and complications. Ann Surg Oncol 7:593–600
46. de Baere T, Elias D, Dromain C, Din MG, Kuoch V, Ducreux M, Boige V, Lassau N, Marteau V, Lasser P, Roche A (2000) Radiofrequency ablation of 100 hepatic metastases with a mean follow-up of more than 1 year. Am J Roentgenol 175:1619–1625
47. Curley SA, Izzo F, Ellis LM, Nicolas Vauthey J, Vallone P (2000) Radiofrequency ablation of hepatocellular cancer in 110 patients with cirrhosis. Ann Surg 232:381–391
48. Gervais DA, McGovern FJ, Wood BJ, Goldberg SN, McDougal WS, Mueller PR (2000) Radio-frequency ablation of renal cell carcinoma: early clinical experience. Radiology 217:665–672
49. Mayo-Smith WW, Dupuy DE, Parikh PM, Pezzullo JA, Cronan JJ (2003) Imaging-guided percutaneous radiofrequency ablation of solid renal masses: techniques and outcomes of 38 treatment sessions in 32 consecutive patients. Am J Roentgenol 180:1503–1508
50. Dupuy DE, Zagoria RJ, Akerley W, Mayo-Smith WW, Kavanagh PV, Safran H (2000) Percutaneous radiofrequency ablation of malignancies in the lung. Am J Roentgenol 174:57–59
51. Goetz MP, Callstrom MR, Charboneau JW, Farrell MA, Maus TP, Welch TJ, Wong GY, Sloan JA, Novotny PJ, Petersen IA, Beres RA, Regge D, Capanna R, Saker MB, Gronemeyer DH, Gevargez A, Ahrar K, Choti MA, de Baere TJ, Rubin J (2004) Percutaneous image-guided radiofrequency ablation of painful metastases involving bone: a multicenter study. J Clin Oncol 22:300–306
52. Rosenthal DI, Alexander A, Rosenberg AE, Springfield D (1992) Ablation of osteoid osteomas with a percutaneously placed electrode: a new procedure. Radiology 183:29–33
53. Corby RR, Stacy GS, Peabody TD, Dixon LB (2008) Radiofrequency ablation of solitary eosinophilic granuloma of bone. Am J Roentgenol 190:1492–1494
54. Rybak LD, Rosenthal DI, Wittig JC (2009) Chondroblastoma: radiofrequency ablation--alternative to surgical resection in selected cases. Radiology 251:599–604
55. Neeman Z, Patti JW, Wood BJ (2002) Percutaneous radiofrequency ablation of chordoma. Am J Roentgenol 179:1330–1332
56. Rhim H, Dodd GD 3rd, Chintapalli KN, Wood BJ, Dupuy DE, Hvizda JL, Sewell PE, Goldberg SN (2004) Radiofrequency thermal ablation of abdominal tumors: lessons learned from complications. Radiographics 24:41–52
57. Tsz-Kan T, Man-Kwong C, Shu Shang-Jen J, Ying-Lee L, Wai Man-Wah A, Hon-Shing F (2007) Radiofrequency ablation of recurrent fibromatosis. J Vasc Interv Radiol 18:147–150
58. Ilaslan H, Schils J, Joyce M, Marks K, Sundaram M (2010) Radiofrequency ablation: another treatment option for local control of desmoid tumors. Skeletal Radiol 39:169–173
59. Hong K, Georgiades CS (2010) Radiofrequency ablation: mechanism of action and devices. J Vasc Interv Radiol 21:S179–S186

60. Hui GC, Tuncali K, Tatli S, Morrison PR, Silverman SG (2008) Comparison of percutaneous and surgical approaches to renal tumor ablation: metaanalysis of effectiveness and complication rates. J Vasc Interv Radiol 19:1311–1320
61. Goldberg SN, Grassi CJ, Cardella JF, Charboneau JW, Dodd GD 3rd, Dupuy DE, Gervais DA, Gillams AR, Kane RA, Lee FT Jr, Livraghi T, McGahan J, Phillips DA, Rhim H, Silverman SG, Solbiati L, Vogl TJ, Wood BJ, Vedantham S, Sacks D (2009) Image-guided tumor ablation: standardization of terminology and reporting criteria. J Vasc Interv Radiol 20:S377–S390
62. Erinjeri JP, Clark TW (2010) Cryoablation: mechanism of action and devices. J Vasc Interv Radiol 21:S187–S191
63. Weld KJ, Landman J (2005) Comparison of cryoablation, radiofrequency ablation and high-intensity focused ultrasound for treating small renal tumours. BJU Int 96:1224–1229
64. Callstrom MR, Charboneau JW (2008) Technologies for ablation of hepatocellular carcinoma. Gastroenterology 134:1831–1835
65. Mazaris EM, Varkarakis IM, Solomon SB (2008) Percutaneous renal cryoablation: current status. Future Oncol 4:257–269
66. McTaggart RA, Dupuy DE (2007) Thermal ablation of lung tumors. Tech Vasc Interv Radiol 10:102–113
67. Ritch CR, Katz AE (2009a) Prostate cryotherapy: current status. Curr Opin Urol 19:177–181
68. Ritch CR, Katz AE (2009b) Update on cryotherapy for localized prostate cancer. Curr Urol Rep 10:206–211
69. Littrup PJ, Freeman-Gibb L, Andea A, White M, Amerikia KC, Bouwman D, Harb T, Sakr W (2005) Cryotherapy for breast fibroadenomas. Radiology 234:63–72
70. Littrup PJ, Jallad B, Chandiwala-Mody P, D'Agostini M, Adam BA, Bouwman D (2009) Cryotherapy for breast cancer: a feasibility study without excision. J Vasc Interv Radiol 20:1329–1341
71. Callstrom MR, Atwell TD, Charboneau JW, Farrell MA, Goetz MP, Rubin J, Sloan JA, Novotny PJ, Welch TJ, Maus TP, Wong GY, Brown KJ (2006) Painful metastases involving bone: percutaneous image-guided cryoablation—prospective trial interim analysis. Radiology 241:572–580
72. Erinjeri JP, Maybody M, Avila EK, Chen X, Solomon SB (2010) Minimizing neural injury during radiofrequency ablation and cryoablation of tumors with intraprocedural nerve conduction studies. 34th Annual SIR Annual Meeting, Tampa.
73. Seifert JK, Stewart GJ, Hewitt PM, Bolton EJ, Junginger T, Morris DL (1999) Interleukin-6 and tumor necrosis factor-alpha levels following hepatic cryotherapy: association with volume and duration of freezing. World J Surg 23:1019–1026
74. Chapman WC, Debelak JP, Blackwell TS, Gainer KA, Christman JW, Pinson CW, Brigham KL, Parker RE (2000) Hepatic cryoablation-induced acute lung injury: pulmonary hemodynamic and permeability effects in a sheep model. Arch Surg 135:667–672; discussion 672–663
75. Washington K, Debelak JP, Gobbell C, Sztipanovits DR, Shyr Y, Olson S, Chapman WC (2001) Hepatic cryoablation-induced acute lung injury: histopathologic findings. J Surg Res 95:1–7
76. Seifert JK, France MP, Zhao J, Bolton EJ, Finlay I, Junginger T, Morris DL (2002) Large volume hepatic freezing: association with significant release of the cytokines interleukin-6 and tumor necrosis factor a in a rat model. World J Surg 26:1333–1341
77. Georgiades CS, Hong K, Bizzell C, Geschwind JF, Rodriguez R (2008) Safety and efficacy of CT-guided percutaneous cryoablation for renal cell carcinoma. J Vasc Interv Radiol 19:1302–1310
78. Kujak JL, Liu PT, Johnson GB, Callstrom MR (2010) Early experience with percutaneous cryoablation of extra-abdominal desmoid tumors. Skeletal Radiol 39:175–182
79. Lewis JJ, Boland PJ, Leung DH, Woodruff JM, Brennan MF (1999) The enigma of desmoid tumors. Ann Surg 229:866–872
80. Dalen BP, Meis-Kindblom JM, Sumathi VP, Ryd W, Kindblom LG (2006) Fine-needle aspiration cytology and core needle biopsy in the preoperative diagnosis of desmoid tumors. Acta Orthop 77:926–931

Part II
Special Populations with Desmoid Tumors

Chapter 10
Desmoid Disease in Familial Adenomatous Polyposis

James Church

Contents

Abstract Desmoid disease is a feature of familial adenomatous polyposis, a dominantly inherited syndrome of cancer predisposition due to germline mutations in the tumor suppressor gene *APC*. About 30% of patients with familial adenomatous polyposis develop desmoid disease, especially women, those with a family history of desmoids, those with the extracolonic manifestations of Gardner's syndrome, and those with a mutation 3′ of codon 1440. Most desmoids occur in the abdominal wall or inside the abdomen, usually developing after prophylactic colectomy. They may grow rapidly, causing pain, and bowel or ureteric obstruction. No treatment is predictably effective but options include nonsteroidal antiinflammatory drugs

J. Church (✉)
Department of Colorectal Surgery, Cleveland Clinic Foundation, Cleveland, Ohio 44143, USA
e-mail: church@ccf.org

C. Litchman (ed.), *Desmoid Tumors*,
DOI 10.1007/978-94-007-1685-8_10,

(NSAIDs), antiestrogen drugs, chemotherapy, and excision. While desmoid disease can be lethal, patients usually live in equilibrium with their disease.

Keywords Desmoid disease • Familial adenomatous polyposis

10.1 Introduction

Familial adenomatous polyposis (FAP) is a generalized growth disorder characterized clinically by over a hundred premalignant adenomatous polyps in the large intestine. It is a rare (1 in 8,000 live births), dominantly inherited syndrome, and affected patients, if untreated, will die of colorectal cancer at a young age (average age of cancer diagnosis is 39 years). Because FAP is due to a germline mutation in a tumor suppressor gene, affected patients are prone to tumors in several organs (see Table 10.1). Apart from the large intestine, the most common tumors associated with FAP are duodenal adenomas and carcinomas, and desmoid tumors. These are also the second and third commonest causes of death in FAP [1].

Desmoid tumors in FAP are different than those occurring sporadically in several ways. They are different genetically in that every cell harbors a germline mutation in *APC*, causing inappropriate activation of the Wnt/Wingless signal transduction pathway [2]. Sporadic desmoids also have inappropriate Wnt/Wingless signaling but for different reasons. Perhaps the most important difference between FAP-associated and sporadic desmoids is in the clinical presentation: the tendency of FAP-related tumors to form within the abdomen, in particular in the base of the small bowel mesentery. This location causes problems such as irresectability, enteric fistulas, and bowel obstruction. Because of the difficulty of resection, the complications associated with it, and the high local recurrence rate, medical treatment is often preferred. Unfortunately, there is no single agent that is predictably effective. The natural history of FAP-associated desmoid disease is very variable, with some patients completely untroubled by their desmoid and others dying of their disease [3]. For all these reasons, desmoid disease associated with FAP is a difficult challenge for the physicians faced with it. This chapter will address the challenge of FAP-related desmoid disease.

10.2 Genetics

FAP is caused by loss of function of a key tumor suppressor gene, *APC*. *APC* is a central part of the Wnt/Wingless signal transduction pathway that controls the expression of a series of genes important in cellular growth, division, differentiation, and death. *APC* controls cell growth by forming a complex with actin and GSK to

Table 10.1 Extracolonic manifestations of a germline *APC* mutation seen in patients with familial adenomatous polyposis

	Benign	Malignant
Duodenum	Adenoma	Adenocarcinoma
Stomach	Adenoma Fundic gland polyps	Adenocarcinoma
Pancreas	Adenoma	Adenocarcinoma
Small intestine	Adenoma	Adenocarcinoma
Musculo-aponeurotic tissue	Desmoid Disease	
Adrenal glands	Adenoma	Adenocarcinoma
Thyroid		Papillary cancer
Liver		Hepatoblastoma
Bone	Osteoma	Osteosarcoma
Skin	Epidermoid Cyst	
Teeth	Extra teeth	
Brain		Medulloblastoma

inactivate β-catenin, the protein that passes into the nucleus to activate downstream targets of the pathway. See Chap. 4 for a more detailed discussion of the *APC* gene function. When *APC* is dysfunctional, β-catenin is not inactivated and is free to pass into the nucleus and stimulate growth inappropriately by activation of its target genes. The most common cause of the dysfunction of *APC* is an inactivating mutation that almost always results in a "stop" codon producing truncated APC protein. The size of the truncated protein depends on the site of the mutation, and may result in variable phenotype. Mutations in the middle of the gene tend to be associated with severe disease while mutations at either the 5′ or 3′ end of the gene result in attenuated polyposis [4].Such genotype/phenotype associations noted with polyposis are also seen with desmoid disease. The risk of a FAP patient developing desmoids is higher the more to the right (3′ end) of the gene the mutation is located [5]. When mutations are at the extreme 3′ end of the gene, patients may just have desmoids and no colorectal polyps at all [6].

Gardner's syndrome is a particular combination of adenomatous polyposis (FAP) with certain extracolonic features such as desmoids, epidermoid cysts, osteomas (jaw and skull), and dental abnormalities [7]. Because these benign tumors tend to go together, the presence of an osteoma in a FAP patient signals a high risk of desmoids. Gardner's syndrome is associated with mutations between codons 1440 and 1900 of *APC*.

10.3 Describing Desmoid Disease in FAP

In general, 90% of FAP-related desmoid disease is either intra-abdominal or in the abdominal wall. Less than 10% is extra-abdominal, and these cases are generally those with an extremely 3′ *APC* mutation. While abdominal wall desmoids are almost always mass lesions, intra-abdominal desmoid disease in FAP is a spectrum

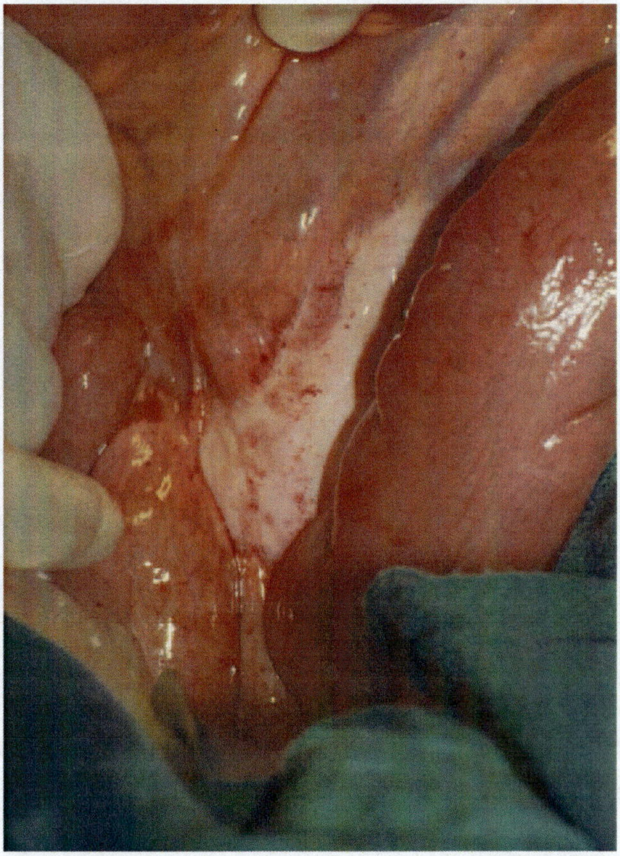

Fig. 10.1 Desmoid reaction: a sheet of hard white tissue on the small bowel mesentery that puckers and distorts adjacent bowel

of lesions ranging from flat, white sheets, or plaques (Fig. 10.1) to large, rapidly growing tumors (Figs. 10.2 and 10.3). The sheet lesions (variously called desmoid reaction or desmoid precursor lesions) are found on the small bowel mesentery or retroperitoneum. They cannot be seen (although they may be suspected) on CT scan or MRI but can still cause problems by their puckering effect on the small intestine and other structures (e.g., ureter). Their presence does not presage future trouble with desmoid tumors [8].

Desmoid tumors may reach large sizes and, when intra-abdominal, tend to occur in the root of the small bowel mesentery.

10.4 Presentation

Usually desmoid disease in FAP patients develops within 5 years of their prophylactic colectomy. The Cleveland Clinic experience shows that 3% of patients will have an unsuspected intra-abdominal desmoid at their initial surgery but 30% of patients having a second abdominal surgery have desmoid disease [8].

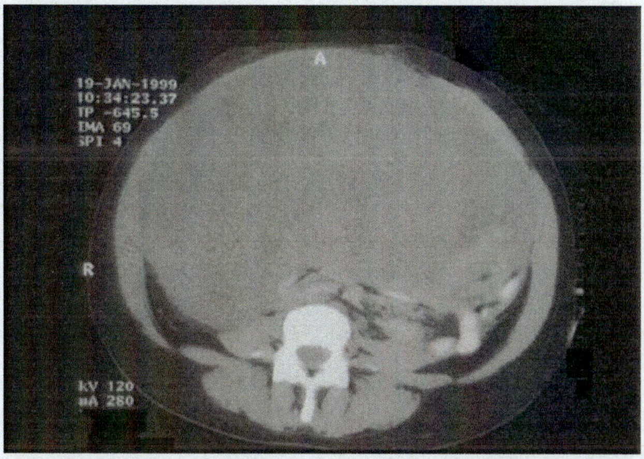

Fig. 10.2 CT scan of a large intra-abdominal tumor

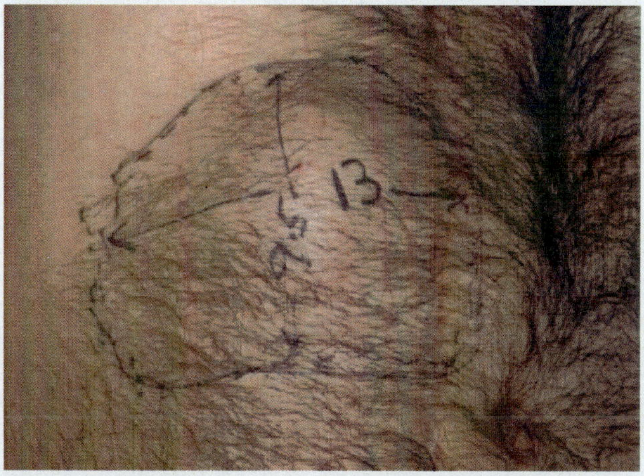

Fig. 10.3 Abdominal wall desmoid tumor

Asymptomatic desmoids are found either on CT scan or at exploratory surgery done for other reasons. Symptomatic patients may present with a mass (most common in abdominal wall desmoids), abdominal pain, and bowel or ureteric obstruction. Many patients have multiple desmoids and we categorize them according to the largest or most symptomatic, as this determines the treatment strategy.

To simplify the clinical management of desmoid disease in FAP we developed a simple staging system that has allowed us to rationalize treatment and to analyze treatment outcomes more meaningfully. This is presented in Table 10.2 [9].

Table 10.2 A staging system for intra-abdominal desmoid tumors in patients with FAP

Stage	Definition
Stage I	Asymptomatic, and <10 cm maximum diameter, and not growing
Stage II	Symptomatic, and <10 cm maximum diameter, and not growing
Stage III	Symptomatic, or bowel/ureteric obstruction, or 10–20 cm, or slowly growing
Stage IV	Severely symptomatic, fistula/hemorrhage, or >20 cm, or rapidly growing

10.5 Treatment of Desmoid Disease

Management of desmoid disease in patients with FAP is difficult. There is no treatment that can be depended upon to work, and there is little guidance in the medical literature about what to try under what circumstances. The range of options includes medical treatment, surgery, radiation, and chemotherapy. We approach the medical treatment of desmoid disease according to the stage of the tumor.

10.5.1 Medical Treatment

10.5.1.1 Stage 1

Stage 1 desmoids are small, stable, and asymptomatic. They are usually found incidentally. It is reasonable to withhold any treatment and simply observe them with a CT scan or MRI in 6 months. While they may grow and their stage may change, this is unlikely. It is also reasonable to treat stage 1 disease with a nonsteroidal, antiinflammatory agent, specifically sulindac. The dose is 150 or 200 mg twice daily. Because of the possibility of gastric irritation common to COX 1 inhibitors, the drug should be taken with food. About 20% of patients cannot tolerate sulindac. A beneficial side effect of sulindac is its effect on polyps, preventing their growth and causing regression in existing polyps in the large and small bowel.

10.5.1.2 Stage 2

Patients with stage 2 desmoids need treatment because they are symptomatic. However the tumors are still relatively small and are not growing quickly. Treatment can therefore begin with sulindac, but usually an estrogen-blocking drug is added. The choices are tamoxifen and raloxifene, both commonly used in treating breast cancer. Most recent data suggests that the tamoxifen dose should be gradually increased from 20 mg a day to 120 mg a day [10]. At this dosage level there may be headaches and menstrual disturbances, and there is increased risk for venous thrombosis. Raloxifene can be started at 120 mg per day, with a lower risk of complications [11]. Occasionally, desmoid growth seems to be encouraged by estrogen blockers.

10.5.1.3 Stage 3

Stage 3 desmoids are significantly symptomatic and need effective treatment with a shorter onset of action. Chemotherapy is the preferred option, usually beginning with the combination of methotrexate and vinorelbine. This combination is well tolerated and is often effective in stopping desmoid growth [12]. An alternative is liposomal doxorubicin (Doxil) which is also relatively well tolerated and effective [13].

10.5.1.4 Stage 4

Stage 4 desmoid disease is life-threatening and very difficult to control. Patients are generally sick from their disease and associated morbidity, such as infection, malnutrition, and chronic pain. These patients are treated with aggressive chemotherapy of the type given to patients with sarcoma (doxorubicin and dacarbazine) if they are able to tolerate it [14]. Doxil is also an option when there are no risk factors for infection. Patients with infected stage 4 desmoids are the most difficult to treat.

10.5.2 Surgery

Abdominal wall desmoid tumors should be resected early in their course when the surgery and the hole left behind are likely to be small. Asymptomatic tumors can be observed but should be treated as soon as they become symptomatic. It is usually possible to resect abdominal wall tumors with clear margins as long as they are not connected to an intra-abdominal tumor (i.e., transabdominal). Because the recurrence rate is about 33%, patients should be treated postoperatively with prophylactic sulindac.

Intra-abdominal desmoids are usually not completely resectable due to their preferred location, the root of the small bowel mesentery. Here they surround the superior mesenteric artery which is the blood supply to the entire small intestine and half of the colon. Resection of a mesenteric desmoid is therefore usually associated with the loss of small bowel. Sometimes it may be necessary to resect such large sections of small bowel that the patient remains dependent on intravenous feeding for the rest of his life [15]. Some desmoid patients have opted for a total small bowel removal with transplant. Early results of this very radical option have been good [16].

When an intra-abdominal desmoid tumor can be surgically removed the recurrence rate is about 50%, whether margins are clear or not [17]. Nonetheless, current dogma is to proceed with surgical resection when the tumor is resectable and is causing symptoms. Desmoid surgery is complicated and difficult, and often involves dealing with bowel that may be attached to the tumor. There are few studies reporting outcomes of this surgery.

10.5.3 Radiation

Desmoid disease is sensitive to radiation, and radiation can be useful where its side effects are likely to be minimal. Unfortunately the small bowel is also radiation sensitive, which means that radiation cannot be used to treat abdominal desmoids.

10.6 Complications of Abdominal Desmoids

10.6.1 Infectious

Desmoid tumors may erode into adjacent structures and cause perforation. When they erode into small bowel, the bacteria in the stool form an abscess. A fistula is created when the abscess is drained. Desmoid-related intestinal fistulas are difficult to treat because the hole in the bowel may be located in the depths of an unresectable desmoid. Patients with desmoid-related fistulas need intravenous feeding (total parenteral nutrition, TPN). Potential surgical treatments include proximal diversion with an ileostomy or jejunostomy, internal bypass, or repair with or without desmoid resection. A general rule of surgery in patients with desmoid disease is not to damage bowel if there is the possibility of a distal obstruction. The obstruction can cause perforation at the suture line.

Desmoids can also be infected without bowel involvement, such as when a desmoid tumor becomes necrotic. The liquefied tumor becomes infected and forms an abscess. Under these circumstances the abscess can be drained without development of a fistula.

10.6.2 Obstructive

Bowel obstruction is the most common complication of intra-abdominal desmoid tumors. Desmoid reaction causes obstruction by puckering adjacent bowel loops, and tumors cause obstruction by puckering and compression. The process is slow, however, and the bowel adapts to a certain extent by dilating. Thus desmoid-related obstruction is rarely acute. Treatment is surgical, by diversion, bypass, or resection. If surgery is not possible, TPN can be used while chemotherapy is given to shrink the tumor and relieve the obstruction.

Ureteric obstruction is also common, found in up to 18% of patients with intra-abdominal desmoid disease. It may present with flank pain from the obstructed kidney, or may be asymptomatic and discovered on CT. Asymptomatic ureteric obstruction, if mild, can be observed and followed. Symptomatic obstruction, or the more moderate to severe degrees of asymptomatic obstruction, is treated with urinary diversion by stent or nephrostomy. Completely obstructed kidneys can be transplanted or removed [18].

10.6.3 Erosion

Occasionally desmoids will erode through an artery or the abdominal wall. These tend to be terminal or near-terminal events. If deemed appropriate the affected arteries can be stented and penetrating tumors can be resected or radiated.

10.6.4 Interfering with Surgery

Intra-abdominal desmoids in patients with FAP may dictate the surgical strategy for treating the FAP itself. Some patients who initially had a colectomy and ileorectal anastomosis may eventually require resection of their rectums. Thirty percent of these patients have intra-abdominal desmoid disease which may prevent construction of an ileal pouch anal anastomosis, the preferred reconstruction after proctectomy. This is the case in about 15% of such patients [19].

10.7 Prevention of Desmoids

Not all patients with FAP are at a similar risk of desmoid disease. Women are more at risk than men. Patients with extra-colonic Gardner's manifestations are at increased risk, as are those with *APC* mutations 3′ of codon 1440, and especially those with a family history of desmoid disease. These factors have been combined into a desmoid risk factor (DRF) that effectively predicts desmoid risk (Table 10.3). Thus patients at high risk of desmoids may have colonic surgery deferred (as long as it is safe to do so), and may be offered different surgical options [20]. The least desmoidogenic surgery is a laparoscopic colectomy and ileorectal anastomosis (IRA), while the most desmoidogenic is a laparoscopic total proctocolectomy and ileostomy [21]. Patients at high risk of desmoid disease should have a laparoscopic IRA.

10.8 Follow-up

When treatment is active and the desmoid is unstable (changing size), follow-up is with a CT scan or MRI scan every 3–6 months. When the desmoid is stable, follow-up can be with yearly clinical examination and occasional scans. In general, about

Table 10.3 Desmoid risk factor

Factors	Points		
	1	2	3
Gender	Male		Female
Family history	–ve	1	>1 relative
Extracolonic manifestations	0	1	>1
Genotype	<1,309	<1,900	<1,900
	With genotype	Without genotype	
Low risk	<7	<6	
Medium risk	7–8	6–7	
High risk	>8	>7	

10–12% of patients with abdominal desmoids will experience disappearance of their tumor. About 7% will die from their tumor. The remaining majority of patients, about 80%, will never be desmoid free but will usually be asymptomatic or minimally symptomatic [3]. There will be times of desmoid growth, and then shrinkage. In general, desmoid disease behaves worst in young women and becomes more benign with increasing age. The desmoid tumors in women who have had children behave in a more benign fashion than in those women who have no children [22].

10.9 Conclusions

Desmoid disease is a benign manifestation of familial adenomatous polyposis that commonly presents after abdominal surgery and can cause severe symptoms due to pressure effects on intra-abdominal structures. Desmoid risk can be predicted based on gender, manifestations of the FAP, genotype and family history, and surgical strategy is predicated on the degree of risk. Treatment is based on stage but surgery is often effective, despite a high local recurrence rate.

References

1. Arvanitis ML, Jagelman DG, Fazio VW, Lavery IC, McGannon E (1990) Mortality in patients with familial adenomatous polyposis. Dis Colon Rectum 33:639–642
2. Lips DJ, Barker N, Clevers H, Hennipman A (2009) The role of APC and beta-catenin in the aetiology of aggressive fibromatosis (desmoid tumors). Eur J Surg Oncol 35(1):3–10
3. Lynch AC, Ozuner G, Church JM (2003) The clinical course of desmoid tumors in familial adenomatous polyposis. Dis Colon Rectum 46:A53
4. Bertario L, Russo A, Sala P et al. (2001) Hereditary colorectal tumours registry. Genotype and phenotype factors as determinants of desmoid tumors in patients with familial adenomatous polyposis. Int J Cancer 95:102–107
5. Eccles DM, van der Luijt R, Breukel C et al. (1996) Hereditary desmoid disease due to a frameshift mutation at codon 1924 of the APC gene. Am J Hum Genet 59:1193–1201

6. Ballhausen WG (2000) Genetic testing for familial adenomatous polyposis. Ann N Y Acad Sci 910:36–47 (Jan)
7. Kaplan BJ (1961) Gardner's syndrome: heredofamilial adenomatosis associated with "soft and hard" fibrous tumors and epidermoid cysts. Dis Colon Rectum 4:252–262
8. Hartley JE, Church JM, Gupta S, McGannon E, Fazio VW (2004) Significance of incidental desmoids identified during surgery for familial adenomatous polyposis. Dis Colon Rectum 47:334–338
9. Church J, Lynch C, Neary P, LaGuardia L, Elayi E (2008) A desmoid tumor-staging system separates patients with intra-abdominal, familial adenomatous polyposis-associated desmoid disease by behavior and prognosis. Dis Colon Rectum 51:897–901
10. Hansmann A, Adolph C, Vogel T, Unger A, Moslein G (2004) High-dose tamoxifen and sulindac as first-line treatment for desmoid tumors. Cancer 100:612–620
11. Tonelli F, Ficari F, Valanzano R, Brandi ML (2003) Treatment of desmoids and mesenteric fibromatosis in familial adenomatous polyposis with raloxifene. Tumori 89:391–396
12. Azzarelli A, Gronchi A, Bertulli R, Tesoro JD, Baratti D, Pennacchioli E, Dileo P, Rasponi A, Ferrari A, Pilotti S, Casali PG (2001) Low-dose chemotherapy with methotrexate and vinblastine for patients with advanced aggressive fibromatosis. Cancer 92(5):1259–1264
13. Bertagnolli MM, Morgan JA, Fletcher CD, Raut CP, Dileo P, Gill RR, Demetri GD, George S (2008) Multimodality treatment of mesenteric desmoid tumours. Eur J Cancer 44(16):2404–2410
14. Lynch HT, Fitzgibbons R Jr, Chong S, Cavalieri J, Lynch J, Wallace F, Patel S (1994) Use of doxorubicin and dacarbazine for the management of unresectable intra-abdominal desmoid tumors in Gardner's syndrome. Dis Colon Rectum 37:260–267
15. Middleton SB, Phillips RK (2000) Surgery for large intra-abdominal desmoid tumors: report of four cases. Dis Colon Rectum 43:1759–1762
16. Chatzipetrou MA, Tzakis AG, Pinna AD, Kato T, Misiakos EP, Tsaroucha AK, Weppler D, Ruiz P, Berho M, Fishbein T, Conn HO, Ricordi C (2001) Intestinal transplantation for the treatment of desmoid tumors associated with familial adenomatous polyposis. Surgery 129(3):277–281
17. Smith AJ, Lewis JJ, Merchant NB, Leung DH, Woodruff JM, Brennan MF (2000) Surgical management of intra-abdominal desmoid tumours. Br J Surg 87:608–613
18. Mignanelli E, Joyce M, Church J (2009) Ureteric obstruction. Dis Colon Rectum 52:811
19. Penna C, Tiret E, Parc R et al. (1993) Operation and abdominal desmoid tumors in familial adenomatous polyposis. Surg Gynecol Obstet 177:263–268
20. Elayi E, Manilich E, Church J (2008) Polishing the crystal ball: knowing genotype improves ability to predict desmoid disease. Dis Colon Rectum 51:802–803
21. Vogel J, Church JM, LaGuardia L (2005) Minimally invasive pouch surgery predisposes to desmoid tumor formation in patients with familial adenomatous polyposis. Dis Colon Rectum 48:662
22. Church JM, McGannon E (2000) Prior pregnancy ameliorates the course of intra-abdominal desmoid tumors in patients with familial adenomatous polyposis. Dis Colon Rectum 43:445–450

Chapter 11
Desmoid Tumor in Children and Adolescents: The Influence of Age

Aaron R. Weiss, Anthony Montag and Stephen X. Skapek

Contents

Abstract Desmoid tumor is a soft tissue neoplasm that can occur in children as well as adults. Formally classified as an intermediate-grade neoplasm, it is known to have a locally invasive growth that can lead to severe and sometimes life-threatening problems. The historical standards of therapy for desmoid tumor center on surgical resection, with or without radiation therapy. However, depending on the site or size of the disease, surgical resection may substantially compromise form

S. X. Skapek (✉)
Department of Pediatrics, Section of Hematology/Oncology and Stem Cell Transplantation, The University of Chicago, Chicago, 60637 IL, USA
e-mail: sskapek@peds.bsd.uchicago.edu

C. Litchman (ed.), *Desmoid Tumors*,
DOI 10.1007/978-94-007-1685-8_11, © Springer Science+Business Media B.V. 2012

or function, making its use especially problematic in children who may be physically and psychologically immature. Further, there is some evidence that radiation is less effective against desmoid tumor in children, as compared to adults with this disease. As such, the treatment of a child with desmoid tumor may present unique problems. In this chapter, we review the pathology, biology, clinical presentation, and treatment of children with desmoid tumor as we highlight the similarities and differences from desmoid tumor in adults.

Keywords Childhood fibromatoses • Juvenile desmoid tumor • Clinical trials • Chemotherapy

11.1 Introduction

The nomenclature of fibroblastic lesions in childhood is somewhat confusing and has changed over the last several decades. The larger category of fibromatoses in childhood includes such benign lesions as infantile digital fibromatosis, fibrous hamartoma of infancy, and fibromatosis coli [14] as well as a more aggressive entity variously described as aggressive fibromatosis, infantile fibromatosis, and deep fibromatosis (desmoid tumor) [20]. More recently, infantile fibromatosis has been recognized to include lipofibromatosis, which occurs in young children and has a less mature fibroblastic phenotype, and a desmoid-type fibromatosis which is the childhood counterpart to adult-type fibromatosis [58, 85]. Throughout this chapter, we focus our discussion on the latter neoplasm which we refer to as "desmoid tumor".

Much of our understanding of pediatric desmoid tumor is extrapolated from the adult literature because of the rarity of the neoplasm in children and the paucity of large, pediatric series. For this reason, it has been widely accepted that desmoid tumor in children and adults shares more similarities than differences; thus, pediatric-specific management guidelines are not well-established. Here we review the current knowledge regarding the epidemiology, pathophysiology, clinical characteristics, management, and outcome of desmoid tumor in childhood and adolescence. We focus on the biology and phenotypes that are distinct from the adult form of the disease, and we conclude with statements regarding how therapy of children with desmoid tumor may differ from adults with the disease.

11.2 Epidemiology

Desmoid tumor in childhood is extremely rare, representing less than 0.1% of all cancers. The overall incidence of desmoid tumor in all age groups is estimated to be two to four new diagnoses per one million people per year [2, 36, 54]. However, the specific incidence in children is difficult to ascertain due to the paucity of pediatric series. Even the largest series only involve 60–90 children [24, 51]. As will be discussed further below (Sect. 11.3), most children with desmoid tumor appear to have a sporadic form of the disease with no known predisposing factors. Desmoid tumor incidence peaks in individuals from 6 to 15 years of age, and again between puberty and 40 years of age in women [28, 67]. Recent studies in children have suggested a slight male predominance [10, 51], although there may be a female predominance during adolescence [21].

There is some evidence that age at presentation varies with tumors in certain anatomic sites. For example, Buitendijk et al. reviewed published series and showed that the median age at presentation was 3.6 years (range, 0.2–9.9 years) in children with head and neck involvement, while the median age at presentation was 7.8 years (range, birth–15.7 years) in children with desmoid tumor of the trunk or extremity [10]. This finding has been corroborated in other retrospective reports [5, 71, 77].

11.3 Etiology

Much of the information regarding desmoid tumor etiology has been gleaned from relatively small series in children. Nonetheless, certain clinical associations provide some insight into disease biology and pathogenesis.

11.3.1 FAP and Gardner's Syndrome

Perhaps the best described conditions predisposing children (and adults) to desmoid tumor are the clinical syndromes of familial adenomatous polyposis (FAP) and Gardner's syndrome. See Chap. 10 for a more detailed discussion on FAP. Additionally, the average age at diagnosis of desmoid tumor is younger in FAP compared to non-FAP patients (mean, 36 years vs. 42 years) [57].

Sporadic desmoid tumor is much more common in children than FAP/Gardner's syndrome-associated disease. However, desmoid tumor diagnosis can sometimes precede the diagnosis of these syndromes [12, 30]. Gardner's syndrome or FAP has been uncovered in 1–5% of cases of seemingly sporadic desmoid tumor [42, 67]. In two of the larger pediatric series, Gardner's syndrome was reported to occur in 2 of 63 (3%) patients and 2 of 28 (7%) patients [21, 74]. In the latter series, which was a prospective clinical trial, the diagnosis of Gardner's syndrome was based on self-reported history; systematic genetic testing was not performed on all study subjects [74]. As such, these numbers might underestimate the incidence of Gardner's syndrome. In another pediatric series, Meazza et al. analyzed 94 children with desmoid tumor and found that three of the seven with abdominal tumors had Gardner's syndrome [51].

Gardner-associated fibroma (GAF) closely resembles desmoid tumor and may represent a less aggressive form or precursor to desmoid tumor [83]. Thus, the identification of GAF should alert physicians to the possibility of an underlying Gardner's syndrome and to the higher risk of developing classical desmoid tumor.

11.3.2 Adenomatosis Polyposis Coli and β-Catenin

Mutations of the *APC* gene are clearly implicated in desmoid tumor pathogenesis in cases of familial disease. *APC* gene mutations impair the ability of the *APC* protein to restrain β-catenin. With *APC* mutation, β-catenin protein is found in the nucleus, where it indirectly fosters cellular proliferation. Over the last 10 years, it has become increasingly clear that somatic mutations in *APC*, which activate β-catenin, as well as activating mutations in the β-catenin gene itself, are found in sporadic cases of desmoid tumor. Refer to Chap. 4 for a more detailed discussion of the *APC* gene and β-catenin.

APC mutations are found in some sporadic desmoid cases [3, 54, 80]; the relative importance of this in children versus adults is not clear due to relatively limited study. One series with a small number of children compared 16 sporadic desmoids to 4 FAP-associated tumors. Germ-line *APC* mutations were noted in 0 of 16 sporadic cases and 4 of the familial cases [32]. However, somatic *APC* mutations were noted in 12.5% of the sporadic tumors; this finding indicates that at least some sporadic desmoid tumors are still driven by *APC* deregulation in non-germ-line cells. Although none of the somatic *APC* mutations were found in children, the ability to detect such mutations is compromised by the small number of cases tested.

Activation of β-catenin function by somatic mutation of the β-catenin gene seems to be relatively common, even in children. Sharma et al. examined ten patients ranging in age from 12 months to 14 years with desmoid tumor of the head and neck [71]. Tumor specimens from 4 of those 10 displayed β-catenin expression in the nucleus, which is a surrogate marker for β-catenin activation.

Larger studies involving children and adults, however, suggest that β-catenin expression and mutations are quite common. Lazar et al. analyzed tissue from 138 patients (with a median age of 32 years and range from 0.2–78) with sporadic desmoid tumor for β-catenin immunohistochemical staining and mutations [43]. A mutation in exon 3 of the *β-catenin* gene was seen in 85% of cases; nearly all tumors had evidence for nuclear and cytoplasmic staining of β-catenin. Importantly, no mutations were found in the adjacent normal tissue. While males were more likely to harbor a mutation than females, no association was found with age at diagnosis, tumor site, and tumor size. Only three different point mutations were identified. They resulted in the following amino acid substitutions: T41A, S45F, and S45P. Mutations leading to S45F resulted in a statistically significant inferior recurrence-free survival compared to the T41A mutation types and wild type (23% vs. 57% vs. 65%, respectively). Upon multivariate analysis only young age and presence of the S45F codon were significant predictors of time to recurrence. The same mutations were observed in a second series of 76 desmoid tumors [4]. Samples from children and adults were included but not separated for analysis.

11.3.3 Trauma

Local trauma has long been recognized to precede the development of desmoid tumor in approximately 20% of cases in children [5, 21, 64]. This association includes abdominal desmoid tumors arising following surgical trauma in the same region [67], and typically occurs within 5 years of the surgery [13]. Although a cause–effect relationship is not firmly established, the association has suggested an underlying defect in connective tissue regulation during wound healing [13, 21]. Desmoid tumor recurrence following surgery is not absolute, though. For example, in a prospective chemotherapeutic trial of almost 30 children with this disease, nearly all enrolled patients had a central venous catheter placed for chemotherapy administration [74]. However, no child developed a desmoid tumor at the site of surgical trauma over several years of follow-up (Skapek, unpublished experience).

11.3.4 Hormonal Influence

The potential role that hormones play in desmoid tumor pathogenesis has been well described [48, 60, 67, 70, 87]. The influence in children with desmoid tumor has not been as well-studied. A series of 27 desmoid tumors were analyzed for estrogen, progesterone, and androgen receptor expression utilizing immunohistochemical staining. The series included tumors from 7 adolescents and 20 adults [41]. Estrogen, progesterone, and androgen receptors were positive in 2/27 (7%), 8/27 (30%), and 14/27 (50%), respectively. The frequency of receptor expression in the adolescent subset was similar to the adult subset. Other series evaluating the expression of these hormone receptors in children include too few samples to confidently draw conclusions [10, 41].

11.4 Pathology

11.4.1 Histology

The WHO classifies desmoid-type fibromatosis as a benign neoplasm with a propensity for locally invasive growth and local disease recurrence, but without the ability to metastasize. The pathologic diagnosis of desmoid tumor in children is still mostly based on the histologic appearance, which closely resembles that of adults [4]. In contrast to most sarcomas, which typically are separated from surrounding tissue by a pseudocapsule, desmoid tumors have an infiltrating border. Grossly, desmoid tumors are firm, reflecting the large amount of collagen present, in contrast to the soft "fish flesh" consistency of most sarcomas. Histologically, interlacing bundles of long thin spindle cells with uniform pointed nuclei are separated by variable amounts of collagen (Fig. 11.1). The parallel arrangement of the nuclei within

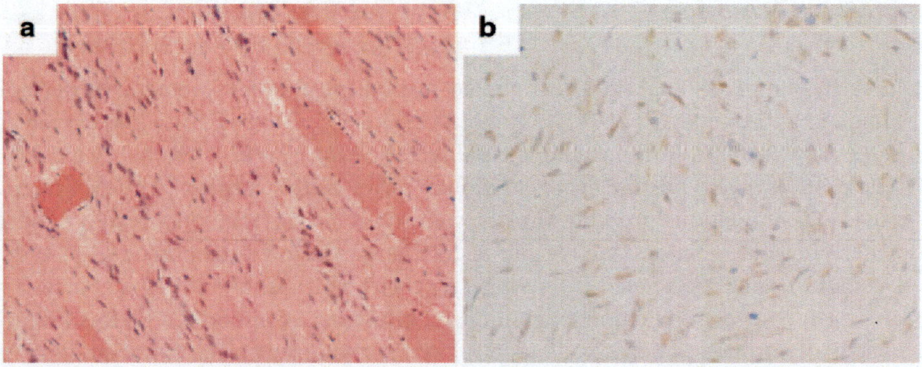

Fig. 11.1 **a** Desmoid-type fibromatosis infiltrating skeletal muscle. Note the low cellularity, pointed fibroblast nuclei and abundant collagen. H&E 200x. **b** Desmoid-type fibromatosis, beta-catenin immunostain. Note nuclear positivity in the fibroblastic spindle cells. Beta-catenin immunostain 400x

a bundle and the amount of collagen resemble tendon or fascia. Mitotic activity is sparse and necrosis is absent. Pediatric desmoid tumors have several differences from their adult counterparts. Higher mitotic rates have been demonstrated in childhood tumors compared to adults [5]. Lesions in children 2 years and older tend to be more cellular [64], and the percentage of tumor cellularity in children has been suggested to be inversely proportional to collagen deposition [13]. Calcification and ossification may be seen in pediatric cases, but rarely in adults [85].

The non-desmoid type of infantile fibromatosis has a variable histologic appearance but in general has a more polygonal and less mature appearing fibroblastic cell type and a less collagenous, frequently more myxoid, matrix. When fat differentiation is a component, the term lipofibromatosis is used. At times, the cellularity may overlap with that of infantile fibrosarcoma, although the latter typically has increased mitotic activity and necrosis is absent. No histologic features, other than positive margins at excision, reliably predict the risk of recurrence for either the desmoid or non-desmoid types of infantile fibromatosis [85].

11.4.2 Immunohistochemistry

Desmoid tumors have a myofibroblastic phenotype, and stain for vimentin, muscle-specific actin, and smooth muscle actin, but lack more specific smooth muscle markers such as desmin and caldesmon. Nuclear immunostaining for β-catenin is observed in approximately 80% of adult [11] and 42% of pediatric desmoid tumors (Fig. 11.1) [81]. Although β-catenin staining is supportive of a diagnosis of fibromatosis, it is seen in other fibroblastic soft tissue tumors including low-grade myofibroblastic sarcoma, superficial fibromatosis, and solitary fibrous tumors [11].

Expression of the tumor suppressor protein, p53, has been reported in desmoid tumor patients [24, 33]. However, there are conflicting reports as to its prognostic significance and actual p53 mutations appear to be rare in fibromatosis [56].

11.4.3 Cytogenetics

Cytogenetic abnormalities in desmoid tumors have not been widely studied, especially in the pediatric population. In the largest analysis performed, De Wever et al. studied 78 cases of fibromatosis, including 27 desmoid tumors, and found a number of cytogenetic abnormalities [16]. The most common findings were trisomies of 8 and 20 and loss of 5q. Interestingly, only 1 of 8 childhood tumors revealed cytogenetic abnormalities compared to 12 of 19 adult tumors. But this is not sufficient evidence to conclude that desmoid tumor in children is molecularly distinct from histologically similar tumors in adults.

11.5 Natural History

The clinical behavior of desmoid tumor is somewhat unpredictable in both the pediatric and adult population. While the majority of tumors will progress and require some form of therapy, some remain stable and a few have been noted to spontaneously regress [34, 68]. As in adults, desmoid tumors in children do not show evidence of metastasis or regional lymph node spread. However, multifocal desmoid tumors have been reported in children, even in the absence of Gardner's syndrome [50, 77, 86]. Mortality from desmoid tumor, though rare, has also been reported in children [51, 85].

11.6 Imaging

Desmoid tumor can be imaged by a variety of different techniques which offer relative advantages or disadvantages. Refer to Chap. 5 for a more complete discussion of imaging techniques. Magnetic resonance imaging (MRI) is generally agreed upon as the best imaging modality in children with desmoid tumor [1, 19, 40, 49]. It can provide excellent definition of soft tissue anatomy and does not involve ionizing radiation.

In the largest pediatric series reviewing MRI and biologic behavior of desmoid tumors, images from 17 children, ages 2 months to 19 years, were analyzed retrospectively [49]. Baseline imaging prior to any therapy was available for ten patients. Nine of the ten primary tumors were isointense to muscle on T1-weighted images, while T2-weighted and STIR images showed mostly high signal intensity.

Contrast enhancement was intense in the majority of the primary tumors. Most tumors displayed enhancement of 80% or more of the tumor volume. McCarville et al. attempted to correlate tumor imaging features with clinical outcome. Involvement of the neurovascular bundle approached significance ($p=0.08$) as a predictor of the presence of residual or recurrent tumor in that four patients with it had gross residual or recurrent tumor following surgical resection. None of the other imaging parameters was a significant predictor of the likelihood of recurrent or residual disease. Further, imaging features did not correlate with the age of the patient.

With respect to therapy-induced signal characteristics, the findings were somewhat variable [49]. All three patients who underwent radiation therapy following surgery had a decrease in the percentage of tumor with hyperintense signal features on T2-weighted or STIR images. MRI features during chemotherapy were evaluated in eight children. While six tumors revealed a decrease in tumor volume, changes in (a) hyperintensity on T2-weighted or STIR images, (b) tumor enhancement, and (c) intensity of enhancement were not consistent.

Attempts were made to correlate changes in MRI features with tumor histology [49]. The tumor with the lowest cellularity and most abundant collagen on histopathologic review had the least enhancement on MRI and less hyperintensity to muscle on T2-weighted and STIR images. In the tumor with the greatest cellularity and rare bands of collagen, the majority of the tumor volume enhanced and displayed increased hyperintensity to muscle on T2- weighted and STIR images. Although tumor margins ranged from sharply defined to infiltrative, margin appearance on MRI did not portend residual or recurrent disease.

Skapek and others retrospectively reviewed imaging characteristics of children treated with systemic chemotherapy [73]. During stable disease, the lesions typically maintained size and MRI imaging characteristics. Some tumors treated prior to surgery with chemotherapy had MRI signal changes suggesting that they became more hypocellular with increased collagen and fibrosis content. These histologic changes were associated with MRI imaging signal changes, with more regions of low signal intensity on T2-weighted sequences [40, 73]. Continued changes in MRI characteristics, suggestive of gradual fibrosis and decreased cellularity, have been demonstrated in a patient even after therapy has been stopped. This patient had no progression of disease 3 years from stopping therapy. Despite this anecdote, it should be noted that similar correlations were not consistently found in the above-mentioned series by McCarville et al. In a separate series, neither MRI signal intensity nor contrast enhancement correlated with tumor behavior, including disease recurrence [69].

11.7 Clinical Presentation

Despite the fact that symptoms may be useful to guide therapeutic decisions for children with desmoid tumor, there is relatively little data formally assessing the presenting symptoms. Those most commonly reported include tumor mass, swelling, pain, weakness, decreased mobility, paresthesia and other neurologic dysfunction, and torticollis. Symptoms may have ranged from days to years prior to diagnosis [71, 73, 74, 77].

Common sites of disease presentation can vary based upon age. While one-third to half of adults typically present with tumors in the abdomen [16, 51, 73], the majority of children and adolescents present with extra-abdominal disease [24, 57, 73]. Infants and young children have a higher propensity toward tumors in head and neck region [5, 24, 57], an uncommon site of disease in adults.

11.8 Management

Multidisciplinary evaluation and treatment is needed to delineate the optimal approach for treating children with desmoid tumor. As in adults, therapeutic options include surgery, radiation therapy, and the use of cytotoxic and noncytotoxic chemotherapy, or a combination of these modalities. While many of the principles are the same in children and adults, some differences relate to the ongoing growth and development of children and potential differences in disease biology.

11.8.1 Surgery

The completeness of initial surgical resection is the most important factor influencing event-free survival following surgery in children with this disease. Disease control after a less than complete surgical resection is the same as that achieved after an intralesional surgery or biopsy [51]. Although there is some variation depending on site of disease, recurrence-free probability at 3 years approximates 15% for patients with positive surgical margins and 70% for those with negative surgical margins in both children and adults [10, 21]. The goals of achieving a complete resection in children, however, must be weighed against complex and sometimes competing issues regarding the child's ongoing growth and physical, cognitive, and emotional development. In this population, multidisciplinary approaches are particularly important for tumors adjacent to or surrounding vital structures.

11.8.2 Radiation

Radiation therapy used in conjunction with surgery has been shown by some investigators to provide better local control, long-term disease stabilization, and preserved function for desmoid tumor in adults [37, 72, 89]. Most agree that effective treatment requires doses of at least 50 Gy [39, 76, 79]. As such, there has been some reluctance to incorporate radiation into the therapy of desmoid tumor in children, especially when disease is localized to challenging anatomic sites such as adjacent to growing bones or joints. Much of the data regarding the use of radiation in children comes from relatively small, retrospective studies.

Merchant et al. retrospectively reviewed cases of 13 children with desmoid tumor treated at St. Jude Children's Research Hospital [53]. Five received radiation therapy immediately following diagnosis. The remaining eight patients received radiation therapy following local recurrence. The median dose to the primary site using external beam radiation was 50 Gy (range, 32–50 Gy). Tumor recurred following radiation therapy in 11 of the 13 patients. The median progression-free survival measured from time of radiation was 19 months (range, 3–135 months). Five of the 13 patients received radiation doses below 50 Gy. The two patients who maintained local control received 50.4 Gy and 56 Gy. Three patients died of disease, and significant morbidity was noted in those surviving. As a result, Merchant et al. concluded that the role of radiation therapy in the primary management of children with desmoid tumor should be reconsidered.

In seeming contrast, several retrospective studies reported somewhat more promising findings. Fourteen of 21 patients were treated with radiation therapy (doses ranged from 50–60 Gy) [36]. Only two of seven patients had local tumor recurrence if they were treated with a gross total resection and had negative margins or positive margins that were radiated. Conversely, 13 of 14 children with other primary treatments failed locally. Similarly, three of the four children receiving adjuvant radiation therapy following gross total resection with positive margins were free of disease as compared to only one of seven children who did not receive radiation in this setting. Findings in this report are similar to those reported in a series of 63 pediatric desmoid cases [21]. Of 11 patients treated with radiation therapy, only four developed recurrent tumor by 3 years follow-up. Of note, tumor recurred in two of the five patients who received doses ≥ 50 Gy.

Radiation therapy is not without risk, particularly in growing children. Postradiation bone fractures, skeletal, and soft tissue growth retardation, tissue fibrosis and/or lymphedema have been noted [51, 53]. Jabbari et al. noted morbidity attributed to radiation in 5 of the 14 patients; this included the development of a papillary thyroid cancer, peripheral neuropathy, pain, and bowel obstruction [36]. Hence, the potential benefits of radiation therapy, even in the context of treating minimal residual disease, must be weighed against the potential adverse effects.

11.8.3 Medical Therapy

Much of what is known about chemotherapy in children with desmoid-type fibromatosis stems from small, single institution, retrospective analyses. Chemotherapy has often been applied in settings where the site or extent of disease makes standard approaches using surgery or ionizing radiation less appealing. For simplicity, we consider the published studies in three groups: cytotoxic chemotherapy, noncytotoxic chemotherapy, and targeted agents.

11.8.3.1 Cytotoxic Chemotherapy

The combination of vinblastine and methotrexate is probably the most widely used systemic therapy for desmoid tumor in children. The combination was first described in eight adults with desmoid tumor [84]. Four of the eight patients had a reduction in tumor size and two additional patients had complete tumor regression. Two retrospective studies were reported by Reich et al. [65] and Skapek et al. [73]. Both series provide anecdotal evidence that "re-treatment" is possible following disease progression after an initial course of vinblastine and methotrexate is discontinued.

To more formally address the combination in the treatment of desmoid tumor in children, the Pediatric Oncology Group (POG) conducted the first, prospective, multiinstitutional trial in children (P9650) [74]. The 26 enrolled patients were less than 19 years old and had primary disease that was deemed unresectable or recurrent disease; vinblastine and methotrexate were administered weekly for 6 months and every other week for an additional 6 months. A measureable response was documented in eight patients while ten patients demonstrated stable disease. Eight additional patients had progressive disease as their best response; as such, approximately two thirds of the patients seemed to derive some benefit from the therapy. Approximately 40% of the children with stable disease remained free of progression at a median of 50 months (range, 33–71 months) after treatment. In the whole group, though, the 1-year progression-free survival was only 58%; the median time to disease progression was 15.9 months (range, 7–35 months) after therapy was stopped. Further, 66% of subjects experienced NCI CTCAE grade 3 or 4 toxicity. This included nausea, vomiting, elevated hepatic transaminases, myelosuppression, and mucositis.

A number of other types of "cytotoxic" therapies have been reported in smaller, retrospective series, some of which included children (Table 11.1). These include vincristine, actinomycin, and cyclophosphamide (VAC) [5, 10, 17, 21, 23, 51, 63, 77, 78, 88]; dacarbazine [27, 51, 59]; dacarbazine with doxorubicin [25]; liposomal doxorubicin [15, 82]; and hydroxyurea [6, 51, 62]. The reported use of doxorubicin and dacarbazine, each given by 96 hour continuous infusion and followed by meloxicam, is particularly intriguing because three of seven patients had complete responses [25]. The relative efficacy of any of these chemotherapeutic approaches is impossible to judge because of the small numbers of patients. However, the potential acute and late effects associated with individual regimens are well-established, even in the pediatric age group.

11.8.3.2 Noncytotoxic Therapy

Several types of noncytotoxic chemotherapeutic approaches have been described for children with desmoid tumor. As was mentioned above, nearly all of the information in children comes from individual cases or very small, retrospective series.

The most widely advocated noncytotoxic approach centers on the use of estrogen antagonists or nonsteroidal antiinflammatory agents, singly or in combination, with

Table 11.1 Series involving children and adolescents with desmoid tumor treated with cytotoxic chemotherapy

Author	Number of patients (No. received chemotherapy)	Age range	Primary/ Recurrent	Chemotherapy	Responses	Follow-up
Goepfert et al. 1982	5 (5)	2 months–4 years	NR	DOX+DTIC	2 CR, 3 PR	NR
Ayala et al. 1986	25 (8)	0–15 years	25/0	DOX+DTIC, VAC	7 PR, 1 SD	2 months–25 years
Delepine et al. 1987	6 (6)	13–23 years	6/0	VAC	2 PR	NR
Raney et al. 1987	6 (6)	3 months–7 years	2/4	VAC	4 CR, 1 PR	1–11 years
Faulkner et al. 1995	63 (6)	0–19 years	3/3	VAC (2) IE (1) AMSA (1) VA, VBL (1) VC, 5-FU, MTX, MH (1)	1 PR 1 PR 1 PR 	1–5 years
Skapek et al. 1998	10 (10)	6–18 years	2/8	VBL/MTX	3 CR, 2 PR, 3 SD, 2 PD	5–37 months
Reich et al. 1999	5 (5)	7–17 years	0/5	VBL/MTX	2 CR, 1 PR, 1 MR, 1 SD	7–76 months
Skapek et al. 2007	27 (27)	7 months–20 years	11/16	VBL/MTX	1 CR, 4 PR, 3 MR, 10 SD, 8 PD	2 months–6 years
Balamuth et al. 2008	18 (18)	1–20 years	NR	HU	8 CR/PR, 7 SD, 3 PD	0–3 years
Constantinidou et al. 2009	11 (11)	3–53 years	0/11	PEG DOX	4 PR, 7 SD	7–39 months
Meazza et al. 2010	94 (45)	1 months–21 years	15/30	VNR/VBL, MTX (19) IVA-VAIA-VAC, DTIC (15) Hormonal, Antiinflammatory (11)	1 CR, 9 PR, 1 MR, 8 SD 2 CR, 5 PR, 6 SD, 2 PD 2 PR, 2 MR, 3 SD, 4 PD	9 months–35 years

DOX doxorubicin, *DTIC* dacarbazine, *VAC* vincristine, actinomycin, and cyclophosphamide, *IE* ifosfamide and etoposide, *AMSA* Amsacrine, *VA* vincristine and actinomycin, *VBL* vinblastine, *VC* vincristine and cyclophosphamide, *5-FU* 5-fluorouracil, *MTX* methotrexate, *MH* methylhydrazine, *HU* hydroxyurea, *PEG DOX* pegylated liposomal doxorubicin, *VNB* Vinorelbine, *IVA* ifosfamide, vincristine, and actinomycin, *VAIA* vincristine, actinomycin, ifosfamide, and doxorubicin, *CR* complete response, *PR* partial response, *MR* marginal response, *SD* stable disease, *PD* progressive disease, *NR* not reported most reports representing adult series that may have included some pediatric patients [8, 31, 41, 55]. Tamoxifen, an estrogen receptor antagonist, has been the most utilized hormonal therapy. Sulindac and diclofenac have been the most common nonsteroidal antiinflammatory drugs studied. Responses in those patients ranged from stable disease to partial response. Correlations among antiestrogen receptor positive and response to antiestrogen therapy have not been clearly demonstrated, especially in the pediatric age group [41]. To more definitively evaluate the benefit of antihormonal and NSAID in children with desmoid tumor, the Children's Oncology Group (COG) conducted a phase II clinical trial (ARST0321) in a patient population similar to that studied in the aforementioned P9650 study. The ARST0321 study was designed to test the efficacy of high-dose tamoxifen and sulindac, each administered orally for up to 1 year. The study closed to accrual in May 2009 and formal data analysis is ongoing. Acute toxicity, although different from P9650, was not insignificant and was perhaps most notable for the development of large ovarian cysts in a subset of the adolescent girls enrolled on the study (SX Skapek, unpublished data from COG Statistics and Data Center).

Interferon-alpha (IFN-α) has been used for the treatment of desmoid tumor. The largest study to date involved 13 patients [45]. Of those, only two were children. One patient received the medication following surgical resection to prevent recurrence and had no evidence of disease at 10 months of follow-up. The other patient received the medication to stabilize progressive disease. This resulted in stable disease at 31 months posttherapy. No other studies involving the use of IFN-α have been performed in children.

11.8.3.3 Targeted Therapy

Data on targeted therapy for desmoid tumor in children is particularly limited. Conceptually, imatinib, a tyrosine kinase inhibitor targeting PDGFR-α, PDGFR-β, and c-*kit*, could be effective in desmoid tumors which express at least some of these target proteins [32]. The largest published study of patients treated with imatinib involved 19 patients, with only two being children [32]. Those two patients demonstrated stable disease for 245 and 615 days following treatment but the disease ultimately progressed in both.

11.8.4 Observation

The concept of watchful waiting as initial "therapy" for desmoid tumor, based on the long-standing observations that desmoid tumor can remain stable for an extended period [68], has found increasing advocacy recently [9, 22]. For example, Bonvalot et al. showed that 3-year event-free survival was similar in patients treated with surgery, medical therapy, or observation only [9]. In another series, which unfortunately excluded children less than 15 years of age, progression-free survival was similar up to 5 years from diagnosis regardless of whether medical therapy or no therapy was given [22]. It should be noted that close to 50% of the patients had progressive disease during the follow-up period. Hence, having more effective therapy may make the expectant management less appealing.

Relatively little is known about the usefulness of expectant management of desmoid tumor in children. A few reports have described stable to regressive disease in children within the setting of either primary or recurrent disease. One report described an infant with desmoid tumor who experienced a spontaneous regression of a primary desmoid tumor without any therapy [34]. Another described an adolescent who demonstrated spontaneous continued tumor regression of a recurrent tumor at 29 months follow-up [47].

11.9 Outcome

Due to the extremely low rate of mortality in children with desmoid tumor, most studies have focused on progression-free survival and recurrence rates as outcome measures. As discussed in detail above, recurrence rate after surgery depends largely on whether the tumor has been completely excised [7, 10, 18, 21]. The association of disease recurrence with margin status seems to be relevant for children on whom surgery is performed for newly diagnosed and locally recurrent disease [21].

Beyond margin status, disease recurrence has also been linked to other clinical, pathology, and molecular variables. Two retrospective series found that chance of getting a complete resection was diminished in those with tumor >5 cm [51, 64]; however, tumor size alone was not predictive of disease recurrence in other series [21, 52]. Tumor involvement of a neurovascular bundle decreased the chance of complete resection, resulting in a greater likelihood of residual or recurrent disease [62, 71]. Ballo et al. found that, in addition to positive surgical margins, age <30 years was associated with a higher risk of disease recurrence [7]. The risk tended to be greater in those with extremity desmoid tumor and those with more than one prior treatment, but this did not reach statistical significance.

Other groups have described a more aggressive disease course and inferior disease-free survival in younger patients [7, 38, 46, 66, 75, 76]. In a multivariate analysis, the relative risk of recurrence in patients <18 years was 2.87-fold greater than in older patients [76]. This same group noted a worse disease-free survival in tumors involving plantar structures of the foot when age was <18 years. In addition to experiencing more recurrences than adults, disease tended to recur at earlier time points in younger patients [69].

Death specifically attributable to local disease progression in children is rare [5, 21, 51, 63, 64]. In a large combined pediatric and adult analysis of 138 patients, 11 deaths were caused by disease progression [61]. The primary sites included the head and neck, chest wall, and abdomen. This suggests that other sites of disease, while producing local morbidity, have a lower risk of death from disease. This is further

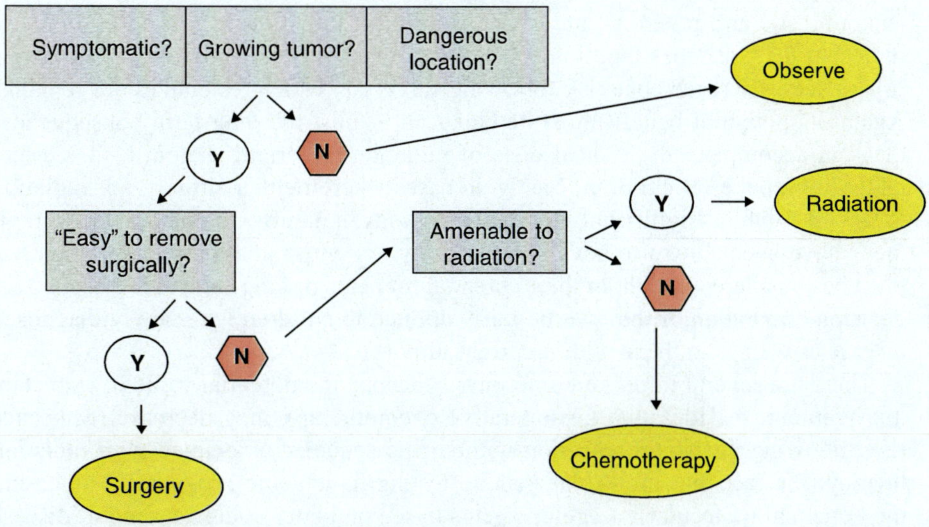

Fig. 11.2 Algorithm for treatment decisions in children with desmoid tumor

supported by the low incidence of mortality from disease progression in children, the majority of which present with extremity primaries [21, 51].

Molecular signatures and an association with outcome have recently been described. DNA mutations that result in the 45F amino acid in β-catenin have been found to be an independent predictor of outcome [43]. Multivariate analysis showed that only young age and presence of the 45F mutation were significant predictors of time to recurrence. Additionally, elevated p53 expression, which often correlates with nonfunctional p53 protein, was also associated with an increased risk of tumor recurrence [24].

11.10 Conclusions

As in adults, desmoid tumor in children represents a biologically and phenotypically heterogeneous disease. Given the relative rarity of the neoplasm and the paucity of published data addressing the issue, one should hesitate to assume that the disease biology is similar in children and adults. Further, the growth and developmental status of children at different ages and their emotional and psychological maturity must be considered as therapeutic options are weighed.

The optimal treatment for children with desmoid tumor depends on numerous factors and some emerging concepts, as depicted in Fig. 11.2. Currently, the application of surgery to cases in which the tumor can be completely resected without compromising form or function is an accepted standard of care. In cases for which treatment is indicated and radiation is felt to be feasible—when considering the anatomic site and potential late effects—ionizing radiation is viewed by many to represent the "next best" option for definitive therapy. This modality also plays a role to decrease recurrence risk following surgery in which residual tumor remains. Again, its potential benefit must be balanced against the long-term consequences that can accompany the typical dose of radiation to certain anatomic sites, especially in prepubertal children. Lastly, in cases where neither surgery nor radiation is feasible without significant potential morbidity, a number of chemotherapy regimens have been shown to have some activity. As with radiation therapy, their use must be considered in light of their potential for acute or long-term side effects. This decision-making algorithm can be fairly applied to children with newly diagnosed disease as well as to those with recurrent tumor.

There are several important emerging concepts: the potential value of expectant management; the idea that postoperative chemotherapy may decrease recurrence risk following near-total resection without the sequelae associated with radiation therapy; the fact that molecular genetic testing have some prognostic value; and the hope that molecularly targeted agents based on better understanding of disease biology may be more effective than the empirical application of cytotoxic and non-cytotoxic agents. All of these concepts should be formally tested in children as well as in adults. The successful completion of two phase II studies in the cooperative group setting in North America establishes that multiinstitutional, prospective clinical trials are feasible for children with this disease. Such prospective studies are more likely to accurately test novel therapeutic approaches, especially if they are conducted as randomized trials. Lastly, given that death from disease is so rare, alternative endpoints such as pain control, functional improvement, and late effects should also be incorporated into the next generations of clinical trials.

References

1. Ahn JM, Yoon HK, Suh YL et al (2000) Infantile fibromatosis in childhood: findings on MR imaging and pathologic correlation. Clin Radiol 55(1):19–24
2. Alebouyeh M, Moussavi F, Tabari AK, Vossough P (2005) Aggressive intra-abdominal fibromatosis in children and response to chemotherapy. Pediatr Hematol Oncol 22(6):447–451
3. Alman BA, Li C, Pajerski ME, Diaz-Cano S, Wolfe HJ (1997) Increased beta-catenin protein and somatic APC mutations in sporadic aggressive fibromatoses (desmoid tumors). Am J Pathol 151(2):329–334
4. Amary MF, Pauwels P, Meulemans E et al (2007) Detection of beta-catenin mutations in paraffin-embedded sporadic desmoid-type fibromatosis by mutation-specific restriction enzyme digestion (MSRED): an ancillary diagnostic tool. Am J Surg Pathol 31(9):1299–1309
5. Ayala AG, Ro JY, Goepfert H, Cangir A, Khorsand J, Flake G (1986) Desmoid fibromatosis: a clinicopathologic study of 25 children. Semin Diagn Pathol 3(2):138–150
6. Balamuth N, Womer R (2008) Successful treatment of pediatric desmoid tumors using hydroxyurea. Connective Tissue Oncology Society Meeting, London
7. Ballo MT, Zagars GK, Pollack A, Pisters PW, Pollack RA (1999) Desmoid tumor: prognostic factors and outcome after surgery, radiation therapy, or combined surgery and radiation therapy. J Clin Oncol 17(1):158–167

8. Benson JR, Mokbel K, Baum M (1994) Management of desmoid tumours including a case report of toremifene. Ann Oncol 5(2):173–177
9. Bonvalot S, Eldweny H, Haddad V et al (2008) Extra-abdominal primary fibromatosis: aggressive management could be avoided in a subgroup of patients. Eur J Surg Oncol 34(4):462–468
10. Buitendijk S, van de Ven CP, Dumans TG et al (2005) Pediatric aggressive fibromatosis: a retrospective analysis of 13 patients and review of literature. Cancer 104(5):1090–1099
11. Carlson JW, Fletcher CD (2007) Immunohistochemistry for beta-catenin in the differential diagnosis of spindle cell lesions: analysis of a series and review of the literature. Histopathology 51(4):509–514
12. Clark SK, Pack K, Pritchard J, Hodgson SV (1997) Familial adenomatous polyposis presenting with childhood desmoids. Lancet 349(9050):471–472
13. Clark SK, Smith TG, Katz DE, Reznek RH, Phillips RK (1998) Identification and progression of a desmoid precursor lesion in patients with familial adenomatous polyposis. Br J Surg 85(7):970–973
14. Coffin CM, Dehner LP, O'Shea PA (eds) (1997) Pediatic soft tissue tumors. Williams & Wilkins, Baltimore, pp 133–159
15. Constantinidou A, Jones RL, Scurr M, Al-Muderis O, Judson I (2009) Pegylated liposomal doxorubicin, an effective, well-tolerated treatment for refractory aggressive fibromatosis. Eur J Cancer 45(17):2930–2934
16. De Wever I, Dal Cin P, Fletcher CD et al (2000) Cytogenetic, clinical, and morphologic correlations in 78 cases of fibromatosis: a report from the CHAMP Study Group. Chromosomes and morphology. Mod Pathol 13(10):1080–1085
17. Delepine N, Delepine G, Desbois JC, Mathe G, Legmann F (1987) Reponse objective du fibrome desmoide a la chimiotherapie (Objective response of desmoid fibroma to chemotherapy). Biomed Pharmacother 41(3):146–148
18. Dormans JP, Spiegel D, Meyer J et al (2001) Fibromatoses in childhood: the desmoid/fibromatosis complex. Med Pediatr Oncol 37(2):126–131
19. Eich GF, Hoeffel JC, Tschappeler H, Gassner I, Willi UV (1998) Fibrous tumours in children: imaging features of a heterogeneous group of disorders. Pediatr Radiol 28(7):500–509
20. Enzinger FM, Weiss SW (1983) Soft tissue tumors, 1st edn. CV Mosby, St. Louis
21. Faulkner LB, Hajdu SI, Kher U et al (1995) Pediatric desmoid tumor: retrospective analysis of 63 cases. J Clin Oncol 13(11):2813–2818
22. Fiore M, Rimareix F, Mariani L et al (2009) Desmoid-type fibromatosis: a front-line conservative approach to select patients for surgical treatment. Ann Surg Oncol 16(9):2587–2593
23. Gansar GF, Krementz ET (1988) Desmoid tumors: experience with new modes of therapy. South Med J 81(6):794–796
24. Gebert C, Hardes J, Kersting C et al (2007) Expression of beta-catenin and p53 are prognostic factors in deep aggressive fibromatosis. Histopathology 50(4):491–497
25. Gega M, Yanagi H, Yoshikawa R et al (2006) Successful chemotherapeutic modality of doxorubicin plus dacarbazine for the treatment of desmoid tumors in association with familial adenomatous polyposis. J Clin Oncol 24(1):102–105
26. Giarola M, Wells D, Mondini P et al (1998) Mutations of adenomatous polyposis coli (APC) gene are uncommon in sporadic desmoid tumours. Br J Cancer 78(5):582–587
27. Goepfert H, Cangir A, Ayala AG, Eftekhari F (1982) Chemotherapy of locally aggressive head and neck tumors in the pediatric age group. Desmoid fibromatosis and nasopharyngeal angiofibroma. Am J Surg 144(4):437–444
28. Goldblum J, Fletcher J (2002) Desmoid-type fibromatosis. International Agency for Research on Cancer Press, Lyon
29. Gurbuz AK, Giardiello FM, Petersen GM et al (1994) Desmoid tumours in familial adenomatous polyposis. Gut 35(3):377–381
30. Halata MS, Miller J, Stone RK (1989) Gardner syndrome. Early presentation with a desmoid tumor. Discovery of multiple colonic polyps. Clin Pediatr (Phila) 28(11):538–540

31. Hansmann A, Adolph C, Vogel T, Unger A, Moeslein G (2004) High-dose tamoxifen and sulindac as first-line treatment for desmoid tumors. Cancer 100(3):612–620
32. Heinrich MC, McArthur GA, Demetri GD et al (2006) Clinical and molecular studies of the effect of imatinib on advanced aggressive fibromatosis (desmoid tumor). J Clin Oncol 24(7):1195–1203
33. Huang PW, Tzen CY (2010) Prognostic factors in desmoid-type fibromatosis: a clinicopathological and immunohistochemical analysis of 46 cases. Pathology 42(2):147–150
34. Humar A, Chou S, Carpenter B (1993) Fibromatosis in infancy and childhood: the spectrum. J Pediatr Surg 28(11):1446–1450
35. Ishizuka M, Hatori M, Dohi O et al (2006) Expression profiles of sex steroid receptors in desmoid tumors. Tohoku J Exp Med 210(3):189–198
36. Jabbari S, Andolino D, Weinberg V et al (2009) Successful treatment of high risk and recurrent pediatric desmoids using radiation as a component of multimodality therapy. Int J Radiat Oncol Biol Phys 75(1):177–182
37. Jelinek JA, Stelzer KJ, Conrad E et al (2001) The efficacy of radiotherapy as postoperative treatment for desmoid tumors. Int J Radiat Oncol Biol Phys 50(1):121–125
38. Kamath SS, Parsons JT, Marcus RB, Zlotecki RA, Scarborough MT(1996) Radiotherapy for local control of aggressive fibromatosis. Int J Radiat Oncol Biol Phys 6:325–328
39. Kiel KD, Suit HD (1984) Radiation therapy in the treatment of aggressive fibromatoses (desmoid tumors). Cancer 54(10):2051–2055
40. Kingston CA, Owens CM, Jeanes A, Malone M (2002) Imaging of desmoid fibromatosis in pediatric patients. Am J Roentgenol 178(1):191–199
41. Lackner H, Urban C, Kerbl R, Schwinger W, Beham A (1997) Noncytotoxic drug therapy in children with unresectable desmoid tumors. Cancer 80(2):334–340
42. Latchford AR, Sturt NJ, Neale K, Rogers PA, Phillips RK (2006) A 10-year review of surgery for desmoid disease associated with familial adenomatous polyposis. Br J Surg 93(10):1258–1264
43. Lazar AJ, Tuvin D, Hajibashi S et al (2008) Specific mutations in the beta-catenin gene (CTNNB1) correlate with local recurrence in sporadic desmoid tumors. Am J Pathol 173(5):1518–1527
44. Lee JC, Thomas JM, Phillips S, Fisher C, Moskovic E (2006) Aggressive fibromatosis: MRI features with pathologic correlation. Am J Roentgenol 186(1):247–254
45. Leithner A, Schnack B, Katterschafka T et al (2000) Treatment of extra-abdominal desmoid tumors with interferon-alpha with or without tretinoin. J Surg Oncol 73(1):21–25
46. Lev D, Kotilingam D, Wei C et al (2007) Optimizing treatment of desmoid tumors. J Clin Oncol 25(13):1785–1791
47. Lewis JJ, Boland PJ, Leung DH, Woodruff JM, Brennan MF (1999) The enigma of desmoid tumors. Ann Surg 229(6):866–872; discussion 872–873
48. Lim CL, Walker MJ, Mehta RR, Das Gupta TK (1986) Estrogen and antiestrogen binding sites in desmoid tumors. Eur J Cancer Clin Oncol 22(5):583–587
49. McCarville MB, Hoffer FA, Adelman CS, Khoury JD, Li C, Skapek SX (2007) MRI and biologic behavior of desmoid tumors in children. Am J Roentgenol 189(3):633–640
50. McDougall A, McGarrity G (1979) Extra-abdominal desmoid tumours. J Bone Joint Surg Br 61-B(3):373–377
51. Meazza C, Bisogno G, Gronchi A et al (2010) Aggressive fibromatosis in children and adolescents: the Italian experience. Cancer 116(1):233–240
52. Merchant NB, Lewis JJ, Woodruff JM, Leung DH, Brennan MF (1999) Extremity and trunk desmoid tumors: a multifactorial analysis of outcome. Cancer 86(10):2045–2052
53. Merchant TE, Nguyen D, Walter AW, Pappo AS, Kun LE, Rao BN (2000) Long-term results with radiation therapy for pediatric desmoid tumors. Int J Radiat Oncol Biol Phys 47(5):1267–1271
54. Miyaki M, Konishi M, Kikuchi-Yanoshita R et al (1993) Coexistence of somatic and germline mutations of APC gene in desmoid tumors from patients with familial adenomatous polyposis. Cancer Res 53(21):5079–5082

55. Mukherjee A, Malcolm A, de la Hunt M, Neal DE (1995) Pelvic fibromatosis (desmoid)—treatment with steroids and tamoxifen. Br J Urol 75(4):559–560
56. Muller E, Castagnaro M, Yandel DW, Wolfe HJ, Alman BA (1996) Molecular genetic and immunohistochemical analysis of the tumor suppressor genes Rb and p53 in palmar and aggressive fibromatosis. Diagn Mol Pathol 5(3):194–200
57. Nieuwenhuis MH, Casparie M, Mathus-Vliegen LM, Dekkers OM, Hogendoorn PC, Vasen HF (2010) A nation-wide study comparing sporadic and familial adenomatous polyposis (FAP) related desmoid-type fibromatoses. Int J Cancer doi:10.1002/ijc.25664
58. Parham DM (1996) Pediatric neoplasia: morphology and biology. Lippincott-Raven, Philadelphia, pp 230–232
59. Patel SR, Evans HL, Benjamin RS (1993) Combination chemotherapy in adult desmoid tumors. Cancer 72(11):3244–3247
60. Picariello L, Fiorelli G, Benvenuti S et al (1997) In vitro bioeffects of the antiestrogen LY117018 on desmoid tumor and colon cancer cells. Anticancer Res 17(3C):2099–2104
61. Posner MC, Shiu MH, Newsome JL, Hajdu SI, Gaynor JJ, Brennan MF (1989) The desmoid tumor. Not a benign disease. Arch Surg 124(2):191
62. Ramirez RN, Otsuka NY, Apel DM, Bowen RE (2009) Desmoid tumor in the pediatric population: a report of two cases. J Pediatr Orthop B 18(3):141–144
63. Raney B, Evans A, Granowetter L, Schnaufer L, Uri A, Littman P (1987) Nonsurgical management of children with recurrent or unresectable fibromatosis. Pediatrics 79(3):394–398
64. Rao BN, Horowitz ME, Parham DM et al (1987) Challenges in the treatment of childhood fibromatosis. Arch Surg 122(11):1296–1298
65. Reich S, Overberg-Schmidt US, Buhrer C, Henze G (1999) Low-dose chemotherapy with vinblastine and methotrexate in childhood desmoid tumors. J Clin Oncol 17(3):1086
66. Reitamo JJ (1983) The desmoid tumor. IV. Choice of treatment, results, and complications. Arch Surg 118(11):1318–1322
67. Reitamo JJ, Scheinin TM, Hayry P (1986) The desmoid syndrome. New aspects in the cause, pathogenesis and treatment of the desmoid tumor. Am J Surg 151(2):230–237
68. Rock MG, Pritchard DJ, Reiman HM, Soule EH, Brewster RC (1984) Extra-abdominal desmoid tumors. J Bone Joint Surg Am 66(9):1369–1374
69. Romero JA, Kim EE, Kim CG, Chung WK, Isiklar I (1995) Different biologic features of desmoid tumors in adult and juvenile patients: MR demonstration. J Comput Assist Tomogr 19(5):782–787
70. Santos GA, Cunha IW, Rocha RM et al (2010) Evaluation of estrogen receptor alpha, estrogen receptor beta, progesterone receptor, and cKIT expression in desmoids tumors and their role in determining treatment options. Biosci Trends 4(1):25–30
71. Sharma A, Ngan BY, Sandor GK, Campisi P, Forte V (2008) Pediatric aggressive fibromatosis of the head and neck: a 20-year retrospective review. J Pediatr Surg 43(9):1596–1604
72. Sherman NE, Romsdahl M, Evans H, Zagars G, Oswald MJ (1990) Desmoid tumors: a 20-year radiotherapy experience. Int J Radiat Oncol Biol Phys 19(1):37–40
73. Skapek SX, Hawk BJ, Hoffer FA et al (1998) Combination chemotherapy using vinblastine and methotrexate for the treatment of progressive desmoid tumor in children. J Clin Oncol 16(9):3021–3027
74. Skapek SX, Ferguson WS, Granowetter L et al (2007) Vinblastine and methotrexate for desmoid fibromatosis in children: results of a Pediatric Oncology Group Phase II Trial. J Clin Oncol 25(5):501–506
75. Sorensen A, Keller J, Nielsen OS, Jensen OM (2002) Treatment of aggressive fibromatosis: a retrospective study of 72 patients followed for 1–27 years. Acta Orthop Scand 73(2):213–219
76. Spear MA, Jennings LC, Mankin HJ et al (1998) Individualizing management of aggressive fibromatoses. Int J Radiat Oncol Biol Phys 40(3):637–645
77. Spiegel DA, Dormans JP, Meyer JS et al (1999) Aggressive fibromatosis from infancy to adolescence. J Pediatr Orthop 19(6):776–784
78. Stein R (1977) Chemotherapeutic response in fibromatosis of the neck. J Pediatr 90(3):482–483

79. Stockdale AD, Cassoni AM, Coe MA et al (1988) Radiotherapy and conservative surgery in the management of musculo-aponeurotic fibromatosis. Int J Radiat Oncol Biol Phys 15(4):851–857
80. Tejpar S, Nollet F, Li C et al (1999) Predominance of beta-catenin mutations and beta-catenin dysregulation in sporadic aggressive fibromatosis (desmoid tumor). Oncogene 18(47):6615–6620
81. Thway K, Gibson S, Ramsay A, Sebire NJ (2009) Beta-catenin expression in pediatric fibroblastic and myofibroblastic lesions: a study of 100 cases. Pediatr Dev Pathol 12(4):292–296
82. Wehl G, Rossler J, Otten JE et al (2004) Response of progressive fibromatosis to therapy with liposomal doxorubicin. Onkologie 27(6):552–556
83. Wehrli BM, Weiss SW, Yandow S, Coffin CM (2001) Gardner-associated fibromas (GAF) in young patients: a distinct fibrous lesion that identifies unsuspected Gardner syndrome and risk for fibromatosis. Am J Surg Pathol 25(5):645–651
84. Weiss AJ, Lackman RD (1989) Low-dose chemotherapy of desmoid tumors. Cancer 64(6):1192–1194
85. Weiss SW, Goldblum JR (eds) (2008) Enzinger and Weiss's soft tissue tumors. Mosby, Philadelphia, pp 275–279
86. Weyl Ben Arush M, Meller I, Moses M et al (1998) Multifocal desmoid tumor in childhood: report of two cases and review of the literature. Pediatr Hematol Oncol 15(1):55–61
87. Wilcken N, Tattersall MH (1991) Endocrine therapy for desmoid tumors. Cancer 68(6):1384–1388
88. Woo SY, HC Doku HD, Chung KD (1984) Fibromatosis of the mandible and mitral valve responding to systemic chemotherapy. Proc Am Soc Clin Oncol 3:78–79
89. Zelefsky MJ, Harrison LB, Shiu MH, Armstrong JG, Hajdu SI, Brennan MF (1991) Combined surgical resection and iridium 192 implantation for locally advanced and recurrent desmoid tumors. Cancer 67(2):380–384

Part III
Considerations for Current and Future Advancement in the Search for a Cure

Chapter 12
Microarrays and High-Throughput Sequencing in Desmoid-Type Fibromatosis and Scar

Robert T. Sweeney and Matt van de Rijn

Contents

Abstract Genome and transcriptome analysis of desmoid-type fibromatosis (DTF) and scar tissue with DNA microarray and high-throughput sequencing (HTS) has yielded abundant data. Given the similar histologic appearance of normal scars, keloids, and DTF, and yet markedly dissimilar invasive and recurrent nature of DTF, it is critical to elucidate the underlying biologic differences contributing to the aggressiveness of DTF. Multiple gene sets and biologic pathways have been found to be enriched in DTF when compared with other noninvasive fibroblastic lesions. Investigation is required to fully characterize the pathogenesis with the hope of identifying novel diagnostic markers and therapeutic targets.

Keywords Microarray • Gene expression profile • High-throughput sequencing • 3SEQ • Comparative genomic hybridization • Cytogenetics • Desmoid-type fibromatosis • Solitary fibrous tumor • Nodular fasciitis • Scar • Keloid

---

R. T. Sweeney (✉)
Department of Pathology, Stanford University Hospital and Clinics, Stanford, CA 94305, USA
e-mail: rtsweeney@stanford.edu

C. Litchman (ed.), *Desmoid Tumors*,
DOI 10.1007/978-94-007-1685-8_12,

12.1 Introduction

Global gene expression analysis emerged in the mid 1990s with DNA microarrays and continues to advance using next generation sequencing. Microarray first provided a high-throughput platform to compare and monitor the expression of many genes in parallel. The massive datasets generated by gene microarray studies created the need for new analytical tools in biostatistics and computational biology to assess them. The first cDNA microarrays described in 1995 evaluated the expression of 45 genes; however, in that paper, authors found it feasible to produce arrays containing 20,000 targets with their technique [14]. The current high-density microarrays contain millions of probes. Prior to DNA microarray technology, only the expression of limited sets of genes and limited regions of the genome could be studied using Southern and Northern blotting as well as polymerase chain reaction. DNA microarrays can be used not only to study gene expression but also for the analysis of chromosomal aberrations and gene copy number variations (comparative genomic hybridization or CGH) [4, 10, 18]. Microarray expression profiling studies have allowed for the characterization of expression signatures for different pathologic entities, tumor microenvironments, and cellular responses to various types of stressors. The large datasets from expression profiling have led to the clustering of genes into broad functional categories (e.g., gene ontology or GO categories) and biologic pathways (e.g., Kyoto Encyclopedia of Genes and Genomes or KEGG pathways). Microarray technology is advantageous because of readily available clustering and statistical software programs as well as affordability. The drawbacks to microarray technique for studying global gene expression include the limitations of predetermined probe sequences. In addition, array systems rely on relative comparisons of expression levels rather than absolute measurements, and they also generally have significant background signal that precludes precise assessment of zero (or near zero) levels of expression. Another limitation of DNA microarray for gene expression studies is that it must be performed on fresh tissue, which can be difficult to obtain for many human diseases.

High-throughput next generation sequencing (HTS) has followed microarray technology for characterizing global gene expression and genome profiling by providing entire whole transcriptome or whole genome sequences. In contrast to DNA microarrays, experiments using HTS do not rely on a fixed platform with known-sequence probes, and it has the advantage of being able to yield data on previously uncharacterized biologic molecules such as miRNA and lncRNA. Like microarray, however, most HTS applications require fresh or frozen tissue, which makes studying rare diseases such as DTF more complicated. The vast majority of human tissue pathology samples in the world are archived in formalin-fixed, paraffin-embedded tissue blocks.

A novel technique, 3SEQ, was recently described that uses HTS for quantitative gene expression profiling in formalin-fixed paraffin-embedded tissue, allowing for quantitative expression profiling of human disease tissue in pathology archives [2]. One advantage to 3SEQ is that all polyadenlyated RNA fragments are sequenced, and these reads can include alternative isoforms of genes, previously unknown genes, nonprotein encoding RNA molecules, and viral or microbial RNA. 3SEQ is currently being applied to DTF samples as well as other fibroblastic lesions such as solitary fibrous tumor, scar, keloids, and Dupuytren's contracture tissue. One disadvantage of HTS is that currently, on a per-experiment basis, the cost is significantly higher than that of gene-array-based studies.

However, there has been a dramatic drop in the cost of sequencing over the past few years. For example, sequencing of the first human genome which was completed in 2001 took 250 people about 13 years to complete, and cost over hundreds of millions of dollars [20]. In 2009, Steven Quake at Stanford University reported that he and two other people sequenced his own genome for less than US $50,000 in a fraction of that time [12, 20]. Competition among several HTS systems is expected to lead to a further drop in cost of high-throughput sequencing. Optimistic estimates for the near future suggest that whole genome sequencing costs may fall below US $1,000 per sample. For the distant future, we may anticipate sequencing costs to fall significantly beyond that.

Both microarray and high-throughput sequencing provide an unbiased approach to genetically characterizing tissues and elucidating biological pathways involved in different diseases and conditions. Both also depend heavily on computational biology, given the enormous number of experimental events taking place to compile the data. Currently, the cost of microarray expression profiling is less than US $100 per sample and therefore provides an affordable method to screen many samples. HTS is more unbiased and sensitive and will be increasingly used as costs decline.

In the study of desmoid-type fibromatosis (DTF), microarray studies of chromosomal aberrations as well as gene expression profiles have generated abundant data. Several studies have shown chromosomal aberrancies in subsets of DTF samples, while the majority of DTF samples are genomically normal. The role of chromosomal aberrations remains under investigation and future studies will likely use high-resolution comparative genomic hybridization to investigate gene copy number variations. In gene expression studies, DTF has been compared with solitary fibrous tumor and nodular fasciitis [1, 17]. Studies have shown that many genes can be up and down regulated in DTF, particularly extracellular matrix remodeling genes and Wnt/β-catenin pathway genes, compared with other similar but less aggressive lesions. As discussed in Chap. 11, adenomatous polyposis coli (APC) gene mutation and *CTNNB1* (gene encoding β-catenin) are often mutated in DTF and genes in the Wnt/β-catenin pathway are upregulated. Most of the global gene expression studies analyzed relatively low numbers of cases and they did not correlate gene signatures with clinical behavior. The major questions of predicting aggressiveness or recurrence in DTF and discovering effective molecular therapies therefore remain unanswered. Quantitative gene expression profiling and new RNA molecule characterization by 3SEQ, which provides access to a much larger number of DTF samples in pathology archives with clinical follow up, can be expected to contribute valuable information to the molecular characterization of DTF.

12.2 Chromosomal Abnormalities in Desmoid-Type Fibromatosis (DTF)

Chromosomal abnormalities in desmoid tumors were reported as early as 1992 based on cells cultured from 26 fresh desmoid tumors and analysis of their metaphase karyotypes [5]. Briefly, this type of cytogenetic analysis is done by disaggregating the cells, growing them in culture, adding a mitotic inhibitor to arrest cells in metaphase, and staining the DNA with Giemsa or Wright stains (also known as "banding") to highlight either gene poor A-T rich regions (G-banding) or gene rich A-T poor regions (R-banding). The chromosomes and their banding patterns are evaluated microscopically on a glass slide. This technique highlights full and partial chromosomal gains, losses, and translocations. In this first study and most subsequent cytogenetic studies, chromosomal abnormalities have been identified in subsets of desmoid tumors but no significant prognostic correlations were made [3, 5, 6, 8, 11, 13]. Also, a substantial portion of desmoid tumors, often reported as the majority, have been found to have no chromosomal abnormalities. The findings of Fletcher et al. in the1995 cytogenetic study of desmoids suggesting that trisomy 8 may be correlated with increased risk of recurrence, but this finding has not been conclusively confirmed by subsequent studies [3, 6, 8, 9, 11, 13]. To date, there are no confirmed chromosomal aberrations with reliable prognostic significance.

By 2003, cytogenetic karyotypes of 122 desmoid tumors had been analyzed, and nearly 50% had shown clonal chromosomal abnormalities with gains in chromosome 8 as the most frequent aberration. In addition, by 2003, 54 desmoid tumors studied by a different analysis called chromosomal microarray analysis demonstrated gains of chromosome 20 and 1q21 as the most frequent aberration. Loss of chromosome 6 and 6q were also seen [8, 11, 13]. Chromosomal microarray analysis (also called comparative genomic hybridization) is a technique to evaluate for chromosomal gains and losses. Briefly, this technique is performed by extracting DNA from sample and normal tissue, differentially labeling the sample and normal DNA with flourophores, and mixing them together; this mix of sample and normal DNA is hybridized to a microarray slide containing thousands of predefined DNA probes. Regional differences in fluorescence between the sample and normal DNA hybridization are indicative of chromosomal aberrations. High-resolution comparative genomic hybridization (HR-CGH) is more sensitive and capable of detecting gene copy number variation.

In 2010, Salas et al. studied 194 fresh-frozen desmoid tumors by chromosomal microarray analysis and reported no correlation between sex, tumor size, initial tumor or recurrent tumor, location, Gardner's syndrome, diagnosis during or within 6 months of pregnancy, and genomic alterations. In this study, 77% of the desmoid tumors were genomically normal which is similar to findings in previous studies [13]. Genomic alterations were identified in 46 tumor samples, of which 40 had gain of chromosome 8 and/or 20q and/or loss of 6q and/or 5q. Other alterations included gains and/or losses in 14 other chromosomes. Twenty-one of the 46 tumors with genomic alterations had more than one aberrancy, and there was no correlation between genomic aberrations and locoregional relapse-free survival (LRFS) or *CTNNB1* (the gene coding for β-catenin) mutation status. The only correlation found was that older patients (median 43.3 years vs. 35.7 years at age of diagnosis) were more likely to have tumors with genetic abnormalities. This study failed to confirm previous reports that trisomy 8 is the most frequent genomic aberration and that it is associated with increased risk of recurrence [3, 9, 13]. Interestingly, as discussed in Chap. 4, the genes known to often be mutated in DTF, *APC* and *CTNNB1*, are located on chromosome 5q21 and 3p21, respectively. Of the 46 tumors in the Salas et al. study with chromosomal aberrations, nine had 5q deletions (eight of which involved 5q21), and four had 3p deletions (two of which involved 3p21). High-resolution array CGH (HR-CGH) for copy number variations was not performed in this study, and, to date, no high-resolution study of gene copy number variation has been performed. Future studies will likely utilize high-resolution CGH or genome sequencing for study, of copy number variation and microdeletion/microduplications as has recently been done with the fibroblastic lesion Dupuytren's contracture [16].

12.3 Transcriptome Changes in Desmoid-Type Fibromatosis

Microarray gene expression studies allow for identification and categorization of differential gene expression between tissue or cell types and the possibility of correlating these findings with diagnoses and prognoses. Briefly, the technique is performed by extracting total mRNA from subject cells and control cells, reverse transcribing it to cDNA, fluorescently labeling the cDNA, and then applying the fluorescently labeled cDNA for hybridization to the chip (solid surface) that contains thousands of nucleotide probes for all human genes arranged in rows and columns (array). The fluorescence differential is evaluated to determine relative gene expression levels [4, 18]. These arrays can be spotted to contain cDNA probes or probes can be built as oligonucelotide sequences on the arrays.

Whatever approach is taken, the arrays can now be used to interrogate the global expression profile for a sample by measuring the relative fluorescence level for each gene represented hybridized on the array used.

The first global gene expression study of DTF was published in 2005, comparing the DTF expression profile to the expression profile of another histologically similar fibroblastic proliferation, called a solitary fibrous tumor (SFT) [20]. Solitary fibrous tumors most often arise from the pleural surface, typically do not invade surrounding tissues, only rarely recur after excision, and generally do not metastasize. However, unlike DTF, a minority of SFTs do have malignant features and do show metastatic behavior, and these are frequently associated with chromosomal alterations. Using microarrays with 42,000 probes representing 36,000 unique gene sequences, ten cases of DTF were compared to 13 cases of SFT. Using unsupervised hierarchical cluster analysis and significance analysis of microarray (SAM), 786 genes were found to be differentially expressed between the two tumor types. Given the fact that both tumors are thought to be derived from fibroblasts, the large number of differentially expressed genes is surprising and suggest that the fibroblasts of origin for these tumors may differ significantly in function. The strongest categories of differential expression were extracellular matrix genes, growth factor genes, and Wnt pathway genes. More specifically, DTF highly expressed fibrotic-response collagen genes such as *COL1A1* and *COL3A1* whereas SFT highly expressed basement membrane collagen genes *COL4A5* and *COL17A1*. Extracellular matrix remodeling genes in the ADAM and MMP family (*MMP23b*, *MMP19*, *MMP11*, *ADAM12*, *ADAM19*, and *ADAMTS1*) were highly expressed in DFT but not in SFT, consistent with the difference in infiltrative behavior of DTF compared SFT. SFT was found to express a few of the ADAM family genes (*ADAM22* and *ADAM23*), which are more likely involved in cell adhesion rather than extracellular matrix remodeling. DTF was also found to highly express pro-fibrotic-response growth factor genes, such as *TGFβ* and *CTGF*, which SFT did not express at the same level.

In this study, distinct DTF and SFT gene signatures were defined from the expression data. As both DTF and SFT are fibroblastic lesions and fibroblasts comprise much of the carcinoma stromal microenvironment, these two signatures were correlated with gene expression data and overall survival in 295 cases of breast carcinoma. The analysis showed that the DTF signature, when present in breast carcinomas, correlated with better prognosis while presence of the SFT signature correlated with worse prognosis. From the DTF and SFT gene expression signatures, two in situ hybridization (ISH) probes representing the DTF signature and one ISH probe and one antibody representing the SFT signature were applied to various normal tissues (including skin, breast, and keloid). The staining patterns showed differential expression of cell types in these tissues, lending support to the idea mentioned above that distinct fibroblastic precursors give rise to DTF and SFT. This study exemplifies how microarray gene expression data can be used not only to characterize the tumors that are used to generate the data but also to further the study of tumor microenvironments; these findings can be extrapolated to other areas of molecular biology and pathology as well.

In 2006, the second microarray global gene expression study of DTF was published, which compared DTF to another nonmalignant myofibroblastic proliferation, nodular fasciitis (NF) [1]. This is an interesting comparison as NF is a self-limiting proliferation of myofibroblasts while DTF is a scar-like lesion that in many cases has slow uncontrolled growth and aggressive recurrence. While DTF and NF showed similar expression profiles of the majority of genes associated with proliferation and metabolism, 335 genes showed significant differential expression. Of these, 89 were more highly expressed in DTF and 246 more highly expressed in NF. The categories of these genes suggested by GO annotation analysis were signal transduction, inflammation, extracellular matrix remodeling, and developmental transcription factors. Wnt/β-catenin pathway genes, including *AXIN2*, *SFRP1*, and *PITX2* among others, were more highly expressed in DTF. *PTK7*, a tyrosine kinase, was also found to be more highly expressed in DTF. Extracellular matrix remodeling genes, *MMP23*,

ADADAMTS9, and *PCSK6*, were more highly expressed in DTF than NF. The genes showing the highest differential expression between DTF and NF encoded matricellular proteins associated with bone formation or cell–matrix interaction. For example, osteoglycin (*OGN*) was more highly expressed in DTF and, similar to SFT, sparc/osteonectin (*SPOCK*) was more highly expressed in NF. Finally, neuronal development genes (*MDK*, *NRGI*, *NPTX2*, and *NEFH*) were found more highly expressed in DTF as compared with NF.

In conclusion, the microarray gene expression profiling studies of DTF have shown that fibrotic response, extracellular remodeling, and Wnt/β-catenin pathway genes are upregulated as compared to similar, although less aggressive, fibroblastic lesions. Furthermore, the expression profile of DTF has been used to further characterize the stromal microenvironment in breast carcinoma. One challenging aspect of microarray studies is that the relative comparison of gene expression that results from one study of DTF vs. SFT cannot be compared well with the expression results of DTF vs. NF. With increased use of HTS platforms in the future absolute expression levels can be compared, even when samples have been studied in different laboratories.

12.4 Transcriptome Changes in Scar, Hypertropohic Scar, and Keloids

Microarray gene expression profiling has been used to characterize various types of scar tissue. Hypertrophic scars are more proliferative than normal scars, but they do not extend beyond the borders of the injury and are not considered invase. Keloids are more proliferative than hypertrophic scars and do extend beyond the borders of the injury with a pushing border. In contrast to DTF, keloids are not invasive. DTF has similar histology to keloids and scar, but are invasive into surrounding tissues. These three lesions (scar, keloid, DTF) therefore display a range of behavior and for that reason form interesting subjects for study that can yield significant insight in the biology of the most aggressive member of this group, DTF.

In 2000, the first cDNA microarray study of scar tissue was published comparing expression of 4,000 genes among normal skin, normal scar, and hypertrophic scar [19]. The study evaluated normal skin from four patients, normal scar from two patients, and hypertrophic scars from three patients. The study found that collagen genes were increasingly expressed from normal skin, to normal scar, to hypertrophic scar. The a-1 chain of collagen III was the most (and a-2 chain of collagen I among the most) overexpressed in normal and hypertrophic scar as compared with normal skin. Interestingly, the a-3 chain of collagen VI and insulin-like growth factor 2 (*IGF-2*) genes were upregulated in hypertrophic scars compared to normal scar and normal skin. Despite prior reports of upregulated *TGFβ* in hypertrophic scar, this study showed no significant differences in growth factor gene expression across all tissue types. Among matrix metalloproteinases and tissue inhibitors of matrix metalloproteinases (TIMP), the only transcriptional change reaching statistical significance was an increase in expression of *TIMP1* in normal scars compared with normal skin. Hypertrophic scars actually showed a decrease in expression of *TIMP1* compared to normal scar, albeit not a statistically significant decrease. These findings are inconclusive and require further evaluation and with a greater sample size to characterize expression differences between scars and hypertrophic scars.

In 2004, a microarray study was published evaluating the gene expression profiles of hypertrophic scar fibroblasts compared with normal fibroblasts before and after exposure to IL-6 [7]. In normal wound healing and scar formation, IL-6 is synthesized by fibroblasts and is known to alter gene and protein expression in fibroblasts. In this study, hypertrophic scar tissue and normal skin were excised from the burn victims who underwent reconstructive surgery; the tissue was then minced and cultured for 3 weeks. Four groups of cultured fibroblasts from the subjects were compared: fibroblasts from normal skin ($n=5$) and from hypertrophic scar ($n=5$), and fibroblasts exposed to 6 h of IL-6 (10 ng/ml) from normal skin ($n=5$) and from hypertrophic scar ($n=5$). Expression of 12,625 genes were compared and showed upregulation of 12 genes and down regulation of 14 genes in hypertrophic scar compared to normal fibroblasts in the absence of IL-6. Treatment of hypertrophic fibroblasts with IL-6 induced upregulation of 21 genes and downregulation of 12 genes. Treatment of normal fibroblasts with IL-6 upregulated 54 genes and down regulated three genes. There were ten genes commonly upregulated and five genes commonly down regulated by IL-6 in hypertrophic scar and normal fibroblasts. In this study and another microarray study of hypertrophic scar, urokinase plasminogen activator is shown to be upregulated compared with normal fibroblasts. Plasmin not only degrades fibrin but also activates matrix metalloproteinases (MMPs) which are involved in extracellular matrix degradation. IL-6 was shown to increase mRNA of *MMP1* and *MMP3* in normal fibroblasts but did not increase transcription of these genes in hypertrophic scar fibroblasts. Additionally, plasmin has also been shown to activate growth factors such as *TGFβ1*, which is a cytokine involved in tissue inflammation and fibrosis.

Unlike hypertrophic scar, keloids extend beyond the boundaries of the original wound or burn; in this sense keloids show a more aggressive behavior than scar and conceptually fall between self-limited scars and the invasive behavior of DTF. In 2010, a metaanalysis of seven microarray studies of keloids showed 25 genes which were up or down regulated in more than one microarray study [15]. Twelve of the 25 dysregulated genes were associated with extracellular matrix (including *COL1A1*, *TGFβRIII*, and *FN1*), eight associated with inflammation/immune regulation, and five associated with apoptosis. The five down regulated genes in keloids compared to control fibroblasts were *HDGF*, *SERPINF1*, *EGFR*, *KRT19*, and TGFβRIII, of which the latter three showed the strongest and most comparable down regulation. However, there are no genes consistently up or down regulated in microarray studies of keloids.

While much progress has been made in expression profiling of DTF and other fibroblast-derived lesions, none of these studies directly compared all possible members of these fibroblast-derived lesions. Therefore, what is lacking is a large study that includes all of these lesions, on a single HTS platform analysis and with clinical follow up. Depending on whether large numbers of fresh DFT samples are available (as in the Salas et al 2010 study) or whether a large number of samples are pooled from pathology archives, RNA-Seq or 3SEQ, respectively, will be useful platforms for comprehensive transcriptome evaluation and comparison. In our experience, large numbers of samples from rare diseases are easiest to obtain from pathology archives; 3SEQ was specifically developed for quantitative expression profiling in archival tissue. Moreover, frozen specimen from some lesions that include scar and other fibroblastic lesions are very difficult to obtain. With 3SEQ, expression profiles among DTF, scar, keloids, and Dupuytren's contracture can now be compared directly.

12.5 3′-End Sequencing for Expression Quantification (3SEQ) in Desmoid-Type Fibromatosis

In 2010, Beck AH et al. published a study comparing two high-throughput platforms for global gene expression (HEEBO microarray and 3′-end next-generation sequencing (3SEQ)) in both fresh and formalin-fixed paraffin-embedded tissue from DFT and SFT samples [2].

Briefly, human exonic evidence-based oligonucleotide (HEEBO) micorarrays consist of 44,544 70-mer oligonucleotide probes that were designed using a transcriptome-based annotation of exonic structure for genomic loci. The probes consist of 30,718 constitutive exonic probes recognizing all known transcripts of a gene, 8,441 alternatively spliced/skipped exonic probes that will recognize exons present in some but not all transcripts of a gene, 196 noncoding RNA probes recognizing nonprotein coding transcripts, 372 B and T cell rearrangement probes recognizing genes that undergo somatic rearrangement, 843 other probes for mitochondrion-derived DNA, and 4,189 various control probes.

In contrast, 3SEQ uses HTS as a novel method for determining global mRNA transcript abundance whereby all polyadenylated transcripts are isolated from total RNA extracted from tissue, reverse transcribed to single-strand cDNA using a linker adapted for the poly-A tail, and then converted to double-stranded cDNA to create sequencing library of all polyadenylated transcripts from the cells. Sequencing 36 base pair reads are then mapped to the 3′ UTR or 3′ end of the 3′-most exon of all expressed genes and genomic sequences of polyadenylated noncoding RNAs (Fig. 12.1). This method was designed specifically for quantifiable gene expression profiling in formalin-fixed paraffin-embedded tissue (FFPET) because formalin fixation randomly fragments the RNA, making microarray evaluation difficult. Until 3SEQ, there has been no accurate technique for quantitative genome-wide expression profiling from FFPET in which RNA has been extensively degraded.

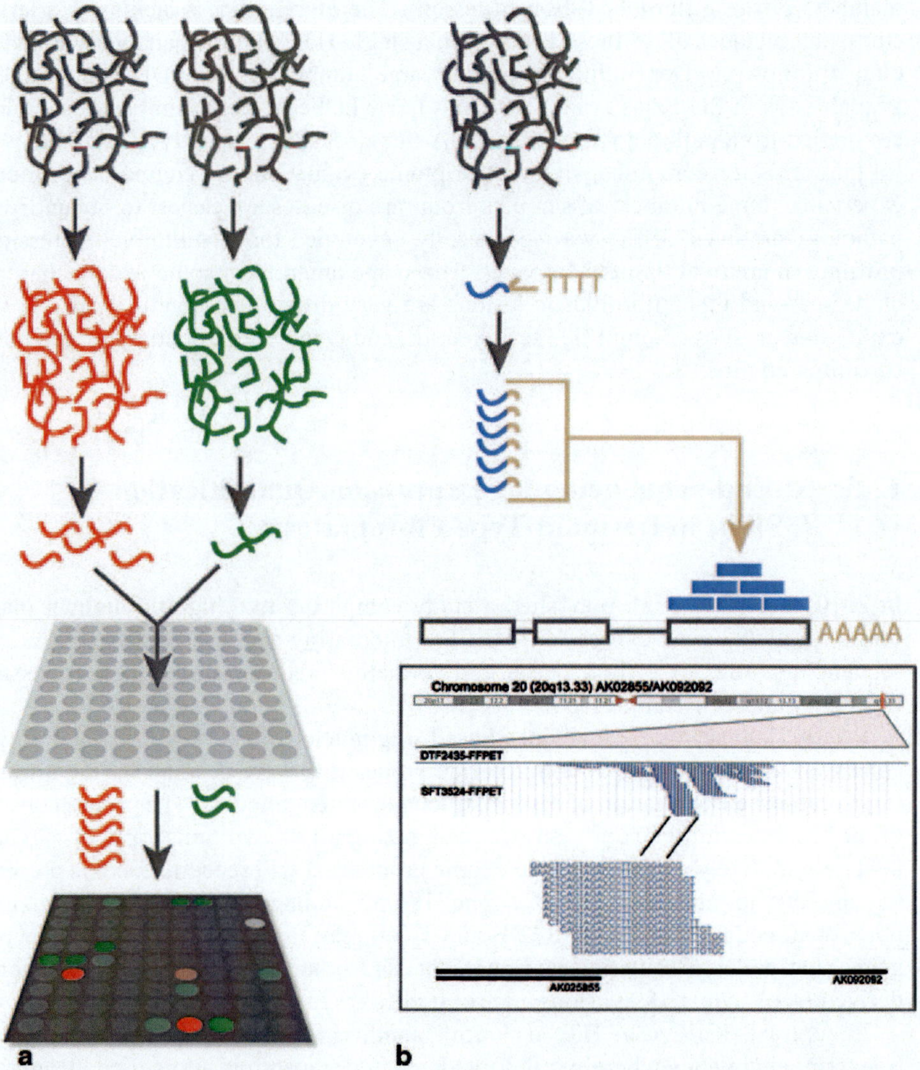

Fig. 12.1 Moving from gene arrays (**a**) to next generation sequencing (**b**). Gene microarrays (**a**) detect the relative abundance for thousands of mRNAs in two differentially labeled preparations. One, derived from a sample of interest (for example a desmoid tumor) is reverse transcribed into cDNA and labeled with a red fluorescent label, while the other is derived from a reference sample and labeled with green fluorescence. Both preparations are then applied to an array on which thousands of probes are spotted. The relative level of red over green fluorescence is a measurement for mRNA in the two starting samples. By keeping the reference sample constant, different desmoid tumors can be compared to each other or to other tumors. In gene expression profiling by 3SEQ (**b**), mRNA molecules are isolated from formalin fixed paraffin embedded tissue (FFPET). The 3′ mRNA fragments are purified through oligo-dT selection, and each fragment is sequenced and mapped to the genome. The number of fragments sequenced for a particular gene is a direct measurement of the level of transcription for that gene. In the example shown, a gene located on chromosome 20 is present in very high levels in a solitary fibrous tumor (SFT3524) but is not detected in a desmoid tumor (DTF2435).

In this study, Beck et al. profiled and compared frozen and FFPE DTF and SFT by HEEBO microarray and 3SEQ. As far as technique sensitivity, analysis showed that 3SEQ identified 9,600 and 8,100 differentially expressed genes and HEEBO identified 4,640 and 69 differentially expressed genes between tumor types on frozen and FFPET, respectively. The findings demonstrated that 3SEQ is an effective technique for gene expression profiling in FFPET (archival pathology samples) and may be particularly helpful for studying rare diseases, such as DTF, in which fresh or frozen tissue is often difficult to obtain.

All four platform-tissue-type combinations identified the Kyoto Encyclopedia of Genes and Genomes (KEGG) pathway extracellular matrix receptor interaction as relatively enriched in DTF. The genes included in this pathway include integrins (*ITGβ1*, *ITGβ5*), collagens (*COL1A1*, *COL1A2*, *COL5A1*, *COL6A2*), glycoproteins (*FN1*, *THBS2*, *SDC1*), and other cell surface proteins. Interestingly, Wnt signaling-related KEGG pathways, known to be critically involved in DTF pathogenesis, were enriched by expression profiles obtained by 3SEQ on both fresh and FFPET but were not identified by HEEBO on either. However, on the other hand, there were three other pathways (glycan structures–biosynthesis 1, axon guidance, and adherens junction) that were identified as enriched in DTF by HEEBO on frozen tissue only; the significance of this finding will need to be addressed in future studies.

The 3SEQ technique is also useful for identifying genes that are expressed at near zero levels in one tissue type while being expressed at measurable levels in the another type. The data produced by high-throughput sequencing have far less background signal than microarray data, making it possible to assess genes exclusively expressed in one type of tissue while expressed at near zero level in other samples. From analysis of 18 K genes that showed at least 25 sequence reads mapped in all samples, 18 genes showed either exclusive expression or 100-fold-increased expression in DTF compared with SFT in both frozen and FFPET data. These 18 genes included several genes known to be expressed in muscle (*MB*, *MYH7*, *TNNI1*, *TNNT1*) as well as in development (*GJB2*, *ACAN*, *DMRT2*, *SLC5A1*, *MYOD1*, and *PAX1*). These findings are suggestive of a myofibroblastic phenotype, which is a known component of DTF, and provide possible targets for further characterizing diagnostic and prognostic markers in DTF. Additionally, the list of exclusively expressed DTF genes includes several poorly characterized transcripts (C20orf58 and DFKZp686J02145) that require further investigation. Importantly these genes were not identified in the experiments using HEEBO arrays as the expression at near zero level in some samples caused them to be filtered out of the dataset.

As sequencing technology advances and its cost declines, 3SEQ will likely provide much needed gene expression profiling for rare tumors, such as DTF and other mesenchymal lesions, which are primarily archived around the world in formalin-fixed paraffin-embedded tissue blocks. The main reason that 3SEQ will be more useful than standard RNA-SEQ for FFPET is that RNA-Seq typically generates nondirectional sequencing libraries of full-length mRNA transcripts, which is not possible in FFPET material where mRNA which has been severely fragmented.

The unidirectional sequencing approach targeting a short region at the 3′ end of the transcript provides a quantitative snapshot at a one-read-per-transcript level for gene expression in FFPET. Further, the low background allows for determination of near zero expression of certain genes rather than the limited, relative comparison of microarray analysis, given its high background signal created by varying degrees of incomplete hybridization.

12.6 Conclusion

DTF is a rare and complicated disease for which the underlying biologic pathways responsible for its invasive and often recurrent nature are being studied with the most advanced molecular biology tools currently available. Over the past two decades cytogenetic and chromosomal microarray studies, which require fresh tissue, have shown numerous chromosomal aberrations in subsets of desmoids tumors; however no etiologic or prognostic correlations have been reliably confirmed. Microarray gene expression studies, also requiring fresh tissue, have compared DTF with two other less aggressive fibroblastic proliferations (SFT and NF) and show increased expression of extracellular matrix remodeling genes (which may be contributory to its invasive nature) and Wnt/β-catenin genes (which are known to be involved in DTF pathogenesis; see Chap. 4). Microarray gene expression studies have tried to characterize genetic profile differences between normal skin, hypertrophic scar, and keloids. These studies found that particular collagens are increasingly expressed in skin, scar, and hypertrophic scar and that urokinase plasminogen activator (plasmin activates extracellular matrix remodeling proteinases) gene expression is upregulated in hypertrophic scar compared to normal scar. Gene expression correlating with the proliferation and extension of keloids beyond the borders of the injury has not been elucidated. To our knowledge, no microarray studies have yet directly compared DTF to these various types of scar tissue.

A recently described HTS technique, 3SEQ, designed specifically for FFPET, is currently being utilized as a sensitive, unbiased, and quantitative gene expression analysis platform to compare DTF, scar, keloid, and Dupuytren's contracture. Unlike microarray, 3SEQ does not rely on predetermined oligonucleotide probes and will sequence any polyadenylated RNA transcripts in the tissue. This may lead to the discovery of new genes or noncoding RNAs. In addition to expression profiling of thousands of genes in DTF, 3SEQ has also already identified two poorly characterized RNA transcripts that require further investigation. With the application of HTS to DTF, more unbiased data will continue to be collected and analyzed to hopefully further characterize the genes and corresponding proteins responsible for the invasive and recurrent nature of the disease. From that point, novel therapeutic targets can start to be identified and tested.

References

1. Bacac M et al (2006) A gene expression signature that distinguishes desmoid tumours from nodular fasciitis. J Pathol 208(4):543–553
2. Beck AH et al (2010) 3′-end sequencing for expression quantification (3SEQ) from archival tumor samples. PloS One 5(1):e8768
3. Brandal P et al (2003) Molecular cytogenetic characterization of desmoid tumors. Cancer Genet Cytogenet 146(1):1–7
4. Bremer M, Himelblau E, Madlung A (2010) Introduction to the statistical analysis of two-color microarray data. Methods Mol Biol 620:287–313
5. Bridge JA et al (1992) Clonal chromosomal abnormalities in desmoid tumors. Implications for histopathogenesis. Cancer 69(2):430–436
6. Bridge JA et al (1999) Trisomies 8 and 20 characterize a subgroup of benign fibrous lesions arising in both soft tissue and bone. Am J Pathol 154(3):729–733
7. Dasu MRK et al (2004) Gene expression profiles from hypertrophic scar fibroblasts before and after IL-6 stimulation. J Pathol 202(4):476–485
8. De Wever I et al (2000) Cytogenetic, clinical, and morphologic correlations in 78 cases of fibromatosis: a report from the CHAMP Study Group. CHromosomes And Morphology. Modern Pathol 13(10):1080–1085
9. Fletcher JA et al (1995) Chromosome aberrations in desmoid tumors. Trisomy 8 may be a predictor of recurrence," Cancer Genet Cytogenet 79(2):139–143
10. Kim YH, Pollack JR (2009) Comparative genomic hybridization on spotted oligonucleotide microarrays. Methods Mol Biol (Clifton, N.J.) 556:21–32
11. Larramendy ML et al (1998) Chromosome band 1q21 is recurrently gained in desmoid tumors. Gene Chromosome Canc 23(2):183–186
12. Pushkarev D, Neff NF, Quake SR (2009) Single-molecule sequencing of an individual human genome. Nat Biotechnol 27(9):847–852
13. Salas S et al (2010) Molecular characterization by array comparative genomic hybridization and DNA sequencing of 194 desmoid tumors. Gene Chromosome Canc 49(6):560–568
14. Schena M et al (1995) Quantitative monitoring of gene expression patterns with a complementary DNA microarray. Science 270(5235):467–470
15. Shih B, Bayat A (2010) Genetics of keloid scarring. Arch Dermatol Res 302(5):319–339
16. Shih BB et al (2010) Genome-wide high-resolution screening in Dupuytren's disease reveals common regions of DNA copy number alterations. J Hand Surg 35(7):1172–1183.e7
17. West RB et al (2005) Determination of stromal signatures in breast carcinoma. PLoS Biol 3(6):e187
18. Whitworth GB (2010) An introduction to microarray data analysis and visualization. Methods Enzymol 470:19–50
19. Blow N (2009) Transcriptomics: The digital generation. Nature 458(7235):239–242
20. Wohlsen M, Quake S, Stanford prof, sequences own entire genome in a week. http://www.huffingtonpost.com/2009/08/10/stephen-quake-stanford-pr_n_255929.html. Last accessed 7 Dec 11

Chapter 13
Desmoid Tumors: Are They Benign or Malignant?

Benjamin Alman

Contents

Abstract The distinction between benign and malignant tumors is classically based on the metastatic potential of a tumor type. While desmoid tumors do not metastasize and as such are classified as benign lesions, their clinical behavior, cellular biology, and molecular etiology all share more characteristics with malignancies than benign processes. Research into these aspects of desmoid tumor biology has the potential not only to develop better treatments for desmoid tumors, but also to shed light into fundamental aspects of tumor biology that will have broad ranging applications. Its classification as a benign process could have implications hampering research, advocacy, and management progress.

Keywords Malignant • Benign • Histology • Cancer stem cells • Invasiveness • Definition

B. Alman (✉)
Department of Surgery, Division of Orthopedics, The Hospital for Sick Children, University of Toronto, Toronto ON, M5G 1L7. Toronto, Canada
e-mail: benjamin.alman@sickkids.ca

C. Litchman (ed.), *Desmoid Tumors*,
DOI 10.1007/978-94-007-1685-8_13,

13.1 Introduction

Definitions are important to help classify disease, but they can sometimes hide the clinical severity of a condition. Tumors are classically categorized as benign or malignant. This classification is based on the potential for a tumor to metastasize [1]. Despite this classical divide, many brain tumors, which do not metastasize but are frequently fatal because of their location, are also classified as malignant. In addition, some tumors that only very rarely metastasize, such as low-grade chondrosarcomas, are classified as malignant [2]. Thus, while the distinction between benign and malignant is clear for many tumor types, for some this distinction is blurred.

13.2 Benign Versus Malignant

Desmoid tumors, also known as aggressive fibromatosis, do not have metastatic potential, but do act locally like a malignant tumor. They are often categorized as locally invasive benign tumors, but this designation belies the rather aggressive clinical behavior of this tumor type. Furthermore, the designation as a benign tumor may hamper advocacy and research efforts. As such, a better understanding of the neoplastic nature, and grouping within the broad range of musculoskeletal tumors is needed. Here we will consider the clinical phenotype, cellular hierarchy, invasive cell behavior, and molecular pathology of desmoid tumors and suggest that they fall into a category between benign musculoskeletal lesions and high-grade sarcomas. Investigations of this tumor type have the incredible potential to shed light onto fundamental aspects of tumor biology.

13.3 Clinical Behavior

From a clinical standpoint, desmoid tumors are quite difficult to manage. Most benign tumors either do not require treatment at all or can be managed by surgical excision alone. In addition, benign tumors very rarely cause substantial morbidity or mortality. In contrast, desmoid tumors do cause significant morbidity and occasional mortality due to impingement upon local structures. Furthermore, they are often treated using a multimodality approach involving surgeons, oncologists, and radiation therapists. This treatment approach is much more similar to that used for sarcomas than for benign lesions. Indeed, current treatments include radiation therapy, traditional chemotherapy, and radical surgical procedures, such as amputation. Treatment results are far from ideal, with recurrence being the rule rather than the exception [3–6]. Thus, from a practical standpoint, treatment for these lesions follows a course similar to that used in malignant tumors, as opposed to a benign lesion. The time and level of concern medical oncologists and radiation therapists place on treating these lesions suggests that they should be classified as something decidedly more aggressive than a benign process.

13.4 Pathology

The cytology of musculoskeletal lesions is used by pathologists to classify musculoskeletal tumors. However, the inconsistent nomenclature and criteria employed by pathologists in classifying these tumors are problematic. This is demonstrated by much of the controversy surrounding malignant fibrous histiocytoma, in which the same tumors are classified different ways by different pathologists, and the diagnosis even changes over time with the same pathologist's evaluation of the lesions. Desmoid tumors are composed of elongated spindle (fibroblast-like) cells surrounded by collagen fibers. They do not contain many mitotic figures. However, in younger children they do contain larger numbers of cells showing evidence of mitosis; this characteristic sometimes makes differentiation between infantile fibrosarcoma and desmoid tumors difficult. Interestingly infantile fibrosarcomas usually have a less aggressive clinical course than do desmoid tumors. Desmoid tumors possess infiltrative capacities to invade into local tissue and vital organs nearby. Morbidity and possibly mortality can result from the impingement of critical organs and obstruction of normal function. The tumors appear to originate from the fascia membrane or musculoaponeurotic planes. Immunohistochemical analysis demonstrated the expression of vimentin, a marker of mesenchymal cells, and lacked the expression of epithelial markers such as E-cadherin, suggesting that aggressive fibromatosis tumors are derived from mesenchymal precursors. These characteristics are the same as many sarcomas, suggesting a commonality with these malignant lesions.

13.5 Molecular Etiology

13.5.1 Familial Forms

Understanding the molecular pathology of desmoid tumors further blurs the distinction between benign and malignant lesions, but has lead to important advances in understanding tumor biology. As discussed in the previous chapters, desmoids can occur as sporadic lesions or they can occur as a manifestation of familial syndromes, including familial adenomatous polyposis (FAP) and hereditary desmoids disease (HDD). It has been observed that aggressive fibromatoses tumors are the first presentation of FAP in some patients [7, 8]. Patients with FAP also develop colon polyps, which have a high chance of going on to become malignant colon cancers. The common molecular etiology of desmoids and colon polyps has raised the possibility that desmoids are malignant precursors. Although progression of a desmoid to a malignant sarcoma has been reported, this is a very rare occurrence, suggesting a fundamental difference between the way the same molecular changes alter cell behavior in different cell types [9–13]. These findings further confound issues of differentiation between benign and malignant lesions, because the exact same molecular event causes a different phenotypic behavior in different cell types.

13.5.2 Clonality

Studies of clonality of desmoid tumors have demonstrated that it is a neoplastic process derived from mesenchymal precursors [14]. Investigation of the clonal nature initially involved the analysis of trisomy 8 and trisomy 20, which are nonrandom clonal aberrations acquired during neoplastic progression. Cytogenic abnormalities, including trisomy 8, trisomy 20, or absence of 5q, have been observed in some cases [15, 16]. By examining the nonrandom inactivation of X chromosome in tumors, it was found that desmoids are a monoclonal disorder; this indicates that tumors derive from a single progenitor cell with a growth advantage and are not composed of normal fibroblasts stimulated by proliferative growth factors [14]. This is a characteristic shared with sarcomas. Another study reported that the inactivation pattern of recurrent fibromatosis tumors was comparable to that of primary tumors, suggesting that recurrent tumors are derived from the same clone as the primary tumor [17], again also a characteristic of sarcomas. Understanding the clonality of this lesion, has guided research towards the examination of the underlying aberrant mechanisms that confer a growth advantage to cells resulting in neoplasia as a whole.

13.5.3 Sporadic Forms

Alteration in β-catenin levels is believed to play a prominent role both in desmoids and in many malignant tumors. A cardinal feature of desmoid tumors is the universal presence of β-catenin protein stabilization; 15% of sporadic tumors contain *APC* mutations, and 60% contain β-catenin mutations [18–28]. This gives desmoid tumors one of the highest reported incidences of β-catenin mutations. These mutations result in β-catenin protein elevation, its nuclear localization, and activation of tcf-mediated transcription. Several groups have confirmed these findings [22, 24–36], and the identification of nuclear β-catenin is in common use as an adjunct in the diagnosis of desmoid tumors [30, 37, 38]. Studies in mice show that β-catenin stabilization can initiate desmoid tumors [39]. β-Catenin is also one of the most frequently activated proteins in cancer, again, showing an overlap between the characteristics of desmoid tumors and malignant processes.

13.6 Cancer Stem Cells

One feature of malignancy that has emerged from research in recent years into a better understanding of cell heterogeneity is the presence of an organized hierarchal structure. Breast, brain, and selected other solid tumors are shown to contain a small subpopulation of cells that initiate tumor formation in immunodeficient mice [40]. This led to the hypothesis that solid tumors contain a subpopulation of tumor-initiating cells (TICs), also termed cancer stem cells [41–43], which are defined by their capacity to self renew and produce the heterogeneous lineage of cells that comprise the tumor (AACR consensus workshop) [44]. As such, this cell population shares properties with stem cells. Only a few such cells would be required to maintain, expand, and disseminate a tumor. This may explain why even after treatment, tumors often persist or recur, as only a few TICs would have to remain to cause disease recurrence. Therefore, targeting the TIC may be a novel approach to eliminate tumors and prevent recurrence [45, 46].

A property of stem cells is their ability to efflux certain dyes such as Hoechst 33342. Cells that efflux this dye are referred to as the side population (SP), as they are the negatively stained cells that fall to the "side" of the majority of cells on a density dot plot during flow cytometry analysis [47, 48]. This property has been used to enrich for progenitor cells in normal brain, muscle, skin, breast, and blood [49, 50]. This feature is conferred partly by expression of ABC family transporters on the progenitor cells which can be blocked by verapamil; this property is used as a control to identify this subpopulation [51]. Tumor-initiating cells have been identified using this technique in desmoid tumors as well as other mesenchymal tumors [52]. Although controversy remains about the true existence of cancer stem cells [53], it is clear that there is cellular heterogeneity within tumors, and the SP represents a group of cells with different biologic behavior, including potential chemoresistance, even if it does not represent a population enriched for true cancer stem cells.

The inherent heterogeneous nature of these tumors coupled with the prospective identification of TICs with enhanced tumor-initiating potential provides strong support that cells within these tumors are organized in a cellular hierarchy; the mesenchymal tumor stem cells are found at the apex, and its differentiated progeny compose the heterogeneous tissue of the tumor body. The biologically distinct properties of these cells, which include a stem-like phenotype, further support this hypothesis. Identification of the signaling pathways in the TICs population that can be manipulated to inhibit tumor growth demonstrates one biologically discreet feature of these cells with important clinical implications for tumor treatment. Thus, the finding that desmoid tumors contain a subpopulation of cells with TIC characteristics not only demonstrates another similarity with malignancies, but also suggests that research into therapeutically targeting these cells will identify improved ways to treat desmoid tumors.

13.7 Cell of Origin

A recent study has identified the cell of origin of desmoid tumors [54]. Desmoid tumors express genes and cell surface markers characteristic of mesenchymal stem cells. In mice that are genetically predisposed to develop desmoid tumors, the number of tumors that form is proportional to the number of mesenchymal stem cells present. In addition, *Sca-1*$^{-/-}$ mice, which develop fewer mesenchymal stem cells, were crossed with mice genetically predisposed to develop desmoid tumors; it was found that mice deficient in *Sca-1* developed substantially fewer desmoid tumors than wild-type littermates. Furthermore, mesenchymal stem cells isolated from mice that are genetically predisposed to develop desmoid tumors induced aberrant cellular growth reminiscent of desmoid tumors, after engraftment to immunocompromised mice. This is the same cell of origin of several sarcoma subtypes [55], showing another similarity between desmoid tumors and sarcomas. These data also suggest that protecting this progenitor cell population might prevent tumor formation in patients harboring a germ line *APC* mutation, in whom desmoids are currently the leading cause of death.

13.8 Conclusion

Desmoid tumors have a clinical behavior similar to a malignancy, exhibit a cellular hierarchy similar to that of sarcomas and have a similar molecular pathology as preneoplastic lesions. Despite the classification as a benign lesion, desmoids share more characteristics with sarcomas than benign lesions. Their classification as a benign process could hamper research funding and public awareness. Despite this, their unique characteristics make them an extremely important tumor for research, not only to identify better treatments for patients with desmoid tumors, but also because research into desmoid tumors will have far-reaching implications into a variety of other tumor types. Given the similarities between desmoid tumors and malignant processes, it may make sense to classify this lesion into the malignant tumor category in order to foster research into this tumor type, improve advocacy efforts, and help patients and physicians gain adequate support for treatment of patients with this difficult to manage lesion (Fig. 13.1).

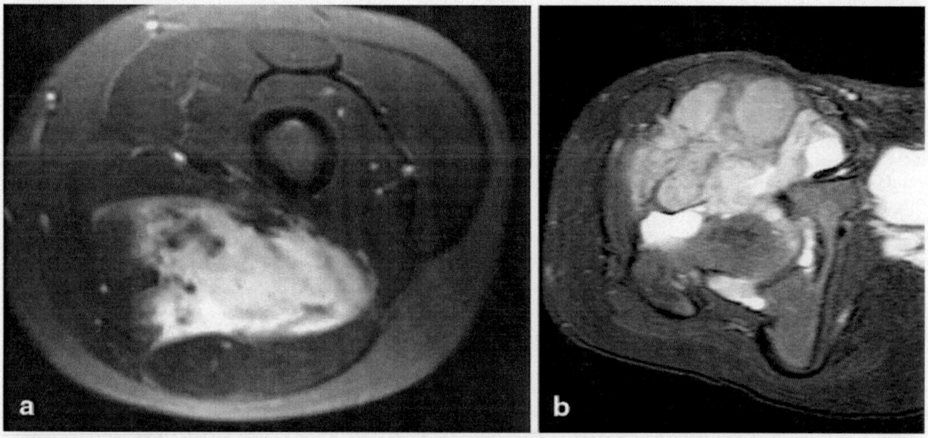

Fig. 13.1 Similarities between desmoids and sarcomas. An MRI image of desmoid (**a**) and a synovial sarcoma (**b**) both in the thigh show similarities in appearance. Both have high signal intensity and show a tumor infiltrating into surrounding tissues. The similarities in local behavior of desmoids and sarcomas blur the distinction between benign and malignant lesions

References

1. Weekes RG, McLeod RA, Reiman HM, Pritchard DJ (1985) CT of soft-tissue neoplasms. Am J Roentgenol 144:355–360
2. Donati D, Colangeli S, Colangeli M, Di Bella C, Bertoni F (2010) Surgical treatment of grade I central chondrosarcoma. Clin Orthop Relat Res 468:581–589
3. Galiatsatos P, Foulkes WD (2006) Familial adenomatous polyposis. Am J Gastroenterol 101:385–398
4. Hosalkar HS, Fox EJ, Delaney T, Torbert JT, Ogilvie CM, Lackman RD (2006) Desmoid tumors and current status of management. Orthop Clin North Am 37:53–63
5. Dormans JP, Spiegel D, Meyer J et al (2001) Fibromatoses in childhood: the desmoid/fibromatosis complex. Med Pediatr Oncol 37:126–131
6. Alman BA, Goldberg MJ, Naber SP, Galanopoulous T, Antoniades HN, Wolfe HJ (1992) Aggressive fibromatosis. J Pediatr Orthop 12:1–10
7. Bandipalliam P, Balmana J, Syngal S (2004) Comprehensive genetic and endoscopic evaluation may be necessary to distinguish sporadic versus familial adenomatous polyposis-associated abdominal desmoid tumors. Surgery 135:683–689
8. Benoit L, Faivre L, Cheynel N et al (2007) 3′ Mutation of the APC gene and family history of FAP in a patient with apparently sporadic desmoid tumors. J Clin Gastroenterol 41:297–300
9. Maher ER, Morson B, Beach R, Hodgson SV (1992) Phenotypic variation in hereditary nonpolyposis colon cancer syndrome. Association with infiltrative fibromatosis (desmoid tumor). Cancer 69:2049–2051
10. Gurbuz AK, Giardiello FM, Petersen GM et al (1994) Desmoid tumours in familial adenomatous polyposis. Gut 35:377–381
11. Eccles DM, van der Luijt R, Breukel C et al (1996) Hereditary desmoid disease due to a frameshift mutation at codon 1924 of the APC gene. Am J Hum Genet 59:1193–1201
12. Scott RJ, Froggatt NJ, Trembath RC, Evans DG, Hodgson SV, Maher ER (1996) Familial infiltrative fibromatosis (desmoid tumours) (MIM135290) caused by a recurrent 3′ APC gene mutation. Hum Mol Genet 5:1921–1924

13. Couture J, Mitri A, Lagace R et al (2000) A germline mutation at the extreme 3′ end of the APC gene results in a severe desmoid phenotype and is associated with overexpression of beta-catenin in the desmoid tumor. Clin Genet 57:205–212
14. Alman BA, Pajerski ME, Diaz-Cano S, Corboy K, Wolfe HJ (1997) Aggressive fibromatosis (desmoid tumor) is a monoclonal disorder. Diagn Mol Pathol 6:98–101
15. Bridge JA, Sreekantaiah C, Mouron B, Neff JR, Sandberg AA, Wolman SR (1992) Clonal chromosomal abnormalities in desmoid tumors. Implications for histopathogenesis. Cancer 69:430–436
16. Fletcher JA, Naeem R, Xiao S, Corson JM (1995) Chromosome aberrations in desmoid tumors. Trisomy 8 may be a predictor of recurrence. Cancer Genet Cytogenet 79:139–143
17. Li M, Cordon-Cardo C, Gerald WL, Rosai J (1996) Desmoid fibromatosis is a clonal process. Hum Pathol 27:939–943
18. Li C, Bapat B, Alman BA (1998) Adenomatous polyposis coli gene mutation alters proliferation through its beta-catenin-regulatory function in aggressive fibromatosis (desmoid tumor). Am J Pathol 153:709–714
19. Alman BA, Li C, Pajerski ME, Diaz-Cano S, Wolfe HJ (1997) Increased beta-catenin protein and somatic APC mutations in sporadic aggressive fibromatoses (desmoid tumors). Am J Pathol 151:329–334
20. Tejpar S, Nollet F, Li C et al (1999) Predominance of beta-catenin mutations and beta-catenin dysregulation in sporadic aggressive fibromatosis (desmoid tumor). Oncogene 18:6615–6620
21. Tejpar S, Li C, Yu C et al (2001) Tcf-3 expression and beta-catenin mediated transcriptional activation in aggressive fibromatosis (desmoid tumour). Br J Cancer 85:98–101
22. Gebert C, Hardes J, Kersting C et al (2007) Expression of beta-catenin and p53 are prognostic factors in deep aggressive fibromatosis. Histopathology 50:491–497
23. Rakheja D, Molberg KH, Roberts CA, Jaiswal VR (2005) Immunohistochemical expression of beta-catenin in solitary fibrous tumors. Arch Pathol Lab Med 129:776–779
24. Bhattacharya B, Dilworth HP, Iacobuzio-Donahue C et al (2005) Nuclear beta-catenin expression distinguishes deep fibromatosis from other benign and malignant fibroblastic and myofibroblastic lesions. Am J Surg Pathol 29:653–659
25. Ng TL, Gown AM, Barry TS et al (2005) Nuclear beta-catenin in mesenchymal tumors. Mod Pathol 18:68–74
26. Saito T, Oda Y, Kawaguchi K et al (2002) Possible association between higher beta-catenin mRNA expression and mutated beta-catenin in sporadic desmoid tumors: real-time semi-quantitative assay by TaqMan polymerase chain reaction. Lab Invest 82:97–103
27. Montgomery E, Lee JH, Abraham SC, Wu TT (2001) Superficial fibromatoses are genetically distinct from deep fibromatoses. Mod Pathol 14:695–701
28. Saito T, Oda Y, Tanaka K et al (2001) Beta-catenin nuclear expression correlates with cyclin D1 overexpression in sporadic desmoid tumours. J Pathol 195:222–228
29. Signoroni S, Frattini M, Negri T et al (2007) Cyclooxygenase-2 and platelet-derived growth factor receptors as potential targets in treating aggressive fibromatosis. Clin Cancer Res 13:5034–5040
30. Jilong Y, Jian W, Xiaoyan Z, Xiaoqiu L, Xiongzeng Z (2007) Analysis of APC/beta-catenin genes mutations and Wnt signalling pathway in desmoid-type fibromatosis. Pathology 39:319–325
31. Bowley E, O'Gorman DB, Gan BS (2007) Beta-catenin signaling in fibroproliferative disease. J Surg Res 138:141–150
32. Ferenc T, Sygut J, Kopczynski J et al (2006) Aggressive fibromatosis (desmoid tumors): definition, occurrence, pathology, diagnostic problems, clinical behavior, genetic background. Pol J Pathol 57:5–15
33. Tajima S, Hironaka M, Oshikawa K et al (2006) Intrathoracic sporadic desmoid tumor with the beta-catenin gene mutation in exon 3 and activated cyclin D1. Respiration 73:558–561
34. Varallo VM, Gan BS, Seney S et al (2003) Beta-catenin expression in Dupuytren's disease: potential role for cell-matrix interactions in modulating beta-catenin levels in vivo and in vitro. Oncogene 22:3680–3684

35. Shitoh K, Konishi F, Iijima T et al (1999) A novel case of a sporadic desmoid tumour with mutation of the beta catenin gene. J Clin Pathol 52:695–696
36. Miyoshi Y, Iwao K, Nawa G, Yoshikawa H, Ochi T, Nakamura Y (1998) Frequent mutations in the beta-catenin gene in desmoid tumors from patients without familial adenomatous polyposis. Oncol Res 10:591–594
37. Amary MF, Pauwels P, Meulemans E et al (2007) Detection of beta-catenin mutations in paraffin-embedded sporadic desmoid-type fibromatosis by mutation-specific restriction enzyme digestion (MSRED): an ancillary diagnostic tool. Am J Surg Pathol 31:1299–1309
38. Carlson JW, Fletcher CD (2007) Immunohistochemistry for beta-catenin in the differential diagnosis of spindle cell lesions: analysis of a series and review of the literature. Histopathology 51:509–514
39. Cheon SS, Cheah AY, Turley S et al (2002) Beta-Catenin stabilization dysregulates mesenchymal cell proliferation, motility, and invasiveness and causes aggressive fibromatosis and hyperplastic cutaneous wounds. Proc Natl Acad Sci U S A 99:6973–6978
40. Reya T, Morrison SJ, Clarke MF, Weissman IL (2001) Stem cells, cancer, and cancer stem cells. Nature 414:105–111
41. Galmozzi E, Facchetti F, La Porta CA (2006) Cancer stem cells and therapeutic perspectives. Curr Med Chem 13:603–607
42. Gudjonsson T, Magnusson MK (2005) Stem cell biology and the cellular pathways of carcinogenesis. Apmis 113:922–929
43. Pardal R, Clarke MF, Morrison SJ (2003) Applying the principles of stem-cell biology to cancer. Nat Rev Cancer 3:895–902
44. Clarke MF, Dick JE, Dirks PB et al (2006) Cancer stem cells--perspectives on current status and future directions: AACR workshop on cancer stem cells. Cancer Res 66:9339–9344
45. Romano G (2005) The role of adult stem cells in carcinogenesis. Drug News Perspect 18:555–559
46. Pierce GB, Speers WC (1988) Tumors as caricatures of the process of tissue renewal: prospects for therapy by directing differentiation. Cancer Res 48:1996–2004.
47. Challen GA, Little MH (2006) A side order of stem cells: the SP phenotype. Stem Cells 24:3–12
48. Goodell MA, McKinney-Freeman S, Camargo FD (2005) Isolation and characterization of side population cells. Methods Mol Biol 290:343–352
49. Hirschmann-Jax C, Foster AE, Wulf GG et al (2004) A distinct "side population" of cells with high drug efflux capacity in human tumor cells. Proc Natl Acad Sci U S A 101:14228–14233
50. Liadaki K, Kho AT, Sanoudou D et al (2005) Side population cells isolated from different tissues share transcriptome signatures and express tissue-specific markers. Exp Cell Res 303:360–374
51. Alison MR (2003) Tissue-based stem cells: ABC transporter proteins take centre stage. J Pathol 200:547–550
52. Wu C, Wei Q, Utomo V, Nadesan P, Whetstone H, Kandel R, Wunder JS, Alman BA (2007) Side population cells isolated from mesenchymal neoplasms have tumor initiating potential. Cancer Res 67:8216–8222
53. Kelly PN, Dakic A, Adams JM, Nutt SL, Strasser A (2007) Tumor growth need not be driven by rare cancer stem cells. Science 317:337
54. Wu C, Nik-Amini S, Nadesan P, Stanford WL, Alman BA (2010) Aggressive fibromatosis (desmoid tumor) is derived from mesenchymal progenitor cells. Cancer Res 70:7690–7698
55. Rubio R, Garcia-Castro J, Gutierrez-Aranda I et al (2010) Deficiency in p53 but not retinoblastoma induces the transformation of mesenchymal stem cells in vitro and initiates leiomyosarcoma in vivo. Cancer Res 70:4185–4194

Chapter 14
The Role of Patient Advocacy Groups in Rare Tumors Such as Desmoid Tumors

Oakleigh Ryan

Contents

Abstract Patient advocacy groups have made huge contributions to facilitating research and improving treatment and its accessibility for rare tumor patients.

By harnessing modern web-based and other communication technologies, these advocacy groups link patients, patrons, medical practitioners and researchers to address the unique problems facing small patient population diseases. This article is a guide to these groups and examines their efforts and results.

Keywords Patient advocacy groups • Rare tumors • Research • Funding • Accessibility

14.1 From a Patient's Perspective

Patient advocacy groups play incredibly important roles in the ongoing battle against rare tumors. But just 10 years ago no patient advocacy group for desmoid tumors existed.

For a desmoid patient today, the world has changed dramatically. I recently sat down to my computer and doing something I often do these days: I searched the Internet for some information. I typed in "desmoid tumors" and the first entry was

O. Ryan (✉)
Whiton House, Janesville, WI 53545, USA
e-mail: Oakleigh@whitonhouse.com

C. Litchman (ed.), *Desmoid Tumors*,

DOI 10.1007/978-94-007-1685-8_14,

for an overview provided by e-Medicine, WebMD's clinical reference repository online. It was useful as a starting point and laid out a basic overview, diagnosis and known treatments [1].

The second and third entries were for the patient advocacy group, Desmoid Tumor Research Foundation or DTRF. From a patient's perspective, I went from reviewing information in a well-organized filing cabinet (e-Medicine) to entering a resource center (DTRF) with faces and names. With one click of my mouse, I found what took me 5 months to unearth in 2002 as a newly diagnosed desmoid patient. The "Find-a-Physician" button on the DTRF home page brought me to a page that shared information about the Sarcoma Alliance for Research through Collaboration (SARC) [2]. The Sarcoma Alliance works with physicians from over 35 institutions in the USA and overseas as part of a collaborative team. The criterion for participation is that the physician must work in a multidisciplinary sarcoma practice with a minimum volume of at least 80 patients. The one-minute search would have taken a patient newly diagnosed with a desmoid tumor, which account for just 0.03% of cancers, from a feeling of loneliness to one of being connected to a network invested with their interest [3]. SOS Desmoide, the DTRF sister organization in Europe, captures its purpose well when it says its aim is to break the patient's isolation [4].

In 2005, Charisse Litchman, MD, Marlene Portnoy, and Jeanne Whiting came together to found DTRF [5]. The disease had impacted each of these women in some way. Their stories varied, but a common thread was that the pathway to effective treatment and information was not an easy one. As is true of so many patient advocacy groups for rare diseases, DTRF was founded due to the passion of people who wanted to make a real difference for those battling the disease.

Mostly everyone has a friend or loved one who has suffered from breast cancer or heart disease, for which patient advocacy groups have played an important role in creating national conversations about what we can do to prevent and fight these diseases. But for those suffering from rare tumors, patients battle not only the disease itself, but also suffer from the general lack of awareness and fundamental knowledge about the tumor itself. As such, advocacy groups are critically important for patients suffering from rare tumors.

There are over 1,200 diseases listed with the National Organization of Rare Disorders [6]. Associated with those diseases are over 2,000 patient organizations and other sources of help. As patients increasingly look to take more control of their disease and social media tools allow more efficient networking and outreach, patient advocacy groups are becoming an important channel of resources, know-how, and passion to fight diseases alongside clinicians and researchers for rare tumors.

According to Conticanet, the Connective Tissue Cancer Network in Europe, "patient advocacy groups are organized in very variable modalities in their structures, goals, organization and means, ranging from small national or even regional organizations, up to international multi-language organizations intervening in a large number of countries" [7]. While patient advocacy groups take many forms, they tend to have impact in three primary areas:

1. Awareness and collaboration
2. Treatment and research
3. Funding, advocacy, and support

14.1.1 Information and Awareness

Perhaps the most fundamental role patient advocacy groups play is one that may be initially the most time-consuming: connecting people, information, and resources to understand and find appropriate treatments for rare diseases. Our healthcare system is by nature complex. Bring in the research end and complexity rises. This complexity can come as a surprise to the new patient, who is inclined to see a simple matter of whether or not there are effective treatments for one's condition.

But treatments and cures start with understanding the basic science of the disease. In other words what do we know about this disease, its causes, mutations, occurrence, and more. The more you know about the basic science the more you can appropriately begin to craft therapies to attack the disease.

However, much of basic research is done in independent laboratories. Two scientists may be working on similar issues but are not necessarily sharing information. Medical and research communities do have vehicles to share important work today, such as the many peer review journals, symposiums, societies and public institutions such as the National Institutes of Health (NIH) that look at developing resources and cures, but in many ways it remains a cottage industry. An article in *Newsweek* in May of 2010 titled "Desperately Seeking Cures" looked at the road from promising scientific breakthroughs to real-world remedies. The article identified a disheartening host of barriers in the United States to getting from basic science to approval of drugs and treatments [8].

A key premise of the article is that while basic research, the starting point for cures, is at least healthy in the USA, for rare tumors this is not necessarily the case. The very rarity of rare diseases works against them, making it hard to attract researchers and clinicians to devote time and work to such efforts [5]. Consequently a critical role for patient advocacy groups is to disseminate information that already exists but is not widely known and to act as a repository for individuals to begin collectively mapping out the disease. "There are thousands of researchers working on exactly the same thing," says Bruce Bloom, whose Partnership for Cures foundation supports research on new uses for existing drugs [8].

One can almost envision building a web. Prior to the work of patient advocacy groups, you might have had a handful of individuals working independently on certain aspects of a rare disease. Enter a patient advocacy group, and these individuals and the knowledge they gain becomes connected and synergistic. Add in the remarkable advances in information technology, the push for electronic health records, and patient access to their own information and you have the potential for a communication transformation around certain diseases.

In an interview, Dr. Charisse Litchman, a DTRF co-founder, shared the following:

> We want clinicians and researchers to know they can come to us and we will help them connect with others. Their time is so valuable. If we can bring a group of dedicated clinicians together in a coherent linked way, we can help unite the individual work to a larger context just by connecting them. What follows is an incredible community of dedicated and passionate clinicians. DTRF was incredibly lucky to have a core of such clinicians ready to create that community [5].

The Connective Tissue Oncology Society (CTOS) is an example in many ways of the power and benefit of bringing clinicians together through the work, in this case, of one patient advocate. The goal of the physician-led society is to advance the care of patients with connective tissue tumors and to increase knowledge of all aspects of the biology of these tumors, including basic and clinical research [9].

But 20 years ago this group did not exist. In 1993, spurred by a lack of communication and therefore suboptimal patient care in managing a threatening sarcoma, a patient of significant means invited a group of physicians and a few others recognized for their interest in sarcomas for a meeting in Florida to discuss the state of knowledge about this group of rare diseases. From this one event came the suggestion to continue the dialogue by forming an organization. Today CTOS is an international group comprised of 400 physicians and scientists from 30 countries with a primary interest in the tumors of connective tissues [9].

As importantly, the formation of CTOS has become a platform for patient advocacy groups to come together as key stakeholders to collaborate and share information and thereby improve their effectiveness. In 2005 the first summit of advocacy groups for sarcomas was held in conjunction with the CTOS Annual Meeting. Fourteen different organizations were represented and agreed to collaborate on issues affecting all sarcoma patients. International Sarcoma Patient Advocacy Network (iSPAN) was founded as a result with one of its primary goals to establish a communication network between all groups. In 2009 iSPAN's directory listed 31 organizations and foundations, and each year the groups continue to meet to discuss current development, issues, and needs affecting sarcoma patients [10].

From a communication perspective, the role of awareness and information dissemination is as important for patients as it is for scientists and clinicians. One of the hardest issues for a patient with a rare tumor is understanding exactly the detail and circumstances of the disease. It is that very lack of information that leaves the patient feeling powerless and unable to make decisions or even to know what questions to ask. In the case of rare diseases, this is often compounded by virtue of the patient's own physician being in a similar situation from a clinical perspective. In optimizing patient care, it is critical that both patient and physician form a collective partnership to tackle the problem at hand.

Patient advocacy groups can provide a simple access to the active and expanding repository of information. In a recent search of the database Cancer Compass, there were posts concerning desmoid tumors [11]. One clearly had the sense of patients "reaching" out for answers to this rare tumor. In two separate instances the patient advocacy group DTRF was identified as a key resource for information and an important starting point.

Perhaps even more fundamental is the help these groups play when a patient is newly diagnosed. The Karen Wyckoff Rein In Sarcoma Foundation (KWRISF) has a simple new patient checklist on its website for newly diagnosed sarcoma patients. The topics include researching doctors, finding a personal advocate, setting up a caring bridge website, and eating right. In the face of what can be a confusing and distressing diagnosis, having information plays a vital stabilizing function for the patient [12].

In the case of the Sarcoma Alliance, their website provides a prominent feature titled "What you need to know." Topics covered include defining a sarcoma and completing online research. This focus, however, is very action-oriented. The alliance has provided a very specific four step process to follow in learning about the specific cancer and treatments that is intended to guide the patient on their pathway to appropriate diagnosis and treatment [13].

While great benefit can be attributed to the role that patient advocacy groups play in collecting, organizing, and disseminating important information concerning rare tumors, most clinicians and patients know that the real battle consists in helping patients receive timely treatment and discovering further treatments and cures. In this mode, patient advocacy groups transition from a "what do we know" mode to "what can we do."

14.1.2 *Treatment and Research*

Perhaps one of the greatest opportunities for patient advocacy groups is identifying and sharing centers of excellence and highlighting the need for patients to seek these centers out. In the instance of rare tumors, surgical removal is a common treatment, especially while options for drug therapies are still being developed. In this case, the number of cases a center sees plays a vital role in building experience that drives excellence, while providing the patient a statistically better outcome.

To that point, another important patient advocacy group, the Liddy Shriver Sarcoma Initiative, focuses on bringing awareness of what are appropriate treatments for sarcomas as one of its primary missions. Sarcomas, cancers of the connective tissue such as nerves and muscles, account for less than 1% of all cancer cases diagnosed in the USA [14]. The initiative was founded by the parents of Liddy Shriver who died at the age of 37 having battled for 2 years against Ewing's sarcoma. In the online, peer-reviewed journal of the Sarcoma Initiative, writer Elizabeth Goldstein-Rice posted an article, "The Importance of Treatment at a Specialty Center for Sarcomas," which highlights a study of sarcoma case records covering a 20-year period by researchers at the University of Miami School of Medicine [15].

Goldstein-Rice cites the above study entitled, "Should Soft Tissue Sarcomas Be Treated at High-Volume Centers? An Analysis of 4205 Patients," [16] which compares patient demographics; tumor type, size and location; and therapy given at low volume (LVC) and high-volume (HVC) medical facilities. Patients seen at HVC's were in more critical condition than those treated at LVC's, having higher-grade tumors and correspondingly worse prognoses. Yet, patients treated at HVC's had better outcomes than their less critical counterparts treated at LVC's. Patients treated at HVC's were offered a broader range of treatment options, including radiation and chemotherapy in addition to surgery. The study states 'a greater proportion of patients treated at HVC received radiation therapy (43% vs. 24.2%, P<0.001) and chemotherapy (14.7% vs. 6.3%, P<0.001).' The addition of radiation and chemotherapy is credited with the better outcomes for these patients. Goldstein-Rice notes that the study shows that "Not only did patients at HVC benefit from the use of a combination of therapies, those who had sarcomas in their extremities were also less likely to have amputations. LVC amputated 13.8% of the time, in contrast to 9.4% at HVC, where doctors have more experience with limb preservation strategies" [16].

From my own perspective, this last point rings especially true and underscores the extraordinary benefit from a patient's perspective of the information being provided by organizations such as the DTRF on identifying sarcoma centers of excellence. I daily thank MD Anderson and my surgeon there for preserving my right arm.

Perhaps most encouraging is that the news is getting out on the importance of where you receive surgery. In a study published in the *Journal of Clinical Oncology* titled "Optimizing Treatment of Desmoid Tumors," researchers noted a nearly three-fold increase in annualized University of Texas MD Anderson Cancer Center (UTMDACC) desmoid referral volume with significantly higher percentages and numbers of primary desmoid tumor referrals when comparing patients treated between 1965 and 1994, and 1995 and 2005. The conclusion drawn from the study was that an "increased awareness" of the complex multidisciplinary management needed for desmoid tumor control may underlie the significantly increased number of referrals to UTMDACC [17]. Having been treated at that institution beginning in 2002, the study has personal meaning.

One of the primary roles of patient advocacy groups is to help ensure there is active and promising research being conducted. This is critical as the research and development process is by its nature inherently challenging. From 1996 to 1999, the US Food and Drug Administration approved 157 new drugs. In the comparable period a decade later—that is, from 2006 to 2009—the agency only approved 74 [8]. The issues behind this decline are numerous. Some of these underlying issues are turf wars for funding, lack of coordination, a mindset of academia to focus on elegant science versus development potential, not to mention the millions of dollars required to go from lab to human clinical trials.

In "Desperately Seeking Cures", Mary Carmichael wrote:

> If we are serious about rescuing potential new drugs from the valley of death, then academia, the NIH, and disease foundations will have to change how they operate. That is happening, albeit slowly. Private foundations such as the MMRF, the Michael J. Fox Foundation for Parkinson's Research, and the Myelin Repair Foundation (for multiple sclerosis) have veered away from the NIH model of 'here's some money; go discover something.' Instead, they are managing and directing scientists more closely, requiring them to share data before it is published, cooperate, and do the non-sexy development work required after a discovery is made [8].

For DTRF for example, they actively work with researchers to ensure access to tissue, overcoming what can be a major obstacle to fundamental research [5]. At the CTOS 16th Annual Conference, the Patient Advocacy Group Session focused on "Success Stories of Patient Groups/Experts Collaboration." Topics included specific research projects underway to broader issues such as building structures of expertise. In these forums one sees the partnering of leaders from patient advocacy groups such as Arthur Beckert of Sarcoma Alliance and Bruce Shriver of Liddy Shriver Sarcoma Initiative with world-renowned physicians and researchers [18].

In fact, patient advocacy groups are taking more active roles in impacting the direction of research and forming very specific research strategies on what to fund. Some of the criteria that are used include:

1. Focusing on early-stage translational research to promoting research at a particular institution
2. Giving enough funds to create meaningful progress in a certain area or focusing on certain researchers
3. Creating links and partnerships with other organizations

The three 2010 grant winners for the DTRF offer a glimpse into the strategies that individual patient advocacy groups develop to support certain research [19]. There is an interesting blend of immediate practicality by screening known therapies to building on more fundamental research that will give a clearer picture of potential targets for therapeutic treatments. A portfolio of research unfolds that is mutually supportive and coordinated versus a simple distribution of funds to individual efforts. In this discernment of what research to support, scientific advisory boards play a critical role and allow the best thinkers to weigh in on potential cures, further strengthening the web that connects individuals around the world in a common pursuit.

In the case of the relatively new Beat Sarcoma patient advocacy group one sees a research relationship being forged with more local academic institutions such as Stanford and UCSF [20]. Likewise the KWRISF partners primarily with the University of Minnesota Masonic Cancer Center. More national organizations such as the Sarcoma Foundation of America (SFA) have taken a broader approach in supporting physicians and scientists from around the world. For example, the Liddy Shriver Sarcoma Initiative funds basic research seed grants [21].

While research increases, the traditional development pathway from research labs to testing in animals for therapeutic benefit and toxicity to then multiple phases of clinical trials in humans takes inordinate amounts of time and money.

While billions of dollars are spent by both the pharma and biotech industries in R&D and the National Institute of Health has a budget of US $ 31 billion, the reality is that the infrequency of rare tumors and diseases tends to work against their funding because the small patient population does not create as loud a clamor for investment as do those diseases that affect millions [8]. This reduced availability of resources makes efficient use of those limited resources all the more critical. In this way, patient advocacy groups play a role similar to what venture capital does for start ups and entrepreneurs: finding, selecting, and funding research that has the most promising potential. The difference is that in this case, the return on investment is saving lives, creating a high-stakes situation.

At the end of the day, however, funding is paramount. Without it, research dries up and with it hope for the future.

14.1.3 *Funding, Support and Advocacy*

One of the key decisions of patient advocacy groups is to decide where to put their efforts in securing more resources. In the case of many groups, the federal government is an important target. Medicare alone accounted for $469.2 billion in spending out of a total of $2.3 trillion spent on healthcare in the USA in 2008. Government spending, including federal, state and local, accounted for 42% of the total sources of funding for the same year [22]. This is expected only to increase.

Each year, hundreds of organizations representing different patient groups seek to meet with federal officials to state their case. This is especially true during the budget and appropriations season. As one can only imagine, the process can be complex, and, in many cases, the education is mutual. In the case of the patient advocacy groups, understanding what committees and subcommittees can impact overall budgets versus specific program funding and regulations is important. Finding congressional members who have a personal experience with the disease is a common and effective approach in gaining advocates for funding. In addition, organizations have become much more focused on matching patients with their own senators or congressmen in patient advocacy group visits to congress.

Additionally, advocacy work can focus on impacting the regulatory environment that affects rare diseases. The SFA was actively involved in the promotion of a "Citizen Petition" that requested the FDA issue a guidance document for the accelerated approval of drugs and biologics that are intended to treat rare cancers [23].

Coverage is also an important issue addressed by advocacy work. Ensuring that treatments are covered under Medicare is critical. Private insurance tends to follow Medicare's lead in approved reimbursement. In the instance of desmoid tumors, it is important that payers recognize that while not classified as malignant, desmoid tumor treatment approaches must be in some cases as aggressive as that for cancerous tumors including treatment at appropriate centers. The bottom line is that while patient advocacy groups are identifying centers of excellence and helping identify and fund new therapies, ensuring that patients have the financial resources to access them through insurance coverage is equally important [5]. In the case of desmoid tumors, the national insurance carrier Cigna has a seven-page section on desmoid tumors on its website including a review of treatments, notation of critical journal articles, and links to resources and organizations including DTRF [3].

At the end of the day, however, patient advocacy groups must be realistic and must focus significant time to raising funds through individuals or organizations. While fundraising has increased significantly and grown in its sophistication through social networking tools, most of the fundraising efforts for rare tumors rely on advocates tapping into a network of their friends, employers, and families to raise awareness and money. Whether it is a run, a golf outing, or some other creative forum, patient advocacy groups are passionately raising money. Funds raised from single events can be for a few thousand dollars to tens of thousands of dollars. Some groups rely on one primary event such as the SFA while others look to a host of smaller engagements.

But this work requires substantial effort, and for those involved, one has to remember that these advocates have their own lives full with jobs and family not to mention their own personal battles. Increasingly founders look to others to help build on their seminal efforts by encouraging further growth across the nation. In the instance of the DTRF the foundation is seeing a growing number of individuals offering to raise money through a wide range of events, an encouraging sign to the founders [5].

Realizing the importance of this activity, various groups offer fundraising tools to encourage others to initiate their own efforts. The National Foundation for Cancer Research (NFCR) has helped kick-start patient advocacy groups by offering a fundraising toolkit. In addition, the NFCR offers a specific contact person to assist those just learning about fundraising and will host a fundraising webpage at the NFCR fundraising portal [24]. Likewise the SFA directs those interested in initiating a fundraiser to their fundraising director promoting events across the country on their website [25].

Ultimately the advocacy and funding role that groups like the DTRF play is part of a bigger picture of a community of patients coming together for taking action on many fronts. Through the development of this community, a support network emerges that can be an incredible asset for any patient. The fear and despair that patients face in battling rare tumors can be and is tempered when one knows you are not alone. It is not surprising that websites and other communication tools of patient advocacy groups are populated with faces. These aren't strangers—these are people with names. The Sarcoma Alliance's website home page greets you with photos of sarcoma survivors and encourages viewers to reach out. The peer-to-peer network will match newly diagnosed patients with another member of the network. The support goes on to include a 24-hour a day chat room on the web with regularly scheduled sessions as well. Finally the support is also financial with funding provided to those who want to seek a second opinion but do not have the financial means to do so [26].

This message is important as patient advocacy groups help patients emerge from being the victims of diseases to part of a group of people who have mobilized to do "something" about their plight.

14.2 Conclusion

That "something" in many cases for patient advocacy groups has been nothing short of amazing. While each group is different, they establish critical beachheads in the battle against their respective diseases in many ways through a methodical multidimensional approach that includes connecting people to information, creating focused attention to critical research projects, or raising money to fund that research.

What makes that possible? Here are organizations whose very founders are going through life altering events, and yet they find the will and resources to put together organizations that have immediate impact on others.

In many cases of the founding of patient advocacy groups, there is a common theme of individuals, faced with an immense challenge, bringing their talents to bear on the fight to cure a rare disease. But more importantly they bring their skills and resources to partner with the very people who need this assistance—our clinicians and researchers. What evolves is a team with players bringing complimentary skills to approach a common problem.

In many ways, patient advocacy groups and their mission of advancing better treatments and improved outcomes for rare tumors serve as a model for the type of partnerships that our healthcare system needs today. No longer is the healthcare picture one of a patient waiting "patiently and compliantly" for the doctor to render a diagnosis. The picture of healthcare must be one where all involved are aligned to a common interest, working together with mutual responsibility and accountability, understanding what is at stake.

A Note of Appreciation Eight years ago I entered a world that approximately 900–1000 people a year enter. I was diagnosed with a desmoid tumor, a rare tumor that most clinicians have never seen or don't even know. I was lucky to have found a path to a center of excellence and best practice treatment. Today because of organizations like DTRF, patients do not have to be dependent on their luck but have incredibly well-organized pathways to appropriate treatment and, most importantly, hope.

References

1. Schwartz R, Trovato M, Lambert PC. Desmoid tumors. (Internet) E-medicine from WebMD. http://emedicine.medscape.com/article/1060887-overview. Accessed 17 Aug 2010
2. Desmoid Tumor Research Foundation (DTRF) (home page on the internet). http://www.dtrf.org/. Accessed 17 Aug 2010
3. Desmoid Tumor (internet) Cigna. http://www.cigna.com/healthinfo/nord1107html. Accessed 5 Sep 2010
4. SOS Desmoide (home page on the internet). http://www.sos-desmoide.asso.fr/rubrique.php3?id_rubrique=23. Accessed 6 Jan 2011
5. Litchman C (2010) Phone interview (29 Aug)
6. National Association of Rare Disorders (home page on the internet). http://www.rarediseases.org/. Accessed 17 Aug 2010
7. Patient Advocacy Groups (internet) Conticanet. http://www.conticanet.eu/html/Advocacy-groups-rub-1-64-77.html. Accessed 6 Jan 2011
8. Carmichael M (2010) Desperately seeking cures. Newsweek. http://www.newsweek.com/2010/05/15/desperately-seeking-cures.print.html. Accessed 19 Aug 2010
9. History of CTOS (internet) The Connective Tissue Oncology Society. http://www.ctos.org/aboutCTOS/. Accessed 9 Sep 2010

10. Directory of Sarcoma Patient Advocacy Organizations and Foundations Brochure (internet) iSPAN. http://www.conticanet.eu/images/illustration/File/Fichiers%20PDF/iSPN.pdf. Accessed 6 Jan 2011
11. Desmoid Tumor Sarcoma (internet) Cancer compass. http://www.cancercompass.com/message-board/message/all,43527,0.htm?mid=310811#310811. Accessed 17 Aug 2010
12. New Patient Checklist (internet) Karen Wyckoff Sarcoma Foundation. http://www.reininsarcoma.org/content/new-patient-checklist. Accessed 6 Jan 2011
13. What is Sarcoma (internet) Sarcoma Alliance. http://www.sarcomaalliance.org/Whatis/whatis9.shtml. Accessed 6 Jan 2011
14. The Sarcoma Learning Center (internet) Liddy Shriver Sarcoma Initiative. http://sarcomahelp.org/sarcoma.html. Accessed 17 Aug 2010
15. Goldstein-Rice E (2008) Electronic sarcoma update newsletter, vol 5, Number 6 (Internet) Liddy Shriver Sarcoma Initiative. http://sarcomahelp.org/learning_center/articles/sarcoma_centers.html. Accessed 17 Aug 2010
16. Gutierrez J, Perez E, Moffat F, Livingstone A, Franceschi D, Koniaris L (2007) Should soft tissue sarcomas be treated at high-volume centers? An analysis of 4205 patients. Ann Surg 245(6)
17. Lev D, Kotilingam D, Wei C, Ballo MT, Zagars GK, Pisters PW, Lazar AA, Patel SR, Benjamin RS, Pollock RE (2007) Optimizing treatment of desmoid tumors. J Clin Oncol 25(13):1785–1791
18. CTOS 16TH Annual Meeting Program (internet). CTOS. http://www.ctos.org/meeting/2010/program.pdf. Accessed 6 Jan 2011
19. DTRF Insider (2010) (Internet) Desmoid Tumor Research Foundation. http://www.dtrf.org/documents/DTRF_spring_2010_email.pdf. Accessed 17 Aug 2010
20. Beat Sarcoma (home page on the internet). http://www.beatsarcoma.org/. Accessed 6 Jan 2011
21. Karen Wyckoff Sarcoma Foundation (KWRISF) (home page on the internet). http://www.reininsarcoma.org/. Accessed 6 Jan 2011
22. National Health Expenditures 2008 Highlights (Internet) U.S. Department of Health and Human Services, Centers for Medicare & Medicaid. http://www.cms.gov/NationalHealthExpendData/downloads/highlights.pdf. Accessed 28 Sep 2010
23. Advocacy (internet). Sarcoma Foundation of America. http://www.curesarcoma.org/index.php/advocacy/. Accessed 6 Jan 2011
24. Start Your Own Fundraiser (internet). National Foundation for Cancer Research. http://www.nfcr.org/index.php?option=com_content&view=article&id=496:start-your-own-fundraiser&catid=3:newsflash&Itemid=209. Accessed 6 Jan 2011
25. Upcoming Fundraisers (internet). Sarcoma Foundation of America. http://www.curesarcoma.org/index.php/upcoming_fundraisers/fundraiser&catid=3:newsflash&Itemid=209. Accessed 6 Jan 2011
26. Sarcoma Alliance (home page on the internet). http://www.sarcomaalliance.org/main.shtml. Accessed 6 Jan 2011

Index

C. Litchman (ed.), *Desmoid Tumors*,
DOI 10.1007/978-94-007-1685-8, © Springer Science+Business Media B.V. 2012